Social Indicators Research Series

Volume 79

This series aims to provide a public forum for single treatises and collections of papers on social indicators research that are too long to be published in our journal *Social Indicators Research*. Like the journal, the book series deals with statistical assessments of the quality of life from a broad perspective. It welcomes the research on a wide variety of substantive areas, including health, crime, housing, education, family life, leisure activities, transportation, mobility, economics, work, religion and environmental issues. These areas of research will focus on the impact of key issues such as health on the overall quality of life and vice versa. An international review board, consisting of Ruut Veenhoven, Joachim Vogel, Ed Diener, Torbjorn Moum, Mirjam A.G. Sprangers and Wolfgang Glatzer, will ensure the high quality of the series as a whole.

More information about this series at http://www.springer.com/series/6548

Graciela H. Tonon

Editor

Teaching Quality of Life in Different Domains

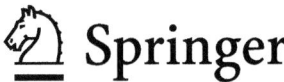 Springer

Editor
Graciela H. Tonon
Master Program in Social Sciences and the Social Sciences Research
Centre (CICS-UP) of the School of Social Sciences
Universidad de Palermo
Buenos Aires, Argentina

ISSN 1387-6570 ISSN 2215-0099 (electronic)
Social Indicators Research Series
ISBN 978-3-030-21550-7 ISBN 978-3-030-21551-4 (eBook)
https://doi.org/10.1007/978-3-030-21551-4

This Springer imprint is published by the registered company Springer Nature Switzerland AG.
The registered company address is: Gewerbestrasse 11, 6330 Cham, Switzerland

To my dear husband, Walter, and my loving sons, Pedro and Erica, who always understand my work and illuminate and enrich my life.
Graciela H. Tonon

Preface

The aim of this book is to present proposals to teach quality of life in different fields. In Chap. 1 entitled "Theory and Methodology in Social Sciences Programs," I present the proposition of quality of life (theoretical/methodological) as a possibility to construct a new outlook on the social field studies and to propose a course that includes the vision of quality of life in a Master/PhD Program in Social Sciences considering that the act of teaching is also a political act, which leads us to say that the role of politics should not only be restricted to the solution of material problems but also to develop an awareness of people's life daily experiences.

In Chap. 2, Dan Weijers discusses the methods, topics, and perspectives that characterize a philosophical approach to teaching well-being or quality of life, focusing especially on how to create and critique a theory of well-being in a methodologically informed way, one that enables students to critique the methods used by a range of well-being and quality-of-life researchers, especially those used by philosophers. The chapter concludes with some suggestions on how to harness the subject matter in a way that creates an engaging undergraduate-level course on well-being and quality of life.

Tobia Fattore in Chap. 3 examines different ways in which well-being and quality of life can be used as pedagogical concepts for teaching Sociology. The chapter begins with a first overview of key philosophical traditions in quality-of-life research for introducing some foundational sociological theories and ways of undertaking social research. Finally the authors canvassed key approaches to researching quality of life which are related to different epistemological approaches in social science research.

In Chap. 4, Daniel T. L. Shek, Xiaoqin Zhu, Diya Dou, Moon Y.M. Law, Lu Yu, Cecilia M.S. Ma, and Li Lin present two programs in response to the results of the research studies that showed worsening mental health conditions such as rising depression and suicidal rates, the increase of adolescent egocentrism, and the declined of empathy and sense of social responsibility among university students in the past decades. To promote holistic development and quality of life in undergraduate students, two credit-bearing leadership subjects were developed at The Hong Kong Polytechnic University (PolyU). The first subject is entitled "Tomorrow's

Leaders," based on the positive youth development (PYD), and the second subject is entitled "Service Leadership."

Chapter 5 is dedicated to the teaching of quality of life in relation with the capability approach. Paul Anand offers new insights into how the capability approach can now make a systematic and transformative contribution to higher education teaching focused on quality of life. The author presents a brief survey of some key distinctive features followed by some suggested areas where capability approach research sheds light on what quality of life requires. The paper suggests such research is particularly useful for discussing the role of opportunities, freedoms, and constraints on the quality of life that individuals achieve and experience, and it highlights potential contributions to quality-of-life teaching by virtue of a capacity to connect structural social and economic drivers to quality-of-life outcomes.

In Chap. 6, written by Takashi Inoguchi, the author describes how political science courses on quality of life may be organized with a syllabus that consists of the following six sections: people's satisfaction with daily life (QOL and daily life satisfaction), people's approval of government conducts especially economic policy (QOL and government economic policy), parents' propensity to nurture their children norms and values (QOL and culture values and norms), QOL and confidence in institutions, QOL-based societal profiling or typology of Asian societies, and Applying QOL studies in Sustainable Development Goals (health, education, and income in East Asia).

Don R. Rahtz, M. Joseph Sirgy, Stephan Grzeskowiak, and Dong-Jin Lee examine in Chap. 7 different ways in which quality-of-life concepts can be integrated into existing marketing coursework. The ultimate goal is to increase the likelihood that students would embrace a QOL orientation in the practice of marketing. The final section ends with a set of suggestions for moving the acceptance of the broader use of QOL-related concepts in marketing departments, the business academy, and both the broader public and private sectors.

Chapter 8 was written by Filomena Maggino who presents the case of *QoLexity* in Italy a post-master program at the University of Florence dedicated to the training of statisticians in the field of quality of life which was conducted for two editions and was closed on 2016.

In Chap. 9, Jon Hall comments how statisticians, economists, and policy makers around the world are working to design and use alternative measures of human progress: measures which focus on outcomes of life quality, rather than simply inputs like economic activity. This chapter discusses some of the ways in which education and training can foster and support this work.

In Chap. 10, Jorge Guardiola proposes Nonviolent Economics as a path for achieving quality of life. This chapter presents an experience of addressing quality of life in an Economic Policy course. The nonviolent approach is the perspective through which quality of life is viewed and is present throughout the whole economics course, with a particular emphasis on the violent component of the economic structure and how to satisfy human needs without using violence against others.

Matías Popovsky in Chap. 11 presents the importance of teaching quality of life using online education, which means conducting a course partially or entirely through the Internet. This chapter aims to discuss the following: the historical context of the education paradigm shift in which this experience is embedded, the educational model for online courses and degree programs at Universidad de Palermo (Argentina), and a proposal of a course to teach quality of life within the framework of this pedagogical model.

Javier Martinez in Chap. 12 presents an approach for teaching and learning quality of life in urban studies. It is contextualized within two higher education courses in an MSc specialization on Urban Planning and Management with a group of international students in the last 10 years. The chapter proposes a reflective and open spiral learning process where students are encouraged to define and operationalize spatial indicators to measure intra-urban quality-of-life variations and to critically use context-sensitive methods such as walking interviews. The teaching described is grounded in the fields of planning, geography, critical cartography, and mixed methods.

Chapter 13 is dedicated on the teaching of quality of life and well-being in Public Health. Chelsea Wesner, Diana Feldhacker, and Whitney Lucas Molitor propose the social ecological model of health as an organizing framework, considering that it is an innovative and integrated approach to teaching that aims to create quality learning experiences. The authors describe how influences of context, social determinants of health, individual factors, culture, and engagement in meaningful activities relate to health, offering learners the possibility to explore factors related to quality of life and well-being. Assignment descriptions and case examples are timely and serve to equip students to meet the demands placed upon health professionals in our modern, globally connected society.

Chapter 14 by Diane E. Mack, Philip M. Wilson, Caitlin Kelley, and Jennifer Mooradian presents how to teach well-being within the context of sports through four evidence-based modules. Defining quality of life and well-being will serve as the focus of the first module. The second module will highlight why consideration of well-being in sport is meaningful. How well-being can be promoted is examined in the third module through consideration of relevant psychological theories and interventions. Finally, the fourth module focuses on distinct groups of athletes including sport participants living with physical and intellectual disabilities, athletes undergoing injury rehabilitation, and current/former athletes transitioning beyond sport.

Finally in Chap. 15, Sabirah Adams, Shazly Savahl, Maria Florence, Kyle Jackson, Donnay Manuel, Mulalo Mpilo, and Deborah Isobell aim to briefly sketch the extent of quality-of-life research relating to children in South Africa and to propose a syllabus for training emerging researchers in conducting QoL research. The chapter identifies and provides a focused discussion on the extent of quality-of-life research within South Africa. The key aspect of the chapter is to propose a syllabus for teaching quality-of-life research with children. In particular five aspects are put forward: contextualizing children and childhood in South Africa, children's QOL and inequalities, theories of children's SWB, methodological considerations, and children's rights and SWB.

My thanks to all the authors from different parts of the world—Africa, Asia, Europe, Latin America, North America, and Oceania—who collaborate with each other their work to make this book a reality. Their committed work allows me to continue learning about the quality of life of people around the world and improve my own quality of life; it is an honor for me to work with all of them.

Buenos Aires, Argentina   Graciela H. Tonon
April 2019

Acknowledgments

To Elsa Zyngman, my Dean at the School of Social Sciences of Universidad de Palermo, Argentina; to Ricardo Popovsky, the President of Universidad de Palermo, Argentina; and to Luis Brajterman, the Academic Secretary of the School of Social Sciences of Universidad de Palermo, Argentina for supporting my work and my initatives.

To Esther Otten, Senior Editor of Sociology and Psychology at Springer, who trusts in my work.

For Alex Michalos, a Great Teacher of the quality-of-life field, whose generosity always opens me new ways to continue working and writing. Many thanks, Alex, for founding all these extraordinary series dedicated to quality of life and for giving me another opportunity to grow in my career.

Graciela H. Tonon

Contents

Chapter 1
The Importance of Teaching Quality of Life Theory and Methodology in Social Sciences Programs

Graciela H. Tonon

Quality of Life

Quality of life is currently defined as a multidimensional concept comprising a number of domains that people consider and evaluate differently according to the importance they attach to each domain in their lives. This definition incorporates both a quantitative-objective approach (what people have and can be observed directly) and a qualitative-subjective approach (what people feel and can be observed indirectly).

As early as in the 1980s, Feinstein (1987) argued that quality of life had become an umbrella term for different indexes depending on the researcher's focus of interest. Subsequently, Dasgupta and Weale (1992) claimed that quality of life not only included the constituents of well-being but also its determinants, and thus connected the personal dimension (the micro level) with the social one (the macro level). In this regard, Diener (2006, p. 154) noted that the early studies on quality of life related it to objective conditions in people's lives, and hence a distinction was drawn with the concept of well-being. Today we can state that the twenty-first century has brought a definition of quality of life that combines and integrates the objective and subjective dimensions.

In addition, quality of life is conditioned by the social structure, considered in terms of demographic features, cultural traits, and psycho-social characteristics of the community and those of its private and public institutions operating within that context (Ferris 2006). Ferris further points out that the demographic foundations and institutional structure of society provide the social environment for an individual's living conditions. In this sense, quality of life is determined by two types of forces: endogenous and exogenous. The former include an individual's mental,

G. H. Tonon (✉)
Master Program in Social Sciences and the Social Sciences Research Centre (CICS-UP) of the School of Social Sciences, Universidad de Palermo, Buenos Aires, Argentina
e-mail: gtonon1@palermo.edu

© Springer Nature Switzerland AG 2020   1
G. H. Tonon (ed.), *Teaching Quality of Life in Different Domains*, Social Indicators Research Series 79, https://doi.org/10.1007/978-3-030-21551-4_1

emotional and psychological responses to his/her living conditions, while the latter refer to the social structure and cultural influences of the community (Ferris 2006).

In sum, we can state that quality of life is the perception each individual has of his/her position in life, within the cultural context and system of values in which he/she lives, in relation to his/her expectations, interests and achievements (Tonon 2015).

Social Sciences

Our approach to the Social Sciences follows Dogan and Pahré's (1993, pp. 15–16) assertion that there is still no consensus about the boundaries of the Social Sciences and that the difficulty in establishing a classification lies in the fact that the various social disciplines are subject to a high degree of fragmentation and that, at the international level, definitions vary depending on the context. According to Gimenez (2003, p. 365), social disciplines are characterised by the porosity of their boundaries, which makes hybridisation[1] between them possible and gives them a familial air, as if they belonged to the same theoretical species.

Thus, social research is currently organised around problems the examination of which requires concepts, methods and techniques from different disciplines (Torres Carrillo 2008); in this respect, we agree with Ortiz (2004, p. 145) that "the boundaries between disciplines cannot be rigid; the opposite would result in a fragmented comprehension of them".

Sotolongo Codina and Delgado Diaz (2006, p. 81) acknowledge that the advance of social knowledge has been less integrated, more piecemeal, more unilateral and slower than it could have been, thus having a less significant impact on actual social situations. In the field of the Social Sciences, the processes of institutionalisation of knowledge and the creation of mechanisms of power have established certain issues and knowledge as dominant discourses in the academic world that have come to be naturalised as notions of truth (Diaz Gomez 2006, p. 225). This shows that the development of the social sciences has historically been based on ideas and organisations – universities and research institutes – providing effective support (Ortiz 2004).

In this regard, it should be noted that the traditional notion of supremacy of the exact and hard sciences over the social sciences – premised on the principle of objectivity of the former, as opposed to the subjectivity of the latter – has seen a shift in recent decades. Along these lines, Torres Carrillo (2008, p. 52) argues that

---

[1] Gimenez (2003, p. 365) states that hybridisation or amalgamation is the merger, recombination or crossing between specialties or fragments of neighbouring disciplines. It does not cover entire disciplines, but only partial sectors of them. The notion of hybridisation is not to be confused with that of multidisciplinarity or pluridisciplinarity, which refers to the mere convergence of monodisciplines around a single object of study, each of them zealously maintaining its own purported boundaries" (Gimenez 2004, p. 268).

nowadays "it is recognised that the social sciences are localised and that the subject and subjectivity are present in all their processes". Along these lines, Sotolongo Codina and Delgado Díaz (2006, p. 52) point to "the historicity of the classical epistemological figure of the object-subject relationship" and in this sense identify a mutation in the statute of the subject, a re-dimensioning of the object and a mutual contextualisation of the subject and the object within a daily praxis context (Sotolongo Codina and Delgado Díaz (2006, p. 52). It is then necessary to create a relationship between each subject (the micro dimension) and society (the macro dimension) that allows passing from the individual to the social and vice-versa (Cipriani 2013).

More than 20 years ago, Wallerstein (1995) pointed out that there were three theoretical-methodological problems to be solved in order to advance in Social Science research: the relationship between the researcher and the research; how to reinsert time and space as constitutive variables in research rather than as mere invariable physical realities within which the social universe exists; and how to overcome the formal separations originated in the nineteenth century between political, economic and socio-cultural issues.

Thus, in the twenty-first century, social scientists must not only be capable of producing and disseminating specialised knowledge but they must also be committed to ethical values and the public interest. These issues play a central role in covering a need in the continuous training of Social Science researchers that may allow them to successfully address contemporary life challenges. In this connection, Weber and Duderstadt (2012, p. 36) argue that "social sciences, arts and humanities are equally important to better understand the conditions for global sustainability, to support thinking differently and to imagine new policies".

Finally, it should be pointed out that although some classifications of the Social Sciences include Sociology, Anthropology and Political Science as the major branches, some other classifications encompass Economics, Geography, History and other disciplines such as Social Communication and International Relations. In recognising the importance of the subjective dimension of social life and personal experiences, social research opens itself up to other languages such as literature, cinema, video, multimedia and theatre as strategies for the construction of knowledge (Torres Carrillo 2008, p. 60).

Whatever approach is adopted to define the Social Sciences, it is worth noting that disciplines can be distinguished from each other not only by their object of study but also by perspectives and ideology.

Teaching in Higher Education: A Socio-political Act

In the history of higher education, a new era has begun; an era in which knowledge is not only necessary to achieve social welfare but is also instrumental in the improvement of every person's quality of life (Duderstadt (2010). Today education is considered an important element of human freedom (Estes and Sirgy 2018, p. 229).

This new trend proposes a switch from formal university degrees, mainly aimed at young students, to a mode of learning that seeks to ensure lifelong education. Thus, continuous learning has become necessary to guarantee work stability and relevance. Societies that deal with accelerating technological change must create a learning society, and education plays an important role in this process (Estes and Sirgy 2018, p. 200).

According to Nussbaum (2012, p. 183) education has had a pivotal role in the initiatives taken by nations in promoting human equality in the past two centuries. It is considered to be particularly central to human dignity, equality and opportunity (Nussbaum 2012, p. 181). Good education requires sensitivity to context, history and cultural and economic circumstances. Attention must be paid to issues of both pedagogy and content, asking whether and how the substance of studies and the nature of classroom interactions relate to citizenship (Nussbaum 2012).

More than four decades ago, Paulo Freire (1973) pointed out that teaching cannot be a mere process of transfer of knowledge from the teacher to the student. It cannot be a mechanical transfer which results in an equally mechanical memorisation. Critical study correlates with an equally critical teaching of a comprehension and realisation of a reading of the word and a reading of the world. In this sense, the task of the teacher is to problematise students with the content that mediates them, rather than disserting about it, giving, delivering, and extending it as if it were something already made, produced, ended and finished (Freire 1973, p. 41).

According to Gimenez (2003, p. 381) "in the face of the proliferation of extra-university institutions in search of information, the only competitive advantage of academia is its capacity to produce knowledge rather than just information". In addition, educational organisations must respond to social dynamics with specific needs and characteristics, in which culture and politics are irreplaceable foundations (Portela Guarin and Murcia Peña 2006, p. 98).

As stated by Nowotny (2010, p. 321), "[w]hile the blurred boundaries of market and state are being redrawn, the social sciences are pressed to integrate knowledge and cultural understandings from other parts of the world and to engage in a fresh dialogue with the Other".

This situation necessarily leads to the gradual yielding of the reductionist model still in force as a certifier of knowledge, towards a model of university that generates a space for the construction of citizenship and democratisation of knowledge, as well as for the improvement of personal quality of life. Moreover, today society and education are the scenarios in which individuals can evolve as persons and citizens in a given social reality.

The Inclusion of Quality of Life as a Concept That Allows an Innovation in the Social Sciences Field

In considering the issue of innovation, we draw on Dogan and Pahre's (1993) definition of innovation as the addition of something new to scientific knowledge, and we hold that such addition must be examined in its development context. Additionally, following Rodríguez Herrera and Alvarado Ugarte (2008, p. 22), we recognise that innovation has a social meaning and therefore consider that none of the persons that take part in this type of processes can be excluded. The importance of innovation thus lies in the praxis that creates a change, and in the fact that such change must be capable of being sustained over time and space (Rodríguez Herrera and Alvarado Ugarte 2008, p. 23).

However, in addition to theoretical and conceptual innovations, innovations can also occur at the methodological level. In other words, innovation also includes the creative application and adaptation of knowledge and technology.

Rodríguez Herrera and Alvarado Ugarte (2008, p. 23) argue that "the originality of innovation lies in the process that helps to make a specific change become a reality". It is thus worth examining the concept of originality and in this respect, we cite Cilleruello (2007, p. 95), who defines originality as that which is not a copy or imitation of something else, but rather a product of creation. This definition highlights the notion of creativity, which is central to any process of innovation. Portela Guarin and Murcia Peña (2006, p. 87) argue that creativity is related to culture, as creating not only involves generating something completely new but it is a social agreement and a creation of symbolic conditions that allow the function or innovation to be valued as such.

In this connection, at the meeting of the American Society for Information Science, Duderstadt (1994), speaking about the University of the twenty-first century, proposed a creative university whose primary activities will shift from a focus on analytical disciplines and professions to those stressing creative activities.

In line with the above statements and as we explain below, we can say that we consider our proposal to include quality of life in Social Science teaching an innovation.

The theoretical proposal of quality of life has had a previous, specific, well-known and considerable development in the fields of health, medicine, psychology and economics, where it gained a prominent place. In this regard, it is worth reflecting on some daily scenes at university when, as we spoke with faculty members of other fields such as education about the importance of studying quality of life, they said that the issue of quality of life is not so much related to education as it is to economics and/or health. This has led us to ask whether they might be confusing the concept of quality of life with that of living conditions or health conditions. It is thus important for those pursuing studies in the Social Sciences – as broadly defined above – to acquire the conceptual and methodological knowledge offered by this proposal, as it will allow them to advance their academic and professional work.

Below we present a concrete case of quality of life teaching in the Social Sciences postgraduate programme.

Syllabus of the Course on Quality of Life and Well-Being of Nations Delivered at the Master's Degree in Social Sciences of Universidad de Palermo, Argentina

The Master's Program in Social Sciences of Universidad de Palermo, Argentina, is an academic programme focused on theory and research that takes account of both of these dimensions within a development context, thus allowing an in-depth examination of the time and space around which the programme is developed.

The introduction of the dimensions of time and space is in line with Passeron's argument, as quoted by Gimenez (2004, p. 275), that the social events that are the object of study of the social sciences have the property that they cannot be divorced from their spatio-temporal context; hence the use of the deictic term making reference to time and place. This is also connected with the above-mentioned view advanced by Wallerstein (1995) that one of the theoretical-methodological problems to be solved in order to advance in Social Science research is precisely how to reinsert time and space as constitutive variables in research.

Since its beginnings, the programme has had an international outlook and drawn on new technologies applied to communication and information in the pedagogical field. These technologies help to develop an academic programme without borders, permanently connected with university institutions and research centres and networks in different parts of the world.

The programme is designed to provide a general and updated understanding of the conceptual and philosophical foundations of the Social Sciences and of current social problems, both nationally and internationally. Students are encouraged to develop a sustained attitude to discover, understand and explain individuals' and groups' life situations, through a critical and cross-cutting exploration of social, cultural, political, economic, historical and geographic issues.

The programme is intended to offer a holistic view of reality, in which the actors – students and faculty – have a central role. It is built on study and the generation of knowledge capable of responding to current challenges with a future projection. In this regard, knowledge holds a prominent place in the syllabus, along with ethical principles based on respect for people and their rights.

In addition, the programme fosters complex and critical thought and commitment to social reality and human diversity through an in-depth exploration of theoretical and methodological aspects with specific practice in Social Science research.

The curricular design of the Master's Program in Social Sciences of Universidad de Palermo is structured around learning goals and techniques to achieve such goals. The programme is organised into courses with an innovative design that, in addition to respecting and integrating the foundational ideas of the Social Sciences, pose new intellectual challenges. In referring to the curriculum, we follow Portela Guarin and Murcia Peña's (2006) definition:

> The curriculum is understood as an instrument of dissemination, reproduction and innovation, based on the various modes of knowledge and appropriation of culture as a form of interpretation, communication, cosmovision, mediation, of constructing the world and as a meaningful horizon, towards the consolidation of subject-world relationships in the process of achieving increased quotas of humanisation. (Portela Guarin and Murcia Peña 2006, p. 92)

This postgraduate programme thus encourages reflection on theoretical issues arising from challenges taking place in this historical stage and integrates new thematic fields such as literature, opera, and studies of the future, risk and audio-visual techniques. Additionally, it offers a comprehensive analysis of contemporary themes such as good living, growing inequality and insecurity.

One of the courses offered by the Master's Program is entitled "Quality of Life and Well-being of Nations".[2]

The course is based on the following goals:

(a) To facilitate the discussion and interpretation of quality of life studies in different social and political contexts.
(b) To make students well acquainted with the methods and techniques used for quality of life research at the micro and macro levels.
(c) To gain in-depth knowledge about well-being and life-satisfaction in the community and in the country.
(d) To gain in-depth knowledge about the construction of "good" nations and societies.
(e) To encourage students to develop a research attitude for the analysis of cases based on Social Science research reports.

The course is organised into the following four thematic units:

---

[2] The course was designed by the author of this chapter, and she is the head lecturer.

Unit I: Quality of Life

Quality of life: origin and evolution of the concept.
Personal well-being and social welfare: the difference of the concepts.
Life satisfaction: concepts and characteristics.
Quality of life of different population groups: children and young people.

Unit II: Community Quality of Life

Quality of life in the community: concepts and characteristics.
The community's well-being: concept and indicators.The community's
   life satisfaction.
The twenty-first century's communities and their definitions.
The communities of Latin American countries: characteristics.

Unit III: Quality of Life and Public Policies

An innovartive way to think the public policy: a view from the quality of
   life measurements.
The satisfaction with democracy: concept and characteristics.
Trust in national institutions.
Citizen's participation in decision makings of public policies.
The well-being of nations.
The use of research results for the decision of public policies.

Unit IV: Methodological Strategies for Quality of Life Research

The PWI for adults and children.
QOL's community indicators.
QOL's indicators for public policy decision making.
Scale of satisfaction with life in the country (ESCVP).
Quality of life and qualitative research methods.
Quality of life and mixed research methods.

References by Unit

Unit I

- Campbell, D., Converse, P., y Rodgers, W. (1976). *The quality of American life*. Nueva York: Russell Sage Foundation.
- Cummins, R. (2016) The Theory of Subjective Well-being Homeostasis: A contribution of understanding life quality. En Maggino, F. (Ed.) *A life devoted to Quality of Life*. Social Indicators Research Series 60. Heilderberg, New York, Dordretch, London. Springer. pp. 61–80.
- Casas, F. (2016) Children, Adolescents and Quality of Life: The Social Sciences Perspective Over Two decades. Maggino, F. *A life devoted to Quality of Life*. Cham, Heilderberg, New York, Dordretch, London. pp. 3–22.

- Diener, E. (2006) Guidelines for National Indicators of Subjective Well-Being and Ill-Being. *Applied Research in Quality of Life 1*:151–157. Dordretch, Heilderberg, London, New York, Springer.
- Estes, R. & Sirgy, J. (Eds.) (2017) *The Pursuit of Human Well-Being. The Untold Global History.* Series International Handbooks of Quality-of-Life, Switzerland, Springer.
- Mieles Barrera, M. & Tonon, G. (2015) Children's quality of life in the Caribbean: a qualitative study en Tonon, G. (Editor) *Qualitative Studies in Quality of Life Methodology and Practice.* Social Indicators Research Series, Vol. 55. Dordretch, Heilderberg, London, New York. Springer. pp. 121–148.
- Savahl, S., Malcolm, CH., Slembrouk, S., Adams, S., Willenberg, I., September, I. (2014) Discourses on Well-Being. *Child Indicators Research* DOI https://doi.org/10.1007/s12187-014-9272-4.
- Sirgy, J., Michalos, A., Ferris, A., Easterlin, R., Patrick, D. & Pavot, W. (2006) The Quality of Life Research Movement: Past. Present and Future. *SIR 76*:343–466.
- Tonon, G. (2012) *Young people's quality of life and construction of citizenship.* SpringerBriefs in Well-being and Quality of Life Research Series. Dordrecht, Heidelberg, London, New York: Springer.
- Tonon, G., Laurito M.J & Benatuil, D. (2018) Leisure, Free time and Well-being of 10 years old Children Living in Buenos Aires Province, Argentina. *Applied Research in Quality of Life,* Springer. First on line March 29, 2018. https://doi.org/10.1007/s11482-018-9612-5
- Toscano, W. & Molgaray, D. (2018) The Research Studies on Quality of Life in South America. *Applied Research in Quality of Life,* Springer. First Online: 27-3-2018.
- Veenhoven, R. (1996) The study of life satisfaction, in: Saris, W.E., Veenhoven, R., Scherpenzeel, A.C. & Bunting B. (eds) *A comparative study of satisfaction with life in Europe.* Eötvös University Press, 1996, pp. 11–48.
- Vittersø J., Røysamb E., Diener E. (2002) The Concept of Life Satisfaction Across Cultures: Exploring Its Diverse Meaning and Relation to Economic Wealth. In: Gullone E., Cummins R.A. (Eds) The Universality of Subjective Wellbeing Indicators. *SIR, vol 16*. Springer, Dordrecht.

Unit II

- Ferris, A. (2006) A theory of social structure and the quality of life. En *Applied Research in Quality of Life Vol 1*. Springer. The Netherlands. Pp. 117–123.
- Jeffres, L. W., Bracken, C. C., Jian, G., & Casey, M. F. (2009). The impact of third places on community quality of life. *Applied Research in Quality of Life, 4*, 333–345.
- Martinez, J., McCall, M. & Preto, I. (2017) Children and Young People's Perceptions of Risk and Quality of Life Conditions in Their Communities: Participatory Mapping Cases in Portugal. Tonon, G. (Editor) *Quality of Life of Communities of Latin Countries*. Cham, Springer. pp. 205–225.

- Phillips, R. & Wong, C. (Editors) (2017) *The Handbook of Community Well-being*. International Handbooks of Quality of Life Series. Cham. Springer.
- Sirgy, M. J., Gao, T., & Young, R. (2008). How does residents' satisfaction with Community Services influence quality of life outcomes? *ARQOL, 3(2),* 81–105.
- Tonon, G. (2017) Rethinking Community Quality of Life in Latin American Countries. Tonon, G. (Editor) *Quality of Life of Communities of Latin Countries*. Cham, Springer. pp. 3–14.
- Tonon, G. (2016) Community Well-Being and National Well-Being: The Opinion of Young People (Chapter 28).Rhonda Phillips and Cecilia Wong (Editors) *Handbook of Community Well-Being Research*. International Handbooks of Quality of Life Series, Springer. pp. 523–530.
- Tonon, G., Mikkelsen, A., Rodriguez de la Vega, L. y Toscano, W. (2017) Neighborhood and housing as explanatory scales of children's quality of life. Castellá Sarriera, J. y Bedin, L. *Psychosocial Well-being in Children and Adolescents in Latin America: Evidence based interventions. Children's Well-being: Indicators and Research Series,* Springer, Switzerland. DOI https://doi.org/10.1007/978-3-319-55,601-7. pp. 91–107

Unit III

- Hagerty, M., Cummins, R., Ferriss, A., Land, K. Michalos, A., Peterson, M. Sharpe, A., Sirgy, J. & Vogel, J. (2001) Quality of life indexes for national policy: review and agenda for research *Social Indicators Research* **55:** 1–96. The Netherlands. *Kluwer Academic Publishers.*
- Macchia, L. & Plagnol, A. (2018) Life satisfaction and confidence in national institutions: Evidence from South America. *ARQOL.* First On-line April 6, 2018.
- Tonon, G. (2014) Satisfaction with democracy. *Encyclopedia of Quality of Life and Well-Being Research,* Michalos, Alex C. (Ed.) 12 volumes. Springer. pp. 1541–1543.
- Tonon, G., (2019) Traditional Academic Presentation of Research Findings and Public Policies. In Pranee Liamputtong (Ed.) *Handbook of Research Methods in Health and Social Sciences.* Volume 1. Heilderberg, New York, New Delhi, Singapore, Hong-Kong. pp. 1–18. First Online: 15 December 2017.
- Veenhoven, R. (2005) Apparent Quality-of-life in Nations: How Long and Happy People Live. *Social Indicators Research, vol 71*, pp. 61–68
- Veenhoven, R. (2009) Well-Being in Nations and Well-Being of Nations. Is There a Conflict Between Individual and Society?. *SIR 91*:5–21 The Netherlands. Springer.
- Veenhoven, R. (2013) The Four Qualities of Life: Ordering concepts and measures of the good life. DellaFave, A (ed) *The Exploration of happiness: Present and future perspectives.* Happiness Studies Book Series, Dordrecht, Netherlands, Springer, pp. 195–226, DOI: https://doi.org/10.1007/978-94-007-5702-8_11.

Unit IV

- Dasgupta, P. y Weale, M. (1992). On measuring quality of life. *World Development 20–1*. pp. 119–131.
- Kajanoja, J. (2002) Theoretical bases for the measurement of quality of life. Gullone, E. y Cummins, R. (eds.) *SIR Vol 16*. The Netherlands. Kluwer. pp. 63–80.
- Maggino, F. (2013) The good society: defining and measuring wellbeing. Between complexity and limit. *Journal de Ciencias Sociales, Año 1, Número 1*. Diciembre pp. 21–41. Universidad de Palermo. Buenos Aires.
- Rees, G., Tonon, G., Mikkelsen, C. & Rodriguez de la Vega, L. (2017) *Urban-rural variations in children's lives and subjective well-being: A comparative analysis of four countries. Children and Youths Service Review, Vol 80 September.* Special Issues Children's Worlds. Elsevier.pp. 41–51. DOI: https://doi.org/10.1016/j.childyouth.2017.06.056
- Sirgy, M., Estes, R & Selian, A. (2017) How we measure well-being: the data behind the history of well-being. In Estes, R. y Sirgy, J. (Eds.) *The pursuit of human well-being: the untold history*. International Handbooks of Quality of Life Series. Cham, Switzerland. Springer. pp. 135–157.
- The International Wellbeing Group (2013) *Personal Wellbeing Index–Adult. Manual.* The Australian Centre on Quality of Life, Deakin University. Melbourne. 5th Edition.
- Tonon, G., (2019) Integrated Methods in Research. En Pranee Liamputtong (Ed.) *Handbook of Research Methods in Health and Social Sciences.* Heilderberg, New York, New Delhi, Singapore, Hong-Kong. First Online: 18 January, 2018.
- Tonon, G. (2015): Relevance of the use of qualitative methods for the study of quality of life, en Tonon, G. (Editor) *Qualitative Studies in Quality of Life Methodology and Practice.* Social Indicators Research Series, Vol. 55. ISBN 978-3-319-13778-0. Dordretch, Heilderberg, London, New York. Springer. pp. 3–21.
- Tonon, G. (2015) The qualitative researcher in the quality of life field en Tonon, G. (Editor) *Qualitative Studies in Quality of Life Methodology and Practice.* Social Indicators Research Series, Vol. 55. ISBN 978-3-319-13778-0. Dordretch, Heilderberg, London, New York Springer. pp. 23–36.
- Tonon, G. (2015) Integration of qualitative and quantitative methods in quality of life studies en Tonon, G. (Editor) *Qualitative Studies in Quality of Life Methodology and Practice.* Social Indicators Research Series, Vol. 55. ISBN 978-3-319-13778-0. Dordretch, Heilderberg, London, New York. Springer. pp. 53–60.

Pedagogical Strategy and Evaluation

The course is grounded in a pedagogical approach that fosters reflection and the integration of theory and practice as the driving force of the pedagogical process. The recognition of students' prior learning allows optimising learning times and integrating knowledge. This generates a space for the exchange of analysis perspectives through a process of critical comment.

In order to successfully complete the course, students have to submit and pass an integrating final paper on one of the topics covered in the course in connection with quality of life. The paper is to be written in the format of an argumentative exercise.

Conclusions

As noted by Martinelli (2010, pp. 287–289) in the *World Social Science Report*, UNESCO, the Social Sciences play different roles in the public sphere: educating students to develop the knowledge and skills required to become researchers, professionals and responsible citizens of democratic societies; producing the empirically tested findings needed for the interpretation and analysis of social phenomena without prejudices; assessing priority issues on the public agenda; contributing as experts to policy-making and to the governance of complex problems.

Duderstadt (2010, p. 425) considers that "education is regarded today as the hope for a significant and satisfactory life", and in that respect, both education and each individual's abilities are increasingly being regarded as the keys to personal quality of life and to the quality of life of society as a whole. Estes and Sirgy (2018, pp. 143–144) express that "Policies designed to improve education, learning, and innovation can enhance the quality of life of people and countries in significant and remarkable ways". In this sense quality of life can be defined considering personal, societal and political dimensions.

Social Sciences are a reflection of the society about itself and a systemathic and controlled exercise of critical autoperception about our times (Lechner 2015, p. 29).

Today, teaching a course about quality of life and well-being in a Master's and in a Ph.D. Programme in Social Sciences can be considered an innovation; however, it must first and foremost be considered to be important and necessary for the training of a social sciences professor and a social sciences researcher.

References

Cilleruelo, E. (2007). Compendio de definiciones del concepto «innovación» realizadas por autores relevantes: diseño híbrido actualizado del concepto. *Revista Dirección y Organización, 34*, 91–98. Recuperado de http://www.revistadyo.org/index.php/dyo/article/view/20/20. 21 de septiembre 2018.

Cipriani, R. (2013). *Sociología cualitativa. Las historias de vida como metodología científica.* Buenos Aires: Editorial Biblos.

Dasgupta, P., & Weale, M. (1992). On measuring quality of life. *World Development, 20*(1), 119–131.

Diaz Gomez, A. (2006). *En Sotolongo Codina, P. y Delgado Diaz, C. La revolución contemporánea del saber y la complejidad social* (pp. 223–232). Buenos Aires: CLACSO Libros.

Diener, E. (2006). Guidelines for national indicators of subjective well-being and ill-being. *ARQOL, 1*(2), 151–157.

Dogan, M., & Pahre, R. (1993). *Las nuevas Ciencias Sociales, La marginalidad creadora.* México: Grijalbo.

Duderstadt, J. (1994). *The University of the 21st century.* Conferencia en The Meeting of the American Society for Information Science. Portland, Oregon, May 23.

Duderstadt, J. (2010). *Una universidad para el Siglo XXI.* Buenos Aires: Universidad de Palermo.

Estes, R., & Sirgy, M. J. (2018). *Advances in well being. Towards a better world.* London: Rowman & Littlefeld International.

Feinstein, A. (1987). Clinimetric perspectives. *Journal of Chronic Diseases, 40*, 635–640.

Ferris, A. (2006). A theory of social structure and the quality of life. *ARQOL, 1*(1), 117–123.

Freire, P. (1973). *Pedagogía del oprimido* (10ª ed.). Buenos Aires: Ed. Siglo XXI.

Gimenez, G. (2003). El debate sobre la prospectiva de las Ciencias Sociales en los umbrales del nuevo milenio. *Revista Mexicana de Sociología, año 65, número 2*, Abril-Junio. México, DF, pp. 363–400.

Gimenez, G. (2004). Pluralidad y unidad de las Ciencias Sociales. En *Estudios sociológicos, Vol. XXII, núm. 2, mayo-agosto*, pp. 267–282. El Colegio de México, A.C. Distrito Federal, México. Retrieved from http://www.redalyc.org/pdf/598/59806501.pdf. November 1, 2018.

Lechner, N. (2015). *Norbert Lechner Obras IV. Política y subjetividad.* Mèxico: FLACSO Mèxico-Fondo de Cultura Econòmica.

Martinelli, A. (2010). *Social science in the public space* (UNESCO, *World Social Science Report*, pp. 287–289). Washington, DC: UNESCO. Retrieved from http://unesdoc.unesco.org/images/0018/001883/188333e.pdf. November 1, 2018.

Nowotny, H. (2010). *Out of science-out of sync* (UNESCO, *World Social Science Report*, pp. 319–322). Washington, DC: UNESCO. Retrieved from http://unesdoc.unesco.org/images/0018/001883/188333e.pdf. November 1, 2018.

Nussbaum, M. (2012). *Crear capacidades. Propuestas para el desarrollo humano.* Barcelona: Paidós.

Ortiz, R. (2004). *Taquigrafiando lo social.* Buenos Aires: Siglo XXI Editores Argentina.

Portela Guarin, H., & Murcia Peña, N. (2006). Repensar el currículo: una perspectiva de deconstrucción mediada por los mundos simbólicos y sus imaginarios. *Revista Latinoamericana de Estudios Educativos (Colombia), vol. 2, núm. 2*, julio-diciembre. pp. 83–102 Universidad de Caldas Manizales, Colombia, recuperado de http://www.redalyc.org/html/1341/134116843005/. October 5, 2018.

Rodriguez Herrera, A., & Alvarado Ugarte, H. (2008). *Claves de la innovación social en América Latina y el Caribe.* Santiago de Chile: CEPAL.

Sotolongo Codina, P., & Delgado Diaz, C. (2006). *La revolución contemporánea del saber y la complejidad social*. Buenos Aires: CLACSO Libros.

Tonon, G. (Ed.). (2015). *Qualitative studies in quality of life methodology and practice* (Social indicators research series, Vol. 55). Heilderberg: Springer.

Torres Carrillo, A. (2008). *Investigar en los márgenes de las Ciencias Sociales* (Folios N° 27, pp. 51–62). Colombia: Universidad Pedagógica Nacional.

Wallerstein, I. (1995). *Abrir las Ciencias Sociales*. Informe de la Comisión Gulbenkian para la reestructuración de las ciencias sociales.

Weber, L. & Duderstadt, J. (Eds.) (2012). *Global sustainability and the responsibilities of universities*. Glion Colloquium Series N° 7. London.

Graciela H. Tonon is Dr. in Political Sciences and Social-worker with Post-doctoral studies in Qualitative Research Methods. She is Professor of Research Methodology in Social Sciences, Methodology in Community Social Work and Quality of life. She is the Director of the Master Program in Social Sciences and the CICS-UP Universidad de Palermo, Argentina. She is the Director of UNI-COM, Universidad Nacional de Lomas de Zamora, Argentina. She received ISQOLS's *Distinguished Service Award for Substantial Service Contributing to a Better Understanding of Quality of Life Studies*. She is the Editor of the *International Handbooks of Quality of Life Series*, Springer and the Director of the *Journal of Ciencias Sociales-UP*. She is Vice president of Publications and Member of ISQOLS' Board of Directors. She is Secretary of the Human Development and Capability Association. Her fields of interest are: Quality of Life, Qualitative Research Methods, Community, Children and Young People, Human Development.

Chapter 2
Teaching Well-Being/Quality of Life from a Philosophical Perspective

Dan Weijers

Introduction

Quality of life is a subject of study that is undeniably relevant to each and every one of us. It is no surprise then, that since humans have been studying anything at all, they have been studying quality of life. Indeed, the original academic subject, philosophy, held quality of life among its few central concerns.

"How should I live?", ancient Greeks would ask before being directed towards Plato's Academy, Epicurus's Garden, or other sanctuaries for critical thinkers. But which sanctuary to choose? The second-century satirist Lucian of Samosata pointed out that each philosophical school had different advice on how to live because they had different views on what it was to live well (Bok 2012; Lucian 2005). The choice of philosophical school was important; much time could be wasted at the feet of any number of hairy-faced ideologues as they revealed their view of the one true path to happiness. And, of course, their mutually exclusive views meant that they could not all be correct.

These days, philosophers refer to the broad investigation of the more theoretical aspects of how we should live as 'normative ethics'. The chief division within normative ethics is between moral theory and well-being. Moral theory is the investigation of what determines the moral rightness or wrongness of actions. It essentially involves identifying and critiquing theories of what we should do, where the normative force of the "should" comes from morality. Well-being, as a subject area in philosophy, is the investigation of what determines how good or bad a life is *for the one living it*. It essentially involves identifying and critiquing theories of what is ultimately good and bad for us, where good and bad are viewed prudentially (i.e., for us, as opposed to for others or for everyone). So, when a philosopher teaches quality of life, they usually understand themselves to be teaching well-being.

D. Weijers (✉)
University of Waikato, Hamilton, New Zealand
e-mail: Dan.Weijers@waikato.ac.nz

© Springer Nature Switzerland AG 2020
G. H. Tonon (ed.), *Teaching Quality of Life in Different Domains*, Social Indicators Research Series 79, https://doi.org/10.1007/978-3-030-21551-4_2

What Does the Term "Well-Being" Refer to in Philosophy?

Conceptual clarity is important to philosophers. We tend to go on a bit, so it frustrates us greatly if we discover we have been talking past each other (for, say, the last 2000 years or so). For this reason, every good philosophical course on well-being or quality of life will start with several conceptual clarifications.

Well-Being: The Prudential Good Life

The philosophical understanding of well-being is shared by many academic disciplines, and is usually considered synonymous with welfare, prudential value, and the prudential good life. The concept is variously described, but the shared meaning within the various descriptions is clear: The life of well-being is the life that is good for the one living (Crisp 2017). So, when we ask about a person's well-being, we are asking about whether their life is going well for them.

The "for them" phrase is important because a life can be good in various ways (Feldman 2004, Chap. 1). A life can be morally good, but morality may require sacrificing one's happiness or even one's life for the sake of others. While such a sacrifice might be the right thing to do in the moral sense of "right", it seems antiprudential – bad for the well-being of the one doing the sacrificing. A life might also be good in the sense of making for a good example of human life by being so perfectly average, or aesthetically good in the sense of making for a good story. Neither of these kinds of good life necessitate that the life is prudentially good – valuable to the one living the life. This is most clear for the aesthetically good life; the protagonists of literature's tragedies tend not to live envious lives. The life of King Lear, for example, is not one I would wish for my children, despite the baubles of office that come with being king. So, philosophers of well-being are interested in prudential value, not necessarily moral or aesthetic value.

Well-Being or Quality of Life?

Well-being is the prudential good life, in other words, the life that is good for the one living it. Well-being and quality of life are sometimes understood as synonyms, but this definition of well-being differs from the definition of quality of life provided in the introduction to this book (and reproduced in Box 2.1), which takes a multidimensional and fairly fluid view of what makes life go well. These differences highlight key dissimilarities in specific methodologies and general approaches used when investigating the topic of prudentially good lives.

The philosophical concept of well-being is like an empty cup with the barest semblance of a form. Defining well-being as the prudential good life – the life going well for the one living it – does give some perspective on the concept of interest, but it does very little to answer the question, "How should I live?". In effect, the bare-bones definition of well-being would answer, "You should live well" – an answer that isn't all that informative. For this reason, philosophers of well-being do not stop after merely outlining the cup. We also try to fill the cup with a theory or account of well-being. So, to draw the analogy to its full extent, drinking from the cup would bestow one with the knowledge of what actually makes a life go well for the one living it (not just the meaning of the term "well-being").

Quality of life, as defined in Box 2.1, is multi-dimensional and at least partly subjective; the definition allows the importance of the various aspects of a good life to be decided by each individual for themselves. From a philosopher's perspective, both of these attributes of the definition are up for debate. This is no surprise when you consider that philosophers see one of their main roles as questioning the assumptions underlying important claims and arguments. Indeed, one of the most important questions in the philosophy of well-being is whether there is just one thing that ultimately makes life go well for the person living it or whether there are several things. In other words, when philosophers argue for a theory of well-being, one of the things they must argue for is whether there are many aspects or just one aspect of the prudential good life.

The issue of subjectivity is dealt with in the same way. A philosopher needs to argue for *why* we should think that the prudential good life has any subjective elements. This is not to say that objective elements are assumed. Philosophers need to justify any subjective or objective aspects of their theory of well-being. Hopefully the message is clear; philosophers should argue for their theory without making assumptions, or at least with making as few assumptions as possible. In practice, this leads to lots of extra opportunities to disagree about the fundamental aspects of the issue in question. This attention to detail and pedantry for addressing the fundamentals is doubtless part of the reason why philosophy has made little progress over the millennia, and quality of life researchers have not waited for a philosophical consensus to emerge before bringing empirical methodologies to the subject.

Another important aspect of a philosophical approach[1] to well-being research is that philosophers tend to look first and foremost for universal answers to the question of interest. Given especially the widespread differences in values across cultures, this preference for universal answers may also have slowed the progress of philosophical investigations of well-being. But imagine the relative importance of discovering what makes life go well for an individual, for a group, for every current person, or for every conceivable person. Not often constrained by practicalities, philosophers tend to aim for the "big fish" – the universal theory of something. Philosophers of well-being are no different, tending to either aim for a universal theory of well-being, or sometimes limiting the scope of their inquiry to humankind so as to keep monographs to readable lengths (e.g., Kraut 2007). Of course, the idea that a fundamental truth about well-being is even possible (and so, worthy of investigation) is an assumption, so this idea is also questioned by philosophers!

How to Create a Philosophical Theory of Well-Being

Any philosophical course on well-being or quality of life would be remiss if it did not look carefully at the process of creating a theory of well-being. There are several issues to address, including the assumptions mentioned above, the identification of what has non-instrumental prudential value, and the prudential rationale – the justification of *why* that thing has (or those things have) non-instrumental prudential value. All of these issues should be addressed to adequately provide the characteristic level of clarity we aspire to in philosophy.

Scope

What or who is your theory of well-being for? There are many possibilities. It would be possible for me to make a theory of well-being that was only intended to apply to myself on this particular day. It would also be possible to make a theory of well-being and intend for it to apply to everything, even inert objects of the distant future. For teaching purposes, the most useful limits of analysis are usually at the individual subjective level (getting students to create a theory of well-being that applies to themselves) and at the level of humankind. Other interesting scopes to investigate include all life or all sentient life, and limits to specific cultures or other meaningful sub-populations of human kind.

When teaching well-being and quality of life from a philosophical perspective, I find it useful to get students to think about a theory of well-being for themselves in

---

[1] There is huge diversity within philosophy. The claims in this chapter refer mainly to the philosophical tradition known as Western Analytic Philosophy, which, now prominent in the Anglophone Western world, traces most of its heritage through Europe to Ancient Greece.

the first instance. Then I encourage students to share their theories with each other and see whether they are compatible. These comparisons lead easily to fruitful discussions about the potential for theories of well-being to be generalised in either a restricted or universal way. Another useful endeavour is encouraging students to think about whether their individual subjective theory of well-being could usefully apply to non-human animals, artificial intelligence, or aliens.

Level of Analysis

Whether well-being can only be sensibly analysed at the level of whole lives is another important issue to consider when creating a theory of well-being. It was not uncommon for Ancient Greeks to claim that an individual's well-being cannot be assed until they are dead, or even long after that (Bok 2012). For example, if honour is a component of well-being and one's honour can be affected by the actions of one's children, then my well-being could be affected long after my death because of the misdeeds of my (poorly raised) children.

Philosophy can also make sense of theories of wellbeing that give assessments of the prudential value of parts of lives, even moments of the briefest duration. The theory of well-being that sums units of pleasure and ignores everything else is as amenable to assessments of moments as much as it is to assessments of whole lives.

Philosophy in the Western Analytical tradition tends to focus on individuals as the relevant unit of analysis. In philosophical research on well-being, this means primarily thinking about what makes a life go well for an individual. Other philosophical perspectives, particularly indigenous perspectives and those originating in the East, may focus on groups as the relevant level of analysis. In the well-being context, that means indigenous or eastern philosophers of well-being may investigate what makes life go well for the *group*. This group-centric approach is not to be confused with simply summing the well-being of each individual in the group in order to determine the well-being of the group. Oftentimes, taking a group-centric approach means treating the group as the smallest unit of analysis for at least some aspects of well-being. For example, whether a group is genuinely harmonious could be an emergent property of the group, based on but not fully determined by the relationships between individuals in the group.

A related issue is whether philosophical investigations of well-being at the individual level should accept group-level well-being or the well-being of relevant others as a potential component of an individual's own well-being. For example, some individuals in East Asian cultures would claim that their well-being is party constituted by the well-being of their family members or local community (Joshanloo 2014; Lu and Gilmour 2006). The key issue here is whether the well-being of another can rightly be seen as being a fundamental (non-instrumental) part of what it is for an individual's life to go well for them, as opposed to being a merely instrumental cause of their well-being. The issue of instrumental vs non-instrumental prudential value is discussed in more detail below.

Different levels of analysis in the hard sciences might mean investigating at the sub-atomic, molecular, organism, or species level. These different levels of granularity do not readily apply in the philosophy of well-being, which usually operates at the level of sensible everyday objects and mental states. For example, Philosophical theories of well-being are likely to operate on the level of emotions, desires, beliefs, friendships, material possessions, and so on. This focus does not exclude interesting possibilities such as the reduction of pleasure to a particular function or neurochemical event in the brain. In practice, however, philosophers tend to operate on the level that requires no equipment to test, and can easily be explained to people without scientific expertise.

Identifying What Has Non-instrumental Prudential Value

With the scope and level of analysis established, the next step in creating a theory of well-being is to clearly state what has value. Specifically, the theory should identify everything that has non-instrumental prudential value. "Non-instrumental" and its counterpart "instrumental" are discussed below, and "prudential" was discussed above. These key terms are also defined in Box 2.2 below.

Box 2.2: Key Definitions 2
- *Prudential value*: goodness or badness *for* an entity (usually a person)
- *Prudential good*: something that contributes to prudential value
- *Instrumental good*: something that indirectly contributes to prudential value (via one or more non-instrumental goods)
- *Non-instrumental value*: something that directly contributes to prudential value

---

Instrumental and Non-instrumental Goods

What is good for people? There are countless objects and activities that positively contribute to well-being. However, the vast majority of these objects and activities are only prudentially valuable because they lead to some other prudential good. Take money as an example; money is cross-culturally desired for its value. But money is also the prototypical example of an *instrumental* good – something that *in*directly contributes to well-being (via one or more *non*-instrumental goods). One way to determine whether a good is instrumentally or non-instrumentally prudentially valuable is to closely examine the connection between the good and well-being.

Does money *directly* contribute to our well-being? To answer this question, we have to think carefully about why money is good for us. Money, unlike perhaps life, does not have intrinsic or inherent value – that is, value in and of itself, without reliance on anything outside of itself. Consider how valuable your monetary savings would be if the currency your savings were held in completely collapsed. For example, imagine if everyone in the world decided to immediately disband all currencies and install a new global currency: sheep. Bill Gates and others would immediately fall off the rich lists, only to be replaced by Lance, Andy, Dave, Sharon, and other sheep farmers from rural New Zealand. The current financial system is required for money to have any value at all, so money's value cannot be intrinsic or inherent.

Re-focusing on how money creates prudential value for us, we can see that money is valuable mainly because it allows us to buy things. Whether the buying of stuff is thought of as an opportunity, a freedom, the ability to satisfy desires, or the ability to buy stuff that is itself prudentially valuable, is for the moment irrelevant. The main point is that the prudential value lies not in the money itself, but in what it provides, like freedom, or in the provisions of the goods that it can be used to purchase, like buying a holiday for your family to increase your happiness.

This process of asking ourselves, "But, why is *that* valuable to our well-being?" is repeatable. We can keep asking this question until we reach the end of the line – the point at which we cannot produce an answer for why something is valuable for us, and yet we remain sure it is valuable. On the face of it, this might seem bad; have we just discovered that we value something for no good reason? Philosophers love justifications (arguments and evidence), so discovering that we value something without justification sounds dreadful to us – will we be forced to hand in our pens and our badges if our philoso-boss finds out? Luckily, struggling to justify a value that we are sure is valuable is a sign of the good in question being non-instrumentally valuable (as opposed to being a sign that we should quit our day job).

For example, I often ask my students a simple question: "Why are you here?", and then keep asking them why this or that. Answers tend to follow this pattern (">" separates each level of justification):

To help me pass the course > To get a degree > to get a job > to get (lots of) money > to buy a house and nice things > to provide for my family > because that makes me feel good > ?

The question mark represents the end of the justificatory line. Feeling good seems to be prudentially valuable, but it is not easy to justify *why* it makes my life go better for me. Consultation with others at this point usually reveals that many people agree with the view that feeling good is obviously prudentially valuable. This makes feeling good a plausible candidate for being a non-instrumental prudential good – it directly contributes to well-being, or perhaps, is a component of well-being.

The distinction between instrumental and non-instrumental prudential goods is vital for creating a philosophical theory of well-being. The main real-world purpose of a theory of well-being is to allow for assessments of the prudential value of lives. These assessments are a kind of accounting for prudential value. And, as every good accountant knows, we want to avoid double-counting. The easiest way to avoid double-counting when assessing the prudential value of lives is to count all and only the non-instrumental prudential goods. Notice that this still allows for the value of instrumental goods to be included in the accounting – any instrumental prudential value a good has must be realised through non-instrumental goods. For example, the instrumental value of money might be fully accounted for through the non-instrumental value of the good feelings or happiness the spending of the money brings about.

A further complication is that some goods will be both instrumentally and non-instrumentally prudentially valuable. Consider feeling good. Feeling good may directly contribute to well-being, but feeling good also makes us more likely to be nice to other people, which may lead to stronger or more friendships (Diener and Tay 2017), and friendship has also been suggested as a non-instrumental good (e.g., Finnis 1980). Of course, having many strong friendships might also make us feel good, but as long as friendship also directly contributes to prudential value (over and above any effect is has on how we feel), then friendship is a non-instrumental prudential good as well as an instrumental prudential good. For prudential value accounting purposes, we would add the non-instrumental value of the friendship to the non-instrumental value of the good feelings (caused by the friendships and other features of life).

Of course, a theory that listed all of the instrumental prudential goods would be a very long theory indeed, far too long to be useful. So, a philosophical theory of well-being aims to identify all of the non-instrumental prudential goods.

It should be noted that this approach differs from many attempts to theorise about well-being or the quality of life from a social-scientific perspective. Many scientists investigating well-being attempt to model it, identifying both the components of well-being and potential causes and effects of well-being. This modelling approach achieves several important aims at once. It provides some evidence that the concept is real in the sense that it coheres with other widely supported concepts and can cause changes in those other concepts when it itself changes. Models are also at once an explanation and a prediction depending on the perspective taken (Foss 2014). Having a precise and accurate model of happiness, for example, might allow us to point to what is likely causing someone's current happiness as well as predict how happy they will be if those causes of happiness reach particular levels. Conceptual social scientific models of well-being are usually developed empirically or quickly operationalised and empirically tested.

Philosophers tend not to use empirical methods when developing their theories of well-being, but they often do think about how their theory coheres with other established theories, principles of value, and examples. This aspect of theorising about well-being will be discussed more in section "How to critique a philosophical theory of well-being".

One or Many Things?

Given the task of creating a theory or well-being, a major issue is how many non-instrumental prudential goods there are. The title of this section suggests that the viable options are one (monism) or many (pluralism). Astute readers may notice an assumption here – why not a theory of well-being with zero non-instrumental prudential goods? Excluding this possibility is an assumption (so, well spotted!), but it is a fairly safe one. If nothing has non-instrumental prudential value, then nothing that happens to us can make our lives go better or worse for us. That means there is no prudential difference between being tortured for the rest of your life and living a regular life like you do now! Since our lives do seem to have their ups and downs, then there must be something or somethings that represent that change in prudential value; non-instrumental prudential goods play that role.

With "none" excluded as an option for number of non-instrumental prudential goods, philosophers are usually left to decide between one and many when creating theories of well-being. Conceptually, identifying the number of non-instrumental prudential goods could be approached in two ways. One way is practically difficult; amassing all of the instrumental goods and interrogating them to discover what non-instrumental prudential good or goods they might lead to. This would be difficult to accomplish because of the sheer number of instrumental prudential goods. The second and more common way to work out how many non-instrumental prudential goods should be in a theory of well-being starts by looking at the prototypical goods. Reflecting (usually from an armchair) on what really makes life go well, and then interrogating those reflections, usually leads to a short or very short list of candidate non-instrumental prudential goods.

The final decision on how many of the candidate non-instrumental prudential goods really are non-instrumental prudential goods is determined by attempts to reduce each of the candidate goods to one or more of the other candidate goods. Consider an extension of the friendship example from above. Imagine your armchair reflections and interrogations have resulted in three candidate non-instrumental prudential goods: feeling good, meaning, and friendship. An attempted reduction of friendship to feeling good and meaning requires thinking about the prudentially valuable aspects of friendship and whether in fact that value is all ultimately found in the good feelings and meaningfulness that friendship provides. One way to do this is to imagine a friendship that is neither pleasurable nor meaningful (it doesn't need to be the opposite of pleasurable and meaningful, just perfectly neutral on those values). Would this pleasure-less, meaningless friendship still be prudentially valuable – would it make your life go better for you? Remember that you do not need to explain *why* it would make your life better for you, you just need to assess whether you have a strong feeling about it (because we are trying to assess whether friendship is non-instrumentally prudentially valuable).

If this process leads you to identify more than one non-instrumental prudential good, then you also need to consider how the goods relate to each other and to well-being. It is important to consider whether one of the goods has priority over others. For example, feeling good and engaging in meaningful activities might both be irreducible non-instrumental prudential goods, but perhaps one is much more valuable than the other. Consider also that one non-instrumental prudential good may be required to enable others to contribute to well-being. For example, being alive might be non-instrumentally prudentially valuable and a pre-requisite for feeling good. It also might be the case that a life without any one of the non-instrumental prudential goods cannot be considered a prudentially good life, no matter how much of the other goods is present.

Subjective or Objective?

The terms subjective and objective are frequently used loosely in both philosophy and social scientific work on well-being or quality of life. The terms are defined relevant to a well-being context in Box 2.3 and the important distinction between them is discussed in this section.

Box 2.3: Key Definitions 3

- *Well-being Subjectivism*: it is up to each individual to decide what makes their life go well for them (and only them)
- *Well-being Objectivism*: there is a fact of the matter about what makes lives go well that applies to people regardless of what they believe about prudential value
- *Mixed subjective-objective accounts of well-being*: what non-instrumentally makes life go well includes both subjective and objective components
- *Well-being Subjective-Objective Hybridism*: a life goes well for the one living it if and only if the person believes that what has objective prudential value is valuable for them, and their life includes what has objective prudential value

---

When discussing any matter of value, subjective accounts give complete power to individuals to decide for themselves what has value. Note that this is different to a measure of well-being relying on self-report data. A life satisfaction survey question with a 0–10 response scale elicits a respondent's judgment about their own life, so it is subjective in the sense that the respondent has complete control over how to rate their life on the scale. However, if the answer to that question is used as a measure of well-being (either total well-being or a component of well-being) then the researcher has made the decision about what ultimately makes the respondent's life go well for them – being satisfied with their life. Subjective theories of well-being allow individuals to choose the concepts that count as non-instrumental prudential goods for their own well-being (they do not get to decide for people generally).

Subjective accounts of well-being the potential drawback that they enable people with very unusual beliefs about prudential value to be living the prudential good life despite living what appears to most observers to be a worthless life.

Objective accounts of well-being do not leave the "what?" question of non-instrumental prudential value to individuals; they dictate what ultimately makes life go well for the one living it. Nearly all philosophical theories of well-being are objective in the sense that they are intended to apply to people even when those people do not agree with the theory. For example, the objective "feels good" theory of well-being states that feeling good is good for you *even if* you do not want some of those good feelings or even if you do not think feelings directly contribute to well-being.

The dictatorial nature of objective accounts of well-being is a benefit in terms of being able to overrule people who claim to have wonderful lives despite outward appearances to the contrary. However, the same dictatorial nature may also be viewed as a weakness because it overrides individuals' idiosyncratic perspectives in a way that may not fully respect any fundamental diversity between individuals.

Objective accounts of well-being should not be confused with the objective measures of well-being or quality of life that are extant in the social scientific literature. If a social scientific measure of well-being or quality of life is referred to as being "objective", this is usually meant to mean that there exists a way to check the data produced by the measure, such as a report on the number of jobs available (e.g., Weijers and Morrison 2018). The "objective" label can even be used when the data are self-reported. For example, employment and related employment categories are usually self-reported in social scientific research. These reports are independently verifiable, at least in principle, because we could momentarily disregard research ethics and track down the respondents' employer. Note that is different to measures of subjective well-being, which effectively refer to something so internal to a person that there may be no independent way to verify the data, even in principle.

It is possible to create subjective-objective mixed accounts of well-being. A mixed theory of well-being would identify at least one objective non-instrumental prudential good and yet still allow individuals to have a say over what the other non-instrumental prudential goods are for themselves. Such accounts are not popular among philosophers. The combining of subjective and objective elements seems to allow for contradictions or at least incalculable value trade-offs. There is one exception to this general rule against mixed accounts – hybrid subjective-objective accounts of well-being. Hybrid accounts are usually characterised by the alignment of subjective and objective prudential values, such that individuals value what is truly worthy of value. For example, the hybrid "feels good" theory of well-being will only attribute non-instrumental prudential value to someone's life when the following conditions are met: the person believes that feeling good is a central component of well-being and the person is feeling good (because according to the theory, feeling good is, objectively speaking, a central component of well-being).

Internalist or Externalist?

The terms internalist and externalist are much less common than subjective and objective but explaining them will help untangle some of the confusion around subjective and objective. The terms are defined relevant to a well-being context in Box 2.4 and the important distinctions between them are discussed in this section.

Box 2.4: Key Definitions 4

- *Internalist accounts of well-being*: Only things internal to a life can be non-instrumentally valuable for the one living that life (such as beliefs, health, and the experience of friendship)
- *Externalist accounts of well-being*: Only things external to a life can be non-instrumentally valuable for the one living that life (such as living in reality even when the person doesn't believe they are)
- *Mixed internalist-externalist accounts of well-being*: At least some things external to a life can be non-instrumentally valuable for the one living that life (such as the truth of a person's beliefs, actually having friends, etc.)

Internalist accounts of well-being only consider things internal to the person whose well-being we are assessing. For example, the internal aspects of mental states are considered, but the external objects of our mental states are not. So, for internalist accounts, it matters that I am feeling good, but it does *not* matter what I'm feeling good about – even if I'm feeling good about the suffering of others! Similarly, what I believe about the world outside of myself can be considered, but the truth of what I believe cannot. If I believe I am a good friend, then it doesn't immediately matter for my well-being whether or not I am a good friend (although it will likely come back to bite me in the future when my friends give up on me). Additionally my body and so my health, is internal to me, so it can also be considered by internalist accounts of well-being.

Externalist accounts of well-being only consider things external to me when assessing the prudential value of my life. The internal aspects of my mental states and the functioning of my body are not considered on these accounts. Instead, my well-being rests solely on things that are *not* about me. Perhaps that God is pleased with me or that I live in the real world (even though I do not know or believe these things).

The focus of externalist accounts on all but the person whose life we are evaluating make them unpopular. Much more popular are mixed internalist-externalist accounts of well-being, which include internal and external elements. On a mixed account, feeling good might contribute more prudential value if it is the result of concerted effort, or it might contribute nothing at all if it is the result of morally depraved behaviour.

Prudential Rationale: Justifying Why It Has Prudential Value

While it is important to be clear about the fundamental details of what has value, the most significant part of any theory of well-being is the prudential rationale. Philosophers are loathed to accept anything at face value – we usually demand clear and compelling justifications for all claims, even (and sometimes especially) those considered common-sense. When faced with a new theory of well-being, we want to know *why* we should believe that the proposed goods are non-instrumentally valuable.

Creating convincing prudential rationales is the most difficult part of creating a theory of well-being. Recall from the discussion of instrumental and non-instrumental goods above that providing a direct reason why a good is prudentially valuable may just reveal a more fundamental prudential good. For example, to argue that eating cake is only valuable because it leads to feeling good is to discover that eating cake is an instrumental good and that feeling good may be a non-instrumental good. Applying the same test to feeling good, we might conclude that feeling good *just is* good for us. This identifies feeling good as a potential non-instrumental prudential good, but it hardly justifies it.

Justifying proposed non-instrumental prudential goods requires providing generally compelling reasons – reasons that should be convincing to reasonable people! The justification can be considered successful if many reasonable people accept that the proposed non-instrumental prudential good makes the life of the one living it go better for them even when the good leads to nothing else. In practice, this justification takes a lot of discussion, often including examples and principles of value.

The prudential rationale for the Simple Unrestricted Desire Satisfaction (SUDS) theory of well-being, can be used to illustrate this. The SUDS theory states that the only non-instrumental prudential good is the satisfaction of one's desires (with any and all desires counted, and all desires weighted according to their intensity) (Lukas 2010). The prudential rationale for the SUDS theory of well-being is that getting what you want is good for you (no matter what it is you want). The justification for the theory would likely include discussion of examples of people with things in their lives that are considered to be non-instrumental prudential goods by other theories, but that the person does not desire. For example, if a person does not desire another friend, then according to SUDS, gaining another friend does not directly increase that person's well-being.

Example Philosophical Theories of Well-Being

Combining these components of theories of well-being in different ways permits a huge range of possible philosophical accounts of well-being. Some combinations, although possible, are not popular. The theories of well-being that have proven popular over time are briefly defined in Box 2.5 and discussed below. It should be noted that there are a lot of sub-variants, different specific accounts of well-being that gather under these major headings. Any philosophical course on well-being would discuss many of the sub-variants.

Box 2.5: Main Philosophical Theories of Well-Being

- *Prudential hedonism*: All and only pleasure is non-instrumentally prudentially valuable and all and only pain is non-instrumentally prudentially
  dis-valuable
- *Desire satisfactionism*: All and only desire-satisfaction is non-
  instrumentally prudentially valuable and all and only desire-frustration is
  non-instrumentally prudentially disvaluable
- *Objective list theory*: There are X non-instrumental prudential goods and
  they are… (e.g., pleasure, truth, and friendship)
- *Perfectionism*: The prudential good life is the perfect life – being a perfect
  specimen of the kind of creature you are

Prudential hedonism is the theory of well-being that takes all and only pleasure
to be non-instrumentally prudentially valuable and all and only pain as the opposite (Weijers 2011). The theory essentially says that the happy life is the prudentially good life and that the happy life is one that includes lots of pleasures and few
pains. Important hedonistic variants include Mill's (1861) qualitative hedonism,
which values higher pleasures (cerebral pleasures that are only available to humans)
over lower pleasures (sensual and bodily pleasures that many animals can experience). An important modern variant is Feldman's (2004) attitudinal hedonism,
which understands non-instrumentally prudentially valuable pleasure as a pro-
attitude, such as appreciation or approval, towards states of affairs (as opposed to
understanding pleasure a pleasant sensation – feeling good).

Desire-satisfaction theories of well-being revolve around the idea that getting
what we want is good for us. The basic version, simple unrestricted desire satisfactionism, allows the satisfaction of any and all desires to contribute positively to
well-being (Lukas 2010). Whole life desire-satisfaction theories are only interested
in whether someone's life as a whole matches up to their desires (Kekes 1982). A
few variants also focus on the desires of well-informed others, rather than the individual living the life (e.g., Suikkanen 2011).

Objective list theories of well-being dictate a number of non-instrumental prudential goods that apply to us whether we agree with them or not. Some important
examples include Finnis' list (1980): life, knowledge, play, aesthetic experience,
sociability (friendship), practical reasonableness, and religion (spirituality) and
Parfit's list (1984): Moral goodness, rational activity, and development of abilities,
having children and being a good parent, knowledge, and awareness of true beauty.

Perfectionist theories of well-being hold that achieving well-being is a matter of
perfecting ones' nature. Informed by Aristotle's eudemonia, Hurka's (1993) perfectionism makes claims about the perfect form of humankind based on our natural
capacities. For example, Hurka would argue that knowledge is (at least in part) a
non-instrumental prudential good because knowledge is an aspect of being human
that can be improved upon and perfected. Perfectionist theories are sometimes
classified as a subset of objective list theories because they invariably end up as a
list of objective non-instrumental prudential goods.

How to Critique a Philosophical Theory of Well-Being

The details of a theory of well-being can sometimes be fruitfully critiqued, such as when a theory is arbitrarily limited in scope, but the most important critiques focus on the prudential rationale. The techniques used to critique prudential rationales are effectively the same as the techniques used to justify prudential rationales – discussing examples, principles, and background theories in a way that affects people's judgments about what has non-instrumental prudential value. The examples are usually hypothetical scenarios about people's lives. The principles are usually simple claims about the kinds of things that can or cannot have prudential value. The background theories are the relevant claims that are well-established in some area such that we generally take them to be true. For example, well-received scientific theories about pleasure and pain might be relevant to evaluating the feels good theory of well-being.

Thought Experiments: The Power of Examples

In practice, examples (the key aspect of thought experiments) tend to overpower principles when assessing potential non-instrumental prudential goods. For example, someone might believe "what you don't know can't hurt you", or more specifically the prudential principle the Experience Requirement: For something to affect my well-being, it must affect my experiences. But they might disregard the principle when asked about a scenario, based on Shelly Kagan's deceived businessman thought experiment (1998), about which of two lives is better for the one living it:

Imagine two people with experientially identical lives. They both had the experience of their partners loving them, their colleagues respecting them, and their work being successful until they died painlessly in their sleep at age 65. One of these people had *genuine* experiences throughout their life. The other was *deceived* by their partner and colleagues and their business failed shortly after their death, although none of this affected their experiences in any way. The deceived person was also then ruthlessly slandered after their death, being accused of heinous acts that they did not commit.

Since the deceived person did not experience any of the deception while they lived or the slandering after they died, the Experience Requirement states that those features of the deceived life do not affect the deceived person's well-being. However, most people judge the deceived life as prudentially worse than the non-deceived life. This judgment can only be correct if the Experience Requirement is false. Faced with this contradiction, the power of most people's judgment that the deceived life is prudentially worse than the non-deceived life makes them give up the Experience Requirement.

When faced with powerful thought experiments like the one above, defenders of principles or theories have also criticised some examples for being "intuition pumps" (Dennett 1980). The criticisms often point to aspects of the scenario that might be misleading or biasing readers' judgments about the lives (Weijers 2013). A lot of philosophical scholarship on well-being takes place at this level – creating and responding to examples designed to criticise theories or principles of prudential value. So, a good philosophical course on well-being or quality of life should include information on how to create and critique these examples. A few classic thought experiments on well-being are listed in Box 2.6.

Box 2.6: Key Thought Experiments on Well-Being

- *Kagan's deceived businessman*: Kagan, S. (1998). *Normative Ethics*, Westview Press, pp. 34–36.
- *Nozick's experience machine*: Nozick, R. (1974). *Anarchy, State, and Utopia*, Basic Books, pp. 42–45.
- *Rawls' grass-counter*: Rawls, J. (1971). *A Theory of Justice*, Harvard University Press, p. 432.
- *Sen's happy slave*: Sen, A. (1987/2012), *On Ethics and Economics*, Oxford University Press, pp. 45–46.

Prudential Principles

Although thought experiments tend to rule the roost, prudential principles are also important to discuss in any philosophical course on well-being or quality of life. Prudential principles work well as objections to many theories and they help clarify and focus people's often nebulous ideas about what matters for well-being. Assessing principles of prudential value is also a fun way to hone critical thinking skills. A few important prudential principles can be found in Box 2.7. Many of the key terms discussed above, such as subjectivism, internalism, and monism can also be understood as prudential principles. While the strong versions of these principles are discussed below, weaker versions are also possible. Weaker versions of the prudential principles might, for eaxample, state that the goods in question contribute less prudential value (rather than none) if the specified requirement is not met.

Box 2.7: Key Prudential Principles

- *Desert requirement*: For goods to contribute to well-being, they must be deserved
- *Experience requirement*: For goods to contribute to well-being, they must (in some way) affect the experiences of the relevant individual
- *Reality requirement*: For goods to contribute to well-being, they must be sufficiently embedded in reality
- *Resonance requirement*: For goods to contribute to well-being, they must be subjectively appreciated by the relevant individual

The Desert Requirement states that goods only confer prudential value if they are deserved. This prudential principle may be used to argue that achievement that is not worked for does not contribute to well-being. Similarly, it may be used to argue that pleasure from immoral behaviour does not contribute to well-being.

The Experience Requirement states that goods only confer prudential value if they affect our experiences. This prudential principle may be used to argue that anything that occurs after our death cannot harm us (because we cannot experience it). Similarly, it may be used to argue that being deceived in a way that never affects our experiences does not impact our well-being.

The Reality Requirement states that goods only confer prudential value if they are sufficiently embedded in reality. This prudential principle may be used to argue that illusory experiences of pleasure or success, such as might be had in an experience machine do not contribute to well-being. According to the Reality Requirement, seeming real is not enough, our experiences would have to be actually real for them to contribute to our well-being.

The Resonance Requirement states that goods only confer prudential value if they are subjectively appreciated as valuable. In other words, if we do not resonate with the supposed prudential value of a particular good, then we have reason to doubt the truth of the theory that stipulates that good is prudentially valuable.

How to Teach a Course on Well-Being or Quality of Life from a Philosophical Perspective

There are many ways that a philosophical course on well-being might be constructed. In this section I explain and argue for a particular way to structure the course based on Fink's (2013) advice on creating significant learning experiences. Later in this section, specific assessments and syllabi are presented.

Appropriate Pedagogy for Teaching Well-Being from a Philosophical Perspective

Informed by the work of Fink (2013), the fundamental pedagogical idea underpinning my approach is getting students to practice using the skills and knowledge that constitute the learning objectives (instead of just learning about those skills and theories). Some courses take a relatively passive approach to student learning – students might just read articles (in which philosophers propose and criticise theories of well-being) and then take quizzes on who argued for what. In contrast, I recommend taking a profoundly active approach to student learning. The benefits of active learning are well-known to education researchers. They include:

[engaging] students more deeply in the process of learning… encouraging critical thinking and fostering the development of self-directed learning. … [As well as helping] students to connect the information from the classroom to practice in the outside world. (Van Amburgh et al. 2007, p. 1)

In practice taking a profoundly active approach to student learning means dedicating a lot of class time to activities that demand critical engagement from students. This approach necessarily requires aiming to teach less content during the course than in traditional content-based courses. Some professors may already feel like their students are not learning enough and think that teaching less content will make matters worse. I disagree. Few students are as adept at learning as professors were when they were students. Rushing through complex content robs most students of the time they need to engage deeply with the novel ideas. Little time for engagement with novel ideas means little chance of understanding or recall. So, by planning to cover a lot of content, many content-based courses don't encourage skill development or even their main goal of knowledge acquisition! The learning objectives I have in mind, including the content-based ones, are best realised by slowing down and making space for students to regularly practice using key skills on the content in a supportive environment (Fortune et al. 2007).

Creating a course full of significant learning experiences requires careful construction of the content and assessment. I recommend using a scaffolded learning approach. Scaffolded learning "describes a cluster of instructional techniques designed to move students from a novice position toward greater understanding, such that they become independent learners" (Colter and Ulatowski 2017). To successfully set up the "scaffolding", I suggest planning assignment instructions and lecture notes ahead of time to ensure that my expectations for each assessment are clear and complete. The instructions should include "pro tips", or something similar, informing students of common errors and explaining how to avoid them. Ideally the final assessment should require students to complete a complex task, such as writing a focussed argumentative essay, which they have been practicing throughout the course with different material. I take most of the instructions (scaffolding) away for the final assessment, encouraging them to use the same skills they have already practiced, and think about the feedback they have received on their earlier attempts at the complex task.

Following this process, I can be confident that the learning outcomes have been achieved because students will only pass the course if they have already demonstrated the requisite skills and knowledge in various assessments during the course.

Suggested Learning Objectives and Content for Teaching Well-Being from a Philosophical Perspective

I recommend skill- and content-based learning outcomes, with the main focus on skills. Why emphasise skills over content? That's simple. The Internet provides unparalleled access to the world's experts and their views on the most recent findings about nearly every kind of "fact" imaginable. While professors will always be content experts in their areas of expertise, anyone with good research skills and an Internet connection can become a content expert in any area they choose. However, useful expertise requires skills – the skills of interpretation, appraisal, argumentation, and application (to name but a few).

Given a focus on skills, Fink (2013) suggests asking yourself a key question before writing your learning objectives – what do you want your students to be able to *do* by the end of the course? Pondering this question led me to devise several learning objectives for philosophical courses on well-being, which you can view in Box 2.8. Notice that the learning objectives are focussed on skills in the context of well-being, rather than being restricted to knowledge of theories and arguments about well-being.

> **Box 2.8: Example Learning Outcomes for Teaching Well-Being from a Philosophical Perspective**
> Students who successfully complete the course should be able to:
>
> - Think critically about issues in the theory of well-being
> - Elucidate and analyse complex problems and concepts arising in the theory of well-being
> - Articulate and defend original arguments in support of contentious theses related to well-being
> - Make prudential decisions in personal, professional, and public contexts
> - Be proficient in the distinctive questions and arguments associated with the theory of well-being
> - Communicate information, arguments, and analyses related to well-being effectively in writing and orally
> - Identify and defend what they think ultimately makes their life go well for them and for people in general

Suggested Content for Teaching Well-Being from a Philosophical Perspective

Box 2.9 shows an ordered list of topics that could constitute a philosophical course on well-being. Possible readings for the topics are indicated. The specific content should depend on the instructor's areas of interest and competence, as well as the duration of the course. The order and timing of topics should be developed in conjunction with the type and timing of assessments. The choice of readings should depend on the level of the course.

Box 2.9: Example Topic List for Teaching Well-Being from a Philosophical Perspective

1. Introduction (motivation, learning outcomes, assessment, rules, culture, and a taste of what is to come)
2. Methodology (using simple toy theories and examples)

    (a) Crisp, R. (2017). Well-Being. *The Stanford Encyclopedia of Philosophy*
    (b) Fletcher, G. (2016). "Introduction", in *The Philosophy of Well-Being: An Introduction*. Routledge, pp. 1–7
    (c) Griffin, J. (1988). "Introduction", In *Well-Being: Its Meaning, Measurement and Moral Importance*. Clarendon Press, pp. 1–6

3. Well-being theories: hedonism

    (a) Weijers, D. (2011). Hedonism, *Internet Encyclopedia of Philosophy*
    (b) Nozick, R. (1974). "The experience machine", in *Anarchy, state, and utopia*, Blackwell Publishers, pp. 42–45
    (c) Kagan, S. (1998). Excerpt of "Well-Being", in *Normative Ethics*, Westview Press, pp. 29–36

4. Well-being theories: attitudinal hedonism

    (a) Feldman, F. (2004). "Attitudinal Hedonism", in *Pleasure and the Good Life*, Oxford: Clarendon Press, pp. 55–107

5. Well-being theories: satisfaction accounts

    (a) Kagan, S. (1998). Excerpt of "Well-Being", in *Normative Ethics*, Westview Press, pp. 36–41
    (b) Lauinger, W. (2011). Dead Sea Apples and Desire-Fulfillment Welfare Theories, *Utilitas*, 23, 324–343
    (c) Lukas, M. (2010). Desire Satisfactionism and the Problem of Irrelevant Desires, *Journal of Ethics and Social Philosophy*, 4(2), 1–25

6. Well-being theories: whole-life satisfaction accounts

    (a) Kekes, J. (1982). Happiness, *Mind*, 91, 358–376
    (b) Suikkanen, J. (2011). An improved whole life satisfaction theory of happiness, *International Journal of Wellbeing*, 1(1), 149–166

7. Well-being theories: objective list accounts

    (a) Arneson, R. J. (1999). Human Flourishing Verses Desire Satisfaction, *Social Philosophy and Policy*, 16(1), 113–142
    (b) Fletcher, G. (2013). A Fresh Start for the Objective-List Theory of Well-Being, *Utilitas*, 25, 206–220

(continued)

Box 2.9 (continued)

8. Well-being theories: perfectionism

   (a) Dorsey, D. (2010). Three Arguments for Perfectionism, *Noûs*, 44, 59–79.
   (b) Hurka, T. (1993). "Part 1: The Perfectionist Idea", in *Perfectionism*, Oxford University Press, pp. 9–51

9. Well-being theories: eastern

   (a) Joshanloo, M. (2014). Eastern conceptualizations of happiness: Fundamental differences with western views. *Journal of Happiness Studies*, 15(2), 475–493

10. Well-being theories: indigenous (best made relevant to the nation in which the course is run)

    (a) Durie, M. (2006). *Measuring Māori Wellbeing*. New Zealand Treasury Guest Lecture Series

11. Well-being theories: religious

    (a) Michalos, A. & Weijers, D. (2017). Excerpt of "Western Historical Traditions of Well-Being", in R. Estes and J. Sirgy (eds.), *The Pursuit of Human Well-Being: The Untold Global History*, Springer, pp. 42–45.

12. Well-being theories: from psychology

    (a) Dodge, R., Daly, A. P., Huyton, J., & Sanders, L. D. (2012). The Challenge of Defining Wellbeing, *International Journal of Wellbeing*, 2(3), 222–235
    (b) Hone, L. C., Jarden, A., Schofield, G. M., & Duncan, S. (2014). Measuring flourishing: The impact of operational definitions on the prevalence of high levels of wellbeing, *International Journal of Wellbeing*, 4(1),62–90

13. Well-being theories: from economics and public policy

    (a) Forgeard, M. J. C., Jayawickreme, E., Kern, M. & Seligman, M. E. P. (2011). Doing the right thing: Measuring wellbeing for public policy, *International Journal of Wellbeing*, 1(1), 79–106
    (b) Frey, B. S., & Stutzer, A. (2007). *Should National Happiness Be Maximized?*, University of Zurich Institute for Empirical Research in Economics, Working Paper 306
    (c) Weijers, D. & Mukherjee, U. (2016). *Living Standards, Wellbeing, and Public Policy*, The New Zealand Treasury

(continued)

Box 2.9 (continued)

14. Science and technology: the science of happiness and well-being

   (a) Layard, R. (2005). "What is happiness?" in *Happiness: Lessons from a new science*, Penguin Books, pp. 11–27
   (b) Huppert, F. A. (2014). "The State of Wellbeing Science: Concepts, Measures, Interventions, and Policies". In F. A. Huppert & C. L. Cooper (eds.) *Wellbeing: A Complete Reference Guide, Volume VI*, John Wiley & Sons, pp. 1–49

15. Science and technology: Ways to increase well-being

   (a) Walker, M. (2011). Happy-people-pills for all, *International Journal of Wellbeing*, *1*(1), 127–148
   (b) Sin, N. L., & Lyubomirsky, S. (2009). Enhancing Well-Being and Alleviating Depressive Symptoms with Positive Psychology Interventions: A Practice-Friendly Meta-Analysis, *Journal of Clinical Psychology*, 65(5), 467–487

16. Science and technology: Dystopic futures and the dark side of happiness

   (a) Huxley, A. (1932). *Brave New World*. London: Vintage, 1998

The very first thing I do when teaching courses on the philosophy of well-being is to motivate the importance of the course and set the ground rules and culture of the course. The scaffolded learning approach underpinning my teaching requires students to practice skills during class, in front of their peers. If that is not scary enough, the skills philosophers aim to develop in students require students to argue with each other and justify their own views in a way that is epistemically motivating for people who might not share the same background beliefs.

Since I genuinely want my students to achieve the learning outcomes, and because I know that practicing skills is the best way to develop them (e.g., Fortune et al. 2007), I go to great lengths to create a supportive environment for learning. I dedicate ample time in the first week of lectures to creating a positive classroom culture. I use an inclusive and collaborative approach to get students to demand a respectful attitude from each other and from me. I also stress that mistakes are very normal in philosophy, and that being shown to be wrong is actually a kind of blessing in disguise. To paraphrase Socrates: If we genuinely want to learn, then being proven wrong is helpful because it moves us closer to the truth. Most importantly, I do my best to enact and enforce the collaboratively established values of the class. The main way I do this is though dealing with student contributions during lectures in a respectful and constructive manner.

With the learning outcomes in mind, it is clear that knowledge of the philosophical methods of well-being is essential for success in the course. As such, I recommend starting with a discussion of the methods immediately after motivating the course and setting the ground rules and culture. The methods discussed in this section should be referred back to throughout the course because it is the skilled application of these methods that constitute the majority of the learning outcomes.

When discussing each type of well-being theory, important sub variants should be discussed. I find it can be fun to discuss at least one ancient version of each major theory, but I focus on contemporary accounts because my learning outcomes are more geared toward answering questions about well-being here and now, as opposed to answering questions about exactly what a particular historical figure believed to be true about well-being. Although I discuss various accounts and objections from the literature, I make lots of time during class for students to attempt to generate their own accounts and objections so that they get to practice the core learning objectives.

The final topics in the course help students realise how a deeper understanding of well-being can be applied to their current and future lives, and society more broadly. I find that students respond well to topics on science and technology, especially related to positive psychology and dystopic futures. Some instructors might also want to focus heavily on economics and public policy later in the course, especially given that well-being research is now having a major impact on public policy (Weijers and Morrison 2018).

Suggested Assessments for Teaching Well-Being from a Philosophical Perspective

Assessments should be thought of broadly. Not all assessments need to contribute to a student's final grade for the course. Indeed, an effective scaffolded learning approach will include many no- and low-stakes assessments that allow students to assess their own learning in preparation for more important assessments.

In a philosophical course on well-being, students should be encouraged to practice generating and critiquing theories of well-being, prudential principles, and thought experiments about the prudential value of lives. The majority of these activities will occur during class in a way that is not assessed (at least not in a major way). I stop several times during an hour-long lecture to get students to discuss in small groups what we are learning about. For example, after explaining a new theory of well-being, I will encourage students to generate their own criticisms of it in small groups before asking them to report back to me on what they came up with.

Small group challenges and competitions can encourage energetic participation from students. For example, I might offer extra credit to the group that came up with the best variant of an objective list theory, or organise a debate between hedonists and perfectionists.

In Box 2.10, I outline a possible schedule of graded assessment tasks. The choice of assessment tasks should be informed by the level of the class, the size of the class, and the pedagogical preferences of the instructor.

Box 2.10: Example Graded Assessment Schedule for Teaching Well-Being from a Philosophical Perspective
1. Quizzes (2 multichoice) – 10%
2. Essay 1 – 15%
3. Essay 2 – 20%
4. Essay 3 – 25%
5. Journal – 30%

I use quizzes to encourage students to take and organise notes on the basic concepts, so they have them to refer to when attempting the more significant assessments. I set quizzes early in the course to get students in the habit of doing work for the class outside of class time from the beginning. Quizzes can also be unscheduled so that students do not know when they will occur. This encourages attendance at class and regular homework.

The first essay should be fairly short and worth relatively few marks. In line with the scaffolded learning approach, a lot of instructions should be provided for the first essay. For a lower division undergraduate class, I would set one simple task for the essay, such as evaluating a criticism of a theory of well-being. For example, I might ask students to write about whether the deceived businessman thought experiment is a powerful objection to prudential hedonism. Students are assessed on their ability to explain the relevant theory and objection as well their ability to critically evaluate the objection.

Each essay after the first would be longer and more demanding. New instructions may be added as old instructions are removed. In the second essay, I might ask students to generate their own criticisms of a theory that we had not discussed in detail in class. The idea is for students to apply the skills they have learned so far to new material by themselves. If they can do this, then it is clear evidence that they have already achieved some of the learning outcomes.

In the final essay, I often let students generate their own theory of well-being and defend it from the strongest criticisms they or I can think of. The prior practice critiquing other theories helps students self-critique their theory as they think about its specific details.

When I set journal assignments, I pre-write all of the journal questions before the course and encourage the students to always have their journal with them when they come to class. Each lesson, I will refer to specific questions in the journal so that students can take their own notes. The questions relate directly to the skills and knowledge required for the learning outcomes as well as the upcoming assessments. During the hedonism topic, for example, journal questions include "Which variant of hedonism is the strongest? Why?" and "What is the strongest objection against this kind of hedonism? How would you respond to it?". I can also read student's journals to assess their learning during the course to check whether key concepts and skills have been learnt.

Tips for Teaching Well-Being from a Philosophical Perspective

Creating a course that requires students to take an active approach to their learning works very well in a philosophical course on well-being. Most students will be intrinsically interested in thinking about what makes life go well for people because they have a life and they are interested in it going well for them! So, do not miss the opportunity to organise activities and assessments that allow students to think critically about prudential value and how it relates to their own lives. This can be easily achieved in the early topics by getting students to think about which theory of well-being resonates best with them and what they can learn from each theory about something that might be valuable in their lives. In the second part of the course, students can be encouraged to apply what they have learnt to how they should conduct themselves. For example, they may want to carry out some positive psychological interventions on themselves or protest against policies that seem detrimental to well-being.

Further Readings to Consider Using for Teaching Well-Being from a Philosophical Perspective

For undergraduate courses on well-being from a philosophical perspective, the following monographs might be suitable:

Fletcher, G. (2016). *The Philosophy of Well-Being: An Introduction*, Routledge.
Mulnix, J. W., & Mulnix, M. J. (2015). *Happy Lives, Good Lives: A Philosophical Examination*, Broadview Press.

These collections might also be useful:

G. Fletcher, G. (ed.). (2015). *The Routledge Handbook of the Philosophy of Well-Being*, Routledge.
Mulnix, J. W., & Mulnix, M. J. (Eds.). (2015). *Theories of Happiness: An Anthology*, Broadview Press.

Readers are also welcome to contact the author for further reading suggestions, including for a more historical approach to the subject.

References

Arneson, R. J. (1999). Human flourishing verses desire satisfaction. *Social Philosophy and Policy, 16*(1), 113–142.

Bok, S. (2012). Happiness studies in ancient Greece? A 2nd century Skeptic's challenge. *International Journal of Wellbeing, 2*(3), 277–283.

Colter, R., & Ulatowski, J. (2017). The unexamined student is not worth teaching: Preparation, the zone of proximal development, and the Socratic model of scaffolded learning. *Educational Philosophy and Theory, 49*(14), 1367–1380.

Crisp, R. (2017). Well-being. In E. N. Zalta (Ed.), *The Stanford Encyclopedia of Philosophy* (Fall 2017 Edition). Retrieved October 16, 2018, from: https://plato.stanford.edu/archives/fall2017/entries/well-being/

Dennett, D. (1980). The milk of human intentionality. *Behavioral and Brain Sciences, 3*(3), 428–430.

Diener, E., & Tay, L. (2017). Chapter 6: A scientific review of the remarkable benefits of happiness for successful and healthy living. In *Happiness: Transforming the development landscape* (pp. 90–117). The Centre for Bhutan Studies and GNH.

Dodge, R., Daly, A. P., Huyton, J., & Sanders, L. D. (2012). The challenge of defining wellbeing. *International Journal of Wellbeing, 2*(3), 222–235.

Durie, M. (2006). *Measuring Māori wellbeing* (New Zealand Treasury Guest Lecture Series, 1). Retrieved October 16, 2018, from: http://www.treasury.govt.nz/publications/media-speeches/guestlectures/pdfs/tgls-durie.pdf

Feldman, F. (2004). *Pleasure and the good life*. Oxford: Clarendon Press.

Fink, L. D. (2013). *Creating significant learning experiences: An integrated approach to designing college courses (revised and updated)*. San Francisco: Jossey-Bass.

Finnis, J. (1980). *Natural law and natural rights*. Oxford: Clarendon Press.

Fletcher, G. (2013). A fresh start for the objective-list theory of well-being. *Utilitas, 25*, 206–220.

Fletcher, G. (2016). *The philosophy of well-being: An introduction*. New York: Routledge.

Forgeard, M. J. C., Jayawickreme, E., Kern, M., & Seligman, M. E. P. (2011). Doing the right thing: Measuring wellbeing for public policy. *International Journal of Wellbeing, 1*(1), 79–106.

Fortune, A. E., Lee, M., & Cavazos, A. (2007). Does practice make perfect? Practicing professional skills and outcomes in social work field education. *The Clinical Supervisor, 26*(1–2), 239–263.

Foss, J. (2014). Science, maps, and models. In J. Foss (Ed.), *Science and the world: Philosophical approaches* (pp. 185–204). Peterborough: Broadview Press.

Frey, B. S., & Stutzer, A. (2007). *Should national happiness be maximized?*. University of Zurich Institute for Empirical Research in Economics, Working Paper 306.

Griffin, J. (1988). *Well-being: Its meaning, measurement and moral importance*. Oxford: Clarendon Press.

Hone, L. C., Jarden, A., Schofield, G. M., & Duncan, S. (2014). Measuring flourishing: The impact of operational definitions on the prevalence of high levels of wellbeing. *International Journal of Wellbeing, 4*(1), 62–90.

Huppert, F. A. (2014). The state of wellbeing science: Concepts, measures, interventions, and policies. In F. A. Huppert & C. L. Cooper (Eds.), *Wellbeing: A complete reference guide, volume VI* (pp. 1–49). Hoboken: Wiley.

Hurka, T. (1993). *Perfectionism*. Oxford: Clarendon Press.

Huxley, A. (1932). *Brave new world*. London: Vintage, 1998.

Joshanloo, M. (2014). Eastern conceptualizations of happiness: Fundamental differences with western views. *Journal of Happiness Studies, 15*(2), 475–493.

Kagan, S. (1998). *"Chapter 2: The Good", in his normative ethics* (pp. 25–69). Oxford: Westview Press.

Kekes, J. (1982). Happiness. *Mind, 91*, 358–376.

Kraut, R. (2007). *What is good and why: The ethics of well-being.* Cambridge, MA: Harvard University Press.

Lauinger, W. (2011). Dead sea apples and desire-fulfillment welfare theories. *Utilitas, 23,* 324–343.

Layard, R. (2005). *Happiness: Lessons from a new science.* New York: Penguin Books.

Lu, L., & Gilmour, R. (2006). Individual-oriented and socially oriented cultural conceptions of subjective well-being: Conceptual analysis and scale development. *Asian Journal of Social Psychology, 9*(1), 36–49.

Lucian (2005). "Hermotimus or on Philosophical Schools," in Lucian (2005). In *Lucian: Selected dialogues* (C. D. N. Costa, Trans.). Oxford University Press.

Lukas, M. (2010). Desire Satisfactionism and the problem of irrelevant desires. *Journal of Ethics and Social Philosophy, 4*(2), 1–25.

Mill, J. S. (1861). *Utilitarianism.* Indianapolis: Bobbs-Merrill, 1957.

Parfit, D. (1984). *Reasons and persons.* Oxford: Clarendon.

Sin, N. L., & Lyubomirsky, S. (2009). Enhancing well-being and alleviating depressive symptoms with positive psychology interventions: A practice-friendly meta-analysis. *Journal of Clinical Psychology, 65*(5), 467–487.

Suikkanen, J. (2011). An improved whole life satisfaction theory of happiness. *International Journal of Wellbeing, 1*(1), 149–166.

Van Amburgh, J. A., Devlin, J. W., Kirwin, J. L., & Qualters, D. M. (2007). A tool for measuring active learning in the classroom. *American Journal of Pharmaceutical Education, 71*(5), 85.

Walker, M. (2011). Happy-people-pills for all. *International Journal of Wellbeing, 1*(1), 127–148.

Weijers, D. (2011). Hedonism. In *Internet Encyclopedia of Philosophy.* Retrieved October 16, 2018, from: http://www.iep.utm.edu/hedonism/

Weijers, D. (2013). Intuitive biases in judgements about thought experiments: The experience machine revisited. *Philosophical Writings, 41*(1), 17–31.

Weijers, D., & Morrison, P. (2018). Wellbeing and public policy: Can New Zealand be a leading light for the 'Wellbeing Approach'? *Public Policy Quarterly, 14*(4), 3–12.

Weijers, D. & Mukherjee, U. (2016). *Living standards, wellbeing, and public policy.* The New Zealand Treasury. Retrieved October 16, 2018, from: http://www.treasury.govt.nz/government/longterm/fiscalposition/2016/ltfs-16-bg-lswpp.pdf

Dan Weijers is a Senior Lecturer in the Philosophy Program at the University of Waikato, New Zealand, dedicated to interdisciplinary and open access wellbeing research. Dan has published in a variety of disciplinary areas and co-founded and co-edits the International Journal of Wellbeing. Dan does theoretical, empirical, and experimental research on the good life and collaborates with a range of scholars from different disciplines. He is a multi-award-winning teacher who regularly teaches a course on happiness and wellbeing. The course is interdisciplinary, but deeply grounded in philosophical inquiry. For more information, see: www.danweijers.com.

Chapter 3
Well-Being and Quality of Life as Resources for Teaching Sociology

Tobia Fattore

Introduction

The pursuit of the well-being of individuals and nations is an evaluative measure of how a society functions. Yet, our sense of well-being is highly personal. We feel best positioned to determine what our experience of well-being is, what gives us a sense of well-being and how we might best pursue the achievement of well-being. Consequently, well-being and quality of life provide rich veins for understanding social concepts, processes and movements.

This chapter examines ways in which quality of life research can be used as a pedagogical mechanism for teaching sociology. Sociology concerns itself with many areas of human behaviour and while the scope of sociological analysis is broad, in general sociologists are concerned with examining how things that are taken for granted as natural are socially constructed. They try and make sense of social patterns, routines and orders, to help explain why people act in certain ways under certain circumstances. They also consider the relationship between the individual and their environments, to evaluate how life choices are related to the conditions in which we live, and to understand the extent that we have agency. Sociologists are also interested in how societies change and how social change happens.

Sociological approaches to quality of life share many of the concerns of traditional areas of sociological investigation. In particular, a sociological perspective explores how quality of life is a social construct that reflects what is valued in a society. For example, in some societies material wealth is highly prized and linked to well-being, whereas in others being a morally good person is key to achieving a sense of well-being. Additionally, sociology is interested in how experiences of quality of life are distributed across social groups. Even where there might be consensus about what leading a good life involves, sociologists believe the extent to

T. Fattore (✉)
Department of Sociology, Macquarie University, Sydney, Australia
e-mail: tobia.fattore@mq.edu.au

© Springer Nature Switzerland AG 2020   43
G. H. Tonon (ed.), *Teaching Quality of Life in Different Domains*, Social
Indicators Research Series 79, https://doi.org/10.1007/978-3-030-21551-4_3

which some groups are able to achieve a good life is not random, and can be predicted on the basis of which groups have access to resources that promote quality of life. Furthermore, many sociologists would argue that the way quality of life is defined reflects the interests of powerful groups in society.

To explore what quality of life is and how it is socially distributed, sociologists use systematic methods of empirical investigation to obtain data about the social world. This data can then be assessed to test or build theoretical explanations of social processes. However, because sociologists study individuals and groups with the purpose of understanding society, sociology is different to the natural sciences. This is because human beings are self-aware and are continuously making sense of the world, conferring purpose to their own actions. Sociologists are therefore also interested in understanding the meanings people apply to make sense of their own behaviour. This allows social researchers to ask questions directly to the subject of their research – people.

This chapter canvasses some key areas in which a sociological approach can contribute to understanding quality of life. We overview some foundational philosophies of quality of life to demonstrate how quality of life is a socially contested concept. We use this as a way of introducing three key theoretical traditions in sociology which explain social order and the role of individuals in society in different ways – the Structural-Functionalist, Conflict and Symbolic Interactionist paradigms. We then provide an overview of some key approaches in quality of life studies, to demonstrate how they construct the object of study in different ways. This allows us to explore some of the methodologies sociologists use, to introduce quantitative and qualitative methodologies and methods.

Philosophical Foundations of Well-Being

Section Learning Outcomes

In this section, you will be introduced to some key philosophical approaches to understanding quality of life and will use these to explore some foundational sociological theories. You will:

- Learn about eudemonic and hedonic approaches to well-being.
- Learn that different approaches to well-being are socially constructed and reflect different ideas about what a good society is.
- Be introduced to three key theoretical traditions in sociology – the Structural-Functionalist, Conflict and Symbolic Interactionist paradigms.
- Consider how these different sociological paradigms can unpack quality of life constructs, including assumptions about what is socially valued in a society, the relationship between the individual and social order; and processes of social change.

Eudemonic and Hedonic Well-Being

Research on well-being is derived from two perspectives: 'the hedonic approach, which focuses on happiness and defines well-being in terms of pleasure attainment and pain avoidance; and the eudemonic approach, which focuses on meaning and self-realization and defines well-being in terms of the degree to which a person is fully functioning' (Ryan and Deci 2001, p. 141). These approaches provide alternative conceptions of what constitutes the good life and how to achieve it.

Eudemonic Well-Being

Based in Aristotelian writings, well-being as eudemonia focuses on the good life as the virtuous life. In the *Nicomachean Ethics*, Aristotle discusses how responsibility for the achievement of well-being lies with the individual through intellectual contemplation and the practice of virtue. However not all individuals could achieve a state of well-being, only the more educated men in society and certainly not slaves or women. In Aristotle's view, the educated were responsible for thinking for the masses, a position that fits with conceptions of the state as the vehicle for furthering social well-being. Eudemonia was the end point of both individual self-realization and the responsible practices of the state, achieved through obedience to rules (Gallagher 2010).

The classical philosophical basis of well-being was evident in the European middle-ages, used to buttress the power of the Church. Well-being came to be considered a divine reward for the virtuous, well-lived life, attained through union with God. For example, in Christianity well-being was seen as a goal, achieved by continuous individual effort, obtained in death. We see the notion of divine providence in Max Weber's (1864–1920) explanation of the development of a distinctive form of capitalism in Western societies. In *The Protestant Ethic and the Spirit of Capitalism* (1904), he demonstrated that religious values, especially those associated with Puritanism – such as frugality, hard work and thrift, were critical to capitalist development. Earthly rewards resulting from hard work were both a sign of having a place in the afterlife and an engine for capitalist enterprise.

The eudemonic tradition has been carried forward in **phenomenological and positive psychology traditions**, especially in the work of Rogers (1951, 1961) and Maslow (1987). Their emphasis on personal growth and self-actualization can be likened to Aristotle's concept of the flourishing person. Both emphasize the connection between leading a virtuous life, elaborating a personal morality and having concern for the welfare of others as important to well-being. In contemporary research, the work of Martin Seligman (2011) and Deci and Ryan have also been highly influential. Seligman's work on optimism and flourishing emphasizes not only that happiness is important to well-being, but also virtues associated with engagement, cultivating meaningful relationships, meaningfulness and accomplishment. Deci and Ryan describe the concept of well-being as being about realizing one's true nature by realising one's virtuous capacities (Deci and Ryan 2008, p. 2).

Hedonic Well-Being

Hedonic approaches emphasise well-being as pleasure attainment and pain avoidance and derive from the early Greek philosophy of the **Cyreniacs**. Cyreniacs believed in individual, subjective experience, rather than objective knowledge of the external world, which provides the foundations for quality of life approaches that emphasise subjective experiences as the measure of well-being. While eudemonic approaches are concerned with the achievement of civic virtues, of which only elites could aspire to, hedonic approaches consider that well-being is a fundamental expression of humanness, available to all (Zevnik 2014).

Hedonic principles have been influential for classical political economy and utilitarian philosophy. The eighteenth-century philosopher Jeremy Bentham (1748–1832) is considered the founder of the doctrine of **utilitarianism**. Bentham (1789) argued that 'the hedonistic value of any human action is easily calculated by considering how intensely its pleasure is felt, how long that pleasure lasts, how certainly and how quickly it follows upon the performance of the action, and how likely it is to produce collateral benefits and avoid collateral harms. In emphasising the importance of the 'rational pleasure-maximizing individual', hedonic principles give primacy to 'the sovereignty of the individual in matters of personal welfare. By and large, people know what's best for them and tend to act rationally in the promotion of their interests', given that the individual has 'freedom' and in particular 'the liberty and resources to pursue their various goals however they see fit' (Haybron 2008. p. 21).

This alignment of individual utility with the pursuit of subjective well-being has become a hallmark of hedonic well-being approaches. It is rational for individuals to act in ways that promote their own happiness, or self-interest, and the pursuit of self-interest is therefore a rational principle for organising society.

Using Quality of Life Constructs to Explore the Social

At the core of the eudemonic and hedonic traditions are different ideas about what kinds of behaviours lead to happiness, who is capable of achieving happiness and what behaviours should be socially rewarded. A sociological perspective can provide us with tools to critically evaluate these perspectives, by providing theoretical frameworks that can unpack the assumptions that lie at the heart of these philosophical frameworks. We consider three main theoretical perspectives – Structural Functionalism, Marxism and Symbolic Interactionism, and in so doing demonstrate how different frameworks for understanding quality of life also provide different perspectives on how societies function.

Structural Functionalism: Quality of Life as Fulfilling Social Norms

The emphasis on well-being as virtue suggests society as a harmonious social system. Structural Functionalism is a tradition in sociology that analyses **society as a social system** made up of interconnected parts, that each have a proper function to maintain social stability. Structural functionalism stipulates that social institutions organise the behaviour of individuals into standard patterns. **Institutions** such as the education system, legal system or religious institutions each have a function they perform for the maintenance of society overall or for the functioning of some other institution.

Functionalism emphasises the importance of **moral consensus** for maintaining social order. Moral consensus exists when most people agree on the kinds of values that are worthwhile holding. From a eudemonic perspective, quality of life is linked to living a life which is guided by these social values. It is through developing moral consensus that social structures influence social roles. A **social role** is a behavioural pattern linked to a social institution, for example the role of a teacher and student are linked to the educational institution of the school. Quality of life can therefore be interpreted as the degree to which members of society feel they fulfil these roles. For example Talcott Parsons (1902–1979), who is the considered the founder of structural functionalism, discusses the importance of the 'sick role' to demonstrate how a set of behavioural expectations about how a sick person should behave is institutionalised and becomes a patterned part of social life (Parsons 1951).

Another key proponent of functionalism, Robert Merton (1910–2003), distinguished between social functions and dysfunctions. Merton (1957) pointed out that social processes have many functions. **Manifest functions** are the consequences of a social process that are sought or anticipated, while **latent functions** are the unsought consequences of a social process. Social processes that have undesirable consequences for the operation of society are called dysfunctions. For example, religion has the function of reaffirming people's adherence to important social values, thus contributing to social cohesion. However, religious adherence can also lead to religious conflicts.

Applying this paradigm to the study of quality of life focuses our attention on the:

- Shared dimensions that contribute to a sense of well-being, including the values that contribute to a sense of well-being.
- Implications of 'not fitting in' for experiences of well-being.
- Factors that characterise a well-functioning and harmonious society and those that do not.

Marxism and Conflict Paradigms: Quality of Life as Ideological

While eudemonic concepts of well-being can be used to explore concepts of society as harmonious, inequalities in well-being suggests that societies are characterised by division and competing interests. Karl Marx (1818–1883) was interested in how competing interests within a society explain social order and social change. While Marxism is a body of thought deriving its main ideas from the work of Karl Marx (see Tucker 1978 for a selection of Marx's writings), there are many schools of thought inspired by Marxism, which combine sociological analysis and social reform.

This broad paradigm focuses on struggles between groups, whether that be on the basis of their economic position, gender, religious affiliation, ethnicity, sexual affiliation or some other basis, for power. According to Giddens et al. (2012) **power** is the ability of individuals or members of a group to achieve their aims, even where others oppose them (p. 23). Group interests are sometimes met using direct force, but are usually achieved through the promotion of ideas that serve the interests of dominant groups. This is referred to as **ideology**, and Marxists often discuss the role of social institutions as **ideological apparatuses**. Whereas a functionalist paradigm views the role of institutions as maintaining social harmony, Marxists view this harmony as promoting the interests of the powerful.

From a conflict theoretical perspective quality of life is both (i) unequally distributed; and (ii) reflects the values of dominant groups as to what a good life is. In capitalist systems, because the dominant way of organising social life is through the capitalist market, then the main social division is an economic one, and the main classes around which there is conflict are based on one's economic position – between those who own the means of production (**the bourgeoisie**) and those who sell their labour (**the proletariat**).

Applying this paradigm to the study of quality of life focuses our attention on how:

- Quality of life constructs can reflect the interests of certain groups over others.
- Social inequalities in the distribution of dimensions of quality of life reflect unequal access to resources that support well-being, such as health care, education and work.
- Power and exploitation are key concepts in understanding the distribution of quality of life in society.

Symbolic Interactionism: Quality of Life as Interpersonal Meaning

Structural functionalist and Conflict paradigms focus on the **macro**, or the way societies function at a broad level. However eudemonic and hedonic approaches emphasise subjective practices and personal experiences. The symbolic interactionist paradigm offers an understanding of quality of life that is consistent with this subjective approach, but nonetheless provides a way of thinking about how societies function. Symbolic interactionism views society as a product of the everyday interactions between individuals. People construct the reality of their lives through interactions with others and society is made up of the aggregate of these interactions, whose lives are made meaningful through social interaction.

Symbolic interactionism attempts to understand the processes through which individuals attach meaning to social experiences. Building on Max Weber's theory of sociology as an interpretative discipline (see Gerth and Wright Mills 1958 for a selection of Weber's writings), symbolic interactionism emphasises that an individual's experience of a situation is a subjective process of assigning meaning to an experience, and that this provides the basis for shared, or intersubjective, understanding between individuals.

An important thinker in the symbolic interactionist field is Erving Goffman (1922–1982). According to Goffman, people play social roles in everyday life and attempt to manage the impressions others have of them of their performance. The reactions of others shape an individual's sense of self and therefore performances consist of the joint actions undertaken by individuals in everyday situations. For Goffman (1956), performance involves both an unconscious presentation of self in social situations and a conscious performance for the purposes of 'impression management'.

Applying this paradigm to the study of quality of life focuses our attention on how:

- Individuals define quality of life in ways that are meaningful to them.
- Expressions of well-being are continuously performed as part of social interactions, and the responses of others are important to an individual's sense of well-being.
- Individuals socially construct what a good life means to them and these are generative of and generated from interpersonal interactions.
- General definitions of quality of life may differ markedly from personal definitions of what a good life is.

These three theoretical paradigms and their implications for understanding quality of life are summarised in Table 3.1.

Exercise: Metaphors of Society and Quality of Life

Sociologists Anthony Elliott and Bryan Turner (2015) have provided an overview of how social theory provides metaphors of 'the social'. The three metaphors they identify are:

Society as Structure: this is society constituted as an objective set of relations beyond the control and knowledge of individuals. Market structures are seen as antagonistic to morality and virtue; and social manners and self-control are necessary to protect the foundation of civilization. There is emphasis on problems associated with the disruption of social norms brought about by urbanization and rapid social change. (pp. 815–817)

Table 3.1 Sociological paradigms and quality of life constructs

Theoretical paradigm	Image of society	Key questions	Quality of life as …
Structural functionalism	Harmonious social system	What are the shared factors that contribute to a sense of well-being?	Fulfilling social roles
		What are the implications of 'not fitting in' for experiences of well-being?	
		What social factors characterise a harmonious society?	
Conflict theories	Competing interests and conflict	How do quality of life constructs act as ideological devices for powerful groups?	Contested, ideological and unevenly distributed
		How are the benefits of a good life unequally distributed across society?	
Symbolic interactionism	Aggregate of everyday interactions	How do individuals define quality of life in ways that are meaningful to them?	Subjective experience and interpersonal interaction
		How are constructions of a good life generative of and generated from interpersonal interaction?	
		How do personal definitions of quality of life differ from general definitions of what a good life is?	

Society as Solidarity: emphasises how forms of solidarity cohere into society as a community of sentiment. Solidarity relies upon care, concern, sentiment, affection, tenderness, sympathy and love. In the modern age, social relations are instrumental and contractual, and it is human fellowship that needs protection. This is society held together by thick ties of locality, language, religion and culture. (pp. 818–821)

Society as Creative Process: This is society as "the indeterminate, the ambiguous, pure open-endedness. Society as creation … is built on transactions with the social that exemplify artistry, innovation and the welcoming of change" (pp. 821–822). Social relations are free-flowing and there is an emphasis on individual authenticity and individuality. Society is not 'out there', but generated through the interactions of individuals. (pp. 821–823)

- What concepts of quality of life are embedded in these three metaphors of the social?
- How do these metaphors help us understand the extent to which quality of life is an expression of freedom to live one's life how one wants, of conflict between different groups within society; or of necessity to live according to social rules?
- In what ways do these metaphors relate to eudemonic and hedonic well-being?

Methodologies in Well-Being and Quality of Life Research

Section Learning Outcomes
In this section, you will be introduced to key approaches to studying quality of life and will use these to explore some basic concepts in social research. You will:

- Be introduced to Objective, Subjective and Standpoint approaches to well-being.
- Consider how these approaches produce different kinds of knowledge about quality of life.
- Explore how these approaches assume different epistemological and ontological positions, which influence how research is designed.
- Learn about quantitative and qualitative methodologies and methods.

Researching Quality of Life

In the previous section we discussed how different theoretical paradigms emphasise different constructs of the good life, whether associated with harmonious values, as contested and a source of conflict, or as generated through everyday interactions. Given these diverse constructs, how might we research quality of life?

How a researcher conceptualises quality of life will influence what counts as valid knowledge about quality of life and the appropriate methods that should be used to research quality of life. For example, the view that quality of life is an objective state assumes that it can be measured objectively and quantified. If quality of life is considered a subjective experience, then capturing people's understanding and experiences is more likely to be the approach taken. That is, the theoretical paradigm we adopt is likely to have some influence over what is considered valid knowledge about quality of life and how to research it.

Objective and Subjective Approaches to Measuring Quality of Life and Well-Being

Objective and subjective approaches are two key approaches to researching quality of life. **Objective approaches** measure material indicators of the social conditions of populations or sub-populations, while **subjective approaches** rely on individual assessments of quality of life, including cognitive and affective evaluations of quality of life.

Most measurement frameworks include both objective and subjective measures. An example of monitoring frameworks is Eurostat's *8 + 1 dimensions of Quality of Life* framework. Eurostat is the statistical office of the European Union and their 8 + 1 Framework provides a set of population based measures that cover economic and non-economic aspects of quality of life. These are summarised in the Table 3.2.

Table 3.2 Summary of Eurostat quality of life dimensions

Domain	Sub-dimensions
Material living conditions	Income, consumption and material conditions (deprivation and housing)
Productive or main activity	Quantity of employment, quality of employment and other main activity (inactive population and unpaid work)
Health	Health outcome indicators (e.g. number of healthy life years, subjective assessment of health); chronic diseases, limitations in activity, health determinants (e.g. smoking, fruit and vegetable consumption, exercise); and access to healthcare
Education	Population's educational attainment; self-assessed skills; participation in life-long learning and opportunities for education (rate of enrolment of pupils in pre-primary education)
Leisure and social interactions	Leisure activities including quantity and quality; access to leisure; social interactions including activities with others (frequency of social contacts and satisfaction with personal relationships), volunteering in informal contexts, potential to receive social support; and social cohesion (trust in others)
Economic and physical safety	Physical safety (number of homicides per country, the proportion of those who perceive there is crime, violence or vandalism in area); and economic safety (ability to face unexpected expenses and having or not having arrears, assets)
Governance and basic rights	Trust in institutions and public services; discrimination and equal opportunities; and active citizenship
Natural and living environment	Self-reported exposure to pollution, grime and noise; urban population exposure to air pollution; and noise pollution from neighbours or from the street
Overall experience of life	Life satisfaction (cognitive appreciation), affect (a person's feelings or emotional state, both positive and negative) and eudemonics (a sense of having meaning and purpose in one's life)

Source: https://ec.europa.eu/eurostat/statistics-explained/index.php/Quality_of_life_indicators_-_measuring_quality_of_life

The 8 + 1 Framework is an example of a well-being monitoring framework commonly used by state and non-government actors to monitor the well-being of populations. These frameworks provide an alternative to economic measures of well-being, such as **Gross Domestic Product**, which governments have traditionally relied upon. While economic factors are included, the Eurostat framework also includes leisure, safety, health, political rights and the state of the physical environment as important dimensions of quality of life.

Standpoint Approaches to Understanding Well-Being

One of the critiques of objective and subjective approaches, is that they do not adequately reflect people's evaluations of their own lives. This is because they rely upon quantitative scales of quality of life that are not substantively based on an individual's personal values, views and assessments. Rather, the measures are those deemed important by researchers, to which individuals are asked to respond.

The **standpoint approach** involves an in-depth exploration of what people think and feel about aspects of their life, basing knowledge of what well-being is and how it is experienced, from the actors themselves. This is encapsulated in qualitative research initiatives that work inductively from people's perceptions and experiences as significant inputs about what is important to their sense of well-being.

Standpoint theories have been used to study children's well-being for example (Fattore and Mason 2016; McAuley and Rose 2014). These studies challenge domains typically used in child well-being monitoring frameworks. For example, they demonstrate that the concept of well-being encompasses feelings beyond happiness and satisfaction, but can also be experienced as an interweaving of complex emotions – such as joy with frustration or sadness with happiness. Similar phenomenological contributions exist for a range of well-being areas, including children's experience of health, schooling, use of digital media, material well-being, agency, safety, self-concept and engagement with community.

Table 3.3 provides an example of measures used in objective and subjective well-being approaches and indicators that could be developed from a standpoint approach. The example relates to measures of children's health.

Exercise: Evaluating Research Approaches

What are the benefits and limitations of each of the objective, subjective and standpoint approaches? Consider:

- The appeal of each approach to different stakeholders, including policy-makers, service providers, families and children.
- The comparability of each approach across different geographical, cultural, political and economic contexts.
- The degree to which each approach provides a precise measure.
- The ability of each approach to capture 'authentic' perspectives.

Table 3.3 Objective, subjective and standpoint measures of children's health

Objective	Subjective	Standpoint
Infant mortality rate (the probability of dying before first birthday) per 1000 live births. (Source: White and Sabarwal 2014)	"On a scale from 0 to 10 where zero means you feel very sad, 10 means you feel very happy and the middle of the scale 5 means you feel not happy or sad, how happy are you … with your health?" (Source Cummins and Lau 2005)	Children have the nutritional intake that allows them to engage purposively with daily activities
Proportion of infants 0–5 months who are fed exclusively with breast milk. (Source: World Health Organization 2008)	How satisfied are you with … How you are dealt with when you go to the doctors? (0 = Not at all satisfied through to 10 = Totally satisfied) (Source: ISCIweb 2018)	Children have opportunities to access environments that allow them to engage in everyday health practices associated with positive sensory experiences. (Source: Fattore and Mason 2016)

Using Approaches to Quality of Life Research to Explore Social Research Methodologies

The previous section has demonstrated several approaches used to research well-being. Objective approaches emphasise positive measurement, subjective approaches quantify people's opinions and standpoint approaches focus on people's lived experiences. Each approaches assumes different ways of thinking about what counts as appropriate knowledge of well-being, whether it is something that can be independently observed or whether it is a product of individual perceptions, and the kinds of methods best suited to researching quality of life.

As noted in the introduction, sociologists use systematic methods of empirical investigation to obtain data about the social world. A **research design** is a framework of methods and techniques chosen by researchers that combines components of research in a systematic manner. It includes our **theoretical perspective, methodology**; and **methods**.

Theory as Part of Research Design

Theory provides a conceptual framework for how we think about our data, guides our analysis and frames the kinds of research questions we are interested in studying in the first place. These often align or represent theoretical paradigms, such as Marxism, feminism and postmodernism, For example, if you refer to Table 3.1, you will see that key questions about quality of life vary depending on whether a structural functionalist, Marxist or symbolic interactionist approach is taken.

At a more philosophical level, theory is comprised of:

- **Epistemology**: our theory of knowledge concerned with how the rules of what is counted as knowledge are set. This determines who can and cannot be knowledgeable and what sort of knowledge is valued over others.
- **Axiology**: our theory of values which directs us to questions such as why we have chosen the topic; why we have settled on particular research questions; and how did we decide the topic was worth researching.
- **Ontology**: our theory of being, refers to what is reality and what relationship we have to it.

Quantitative and Qualitative Methodologies

The second main element of a research design is **methodology**, which is "the world-view lens through which the research question and core concepts are viewed and translated into the approach we take to the research" (Walter 2010: 13). There are two main types in social research, quantitative and qualitative. **Methods** are the techniques used to collect data (i.e. social surveys, semi-structured interviews), which are largely determined by the methodology adopted.

Quantitative Methodologies

Quantitative research typically involves counting the opinions, attitudes and behaviours of people, and looking for patterns therein. It often entails asking people specific questions that provide specific data that can be used to make statistically based generalisations. The data collected tends to be analysed using statistical analysis. Quantitative methodologies can be divided into experimental, quasi-experimental and non-experimental research designs.

Experimental designs: seek to determine if a specific treatment influences an outcome under controlled circumstances. A treatment is given to one group and not another and the effects observed. These groups are randomly selected from the population by the researcher. If any observed differences can be attributed to the treatment, then the treatment has a causative effect. What a treatment is depends on the study, for example, it could be exposure to a medication to determine whether it cures an illness, or exposure to a certain news channel to determine whether it influences a person's political attitudes.

Quasi-experiments: involve comparisons between naturally occurring 'treatment' groups, rather than those constructed by the researcher. For example, you might introduce a basic income scheme in one rural community and not in another with similar characteristics, and observe whether there are any differences in community outcomes after 1-year or 5-years.

Non-experimental designs: include correlational studies like survey research. Survey research provides a numeric description of trends, attitudes or opinions of a group, either at one point or at several points of time. While a sample may be randomly selected, there are no comparison groups.

Qualitative Methodologies

According to Yin (2011), qualitative research has several distinct features which include: that its focus is on everyday social contexts that people interact in; that it aims to capture the 'authentic' perspectives of participants; that it explicitly takes contextual factors into account, making context part of the research; that it aims to contribute to theory and concept building; and that it often occurs in complex field settings, which warrant the use of multiple qualitative methods. Some of the main approaches used by qualitative researchers include:

Ethnography: Ethnography involves the study of an intact cultural group in a natural setting over a prolonged period of time. It often involves immersion in the field setting using interviews and observations as the means of collecting data.

Grounded theory: aims to develop a general theory of a process, action or interaction grounded in the views of participants. The process involves reading through texts and identifying themes that emerge without an explicit theoretical framework already in mind.

Case studies: involve exploring an individual, program, event, activity or process in-depth. The focus is on obtaining information about one subject using multiple research techniques. The primary aim is to understand something unique to the case which could then be applied to other cases and contexts.

Phenomenological research: aims to identify the essence of a phenomenon as described by participants. This often involves studying a small number of subjects through prolonged engagement with them to identify patterns and relationships of meaning held by them.

Which strategy or strategies you use will inform your choice of methods, the way you ask questions, the steps in data analysis and the structure of your final narrative.

Exercise: Qualitative Analysis

Below are extracts from two studies asking children about the relationship between physical spaces and safety for their well-being. Both involved in-depth interviews and focus groups. On the left are extracts from a study undertaken in Sydney, Australia. On the left are extracts from a study undertaken in Cape Town, South Africa. In both projects the participants were aged between 8 and 14 years.

Read through the extracts and identify key themes that emerge from each set. You might do this by summarizing what the participants are talking about and from these summaries, identify concepts that could explain what the children are talking about and why they are talking about physical spaces the way they are – for example concepts like security, freedom, danger, risk or beauty (Table 3.4).

- What similarities in themes can you identify from children's discussions between Sydney and Cape Town?
- What differences in themes can you identify from children's discussions between Sydney and Cape Town?
- How do these similarities and differences relate to the context the research was undertaken in?
- On the basis of your analysis, what conclusions can you draw about the relationship between physical spaces, safety and well-being?

Conclusion

In this chapter we have explored how quality of life and well-being are social constructs, how sociological analysis can help us understand how quality of life is related to social conditions and how well-being constructs reflect the social orders that we live in.

Specific philosophical traditions have informed contemporary approaches to quality of life research, and we have used these traditions to discuss different metaphors of the social. Within the vibrant field of quality of life research, differences are also evident in the methodologies and methods employed by researchers and these approaches provide examples of epistemological approaches in social science research.

Many other areas of sociological analysis useful for studying quality of life remain unexplored in this chapter. For example, sociological analysis demonstrates that both subjective and objective quality of life is unequally distributed within societies, being the result of social processes that provide some groups with greater access to valued social resources and denying other groups access to the same

Table 3.4 Extracts from two studies

Sydney, Australia	Cape Town, South Africa
Extract 1	*Extract 1*
Male Participant: Yes, they have more adult stuff and then they have like long buildings [that are okay] for adults to walk past and the children won't be safe and they might die.	Female participant: Of everything that's in the outdoors like the stuff that grew by itself it didn't – it wasn't man made.
Interviewer: Oh, how could that happen?	Female participant: I think of it because I love exploring in the nature and like taking pictures of things that I don't really know much about …
Male Participant: 'Cause the road is big and then they leave it for adults.' Cause they know that adults can walk over. And they don't put any signs for safety. They just put [signs] for adults so then they can walk over.	Female participant: Surfing.
	Female participant: I just like laying on the grass and watch the clouds and the birds and the trees or something.
Interviewer: Do you mean like road problems?	Co-facilitator: … how does that make you feel?
Male Participant: Like roads … they [builders] don't care about children. And then they could just walk over and just get crushed by cars.	Female participant: Relaxed.
Extract 2	*Extract 2*
Female Participant: Yep, well down the road there is a park with equipment … with a slide and things … And me and my friends will just walk down there sometimes and just muck around, fool around … roll around on the grass and muck around. … And because it is an open area, no-one is really going to be able to miss [seeing] it if you are in trouble or anything.	Female participant: My dad says I'm not allowed to go in [the beach] because when we first moved here it was still safe and now my dad says we not allowed if we at home the doors have to be closed and all the windows have to be locked because there are a lot of robberies happening out there.
	Female participant: My mom is very protective of me walking around although lately she has lightened up and like … the other day we walked home for the first time ever.
Source: Fattore and Mason (2016)	Source: Adams et al. (2017)

resources. This can help us understand the effects of inequalities on individual life chances, and also explain some of the reasons why social conflicts occur. Many sociological paradigms not discussed in this chapter could also usefully be applied to analysis of quality of life. For example post-structural approaches could be used to develop an intersectional model that demonstrates how quality of life is a complex interplay of multiple aspects of identity. While we have discussed different methodological approaches to the study of quality of life, we have not explored the benefits of mixed methods approaches. Furthermore, questions of governance and the use of social indicators by national and supra-national organisations, remain unexplored. These and many other topics remain open to intrepid students of sociology.

References

Adams, S., Savahl, S., & Fattore, T. (2017). Children's representations of nature using photovoice and community mapping: Perspectives from South Africa. *International Journal of Qualitative Studies in Health & Well-Being, 12*(1), 1–22.

Bentham, J. (1789). *Introduction to the principles of morals and legislation*. Oxford: The Clarendon Press.

Cummins, R., & Lau, A. (2005). *Personal wellbeing index –school children (PWI-SC)* (English) (3rd ed.). Melbourne: Australian Centre on Quality of Life, School of Psychology, Deakin University.

Deci, E., & Ryan, R. (2008). Hedonia, eudaimonia, and well-being: An introduction. *Journal of Happiness Studies, 9*, 1–11.

Elliott, A., & Turner, B. (2015). Three versions of the social. *Journal of Sociology, 51*(4), 812–826.

Fattore, T., & Mason, J. (2016). *Children and well-being: Towards a child standpoint*. Dordrecht: Springer.

Gallagher, E. (2010). *Aristotle's definition of Eudaimonia*. http://www.academia.edu/514238/Aristotles_Definition_of_Eudaimonia

Gerth, H. H., & Wright Mills, C. (Eds.). (1958). *From Max Weber: Essays in sociology* (translated and edited by). Oxford University Press.

Giddens, A., Duneier, M., Appelbaum, R., & Carr, D. (2012). *Introduction to sociology*. New York: W.W. Norton.

Goffman, E. (1956). *The presentation of self in everyday life*. Edinburgh: University of Edinburgh, Social Sciences Research Centre.

Haybron, D. (2008). Philosophy and the science of subjective well-being. In M. Eid & R. J. Larsen (Eds.), *The science of subjective well-being* (pp. 17–33). New York: The Guilford Press.

ISCIweb. (2018). *Children's worlds: International survey of children's well-being*. http://www.isciweb.org/

Maslow, A. (1987). *Motivation and personality* (3rd ed.). New York: Addison-Wesley.

McAuley, C., & Rose, W. (2014). Children's social and emotional relationships and well-being: From the perspective of the child. In A. Ben-Arieh, F. Casas, I. Frønes, & J. Korbin (Eds.), *Handbook of child well-being: Theories, methods and policies in global perspective* (pp. 1865–1892). Dordrecht: Springer.

Merton, R. K. (1957). *Social theory and social structure*. Glencoe: Free Press.

Parsons, T. (1951). *The social system*. Glencoe: The Free Press.

Rogers, C. (1951). *Client-centered therapy: Its current practice, implications and theory*. London: Constable.

Rogers, C. (1961). *On becoming a person: A psychotherapist's view of psychotherapy*. Boston: Houghton Mifflin Company.

Ryan, R. M., & Deci, E. L. (2001). On happiness and human potentials: A review of research on hedonic and eudaimonic well-being. *Annual Review of Psychology, 52*, 141–166.

Seligman, M. (2011). *Flourish: A visionary new understanding of happiness and well-being*. New York: Free Press.

Tucker, R. (Ed.). (1978). *The Marx-Engels reader* (2nd ed.). New York: Norton.

Walter, M. (Ed.). (2010). *Social research methods*. South Melbourne: Oxford University Press, Australia and New Zealand.

Weber, M. (1904 [1958]). *The protestant ethic and the spirit of capitalism*. New York: Scribner.

White, H., & Sabarwal, S. (2014). *Developing and selecting measures of child well-being* (Methodological Briefs: Impact Evaluation 11). Florence: UNICEF Office of Research.

World Health Organization. (2008). *Indicators for assessing infant and young child feeding practices, part 1, definitions*. Geneva: WHO.

Yin, R. K. (2011). Chapter 5: Doing fieldwork. In *Qualitative research from start to finish* (pp. 109–128). New York: The Guildford Press.
Zevnik, L. (2014). *Critical perspectives in happiness research: The birth of modern happiness.* Dordrecht: Springer.

Tobia Fattore is a senior lecturer in the Department of Sociology, Macquarie University, Australia. His research interests are in the sociology of childhood and sociology of work. He is currently a coordinating lead researcher on the multi-national study *Children's Understandings of Well-being – Global and Local Contexts* which involves a qualitative investigation into how children experience well-being from a comparative and global perspective. He is a Board Member of the International Society for Childhood Indicators.

Chapter 4
Nurturing Holistic Development in University Students Through Leadership Courses: The Hong Kong Experience

Daniel T. L. Shek, Xiaoqin Zhu, Diya Dou, Moon Y. M. Law, Lu Yu, Cecilia M. S. Ma, and Li Lin

Introduction

As university students are pillars of the future society, it is important to nurture the holistic development of university students. Unfortunately, research findings revealed that there are developmental problems in university students. In terms of quality of life, studies showed that emotional problems, suicide, and substance abuse are capturing public attention. For example, in the U.S., Mojtabai et al. (2016) reported that prevalence of depression increased from 8.8% in 2005 to 9.6% in 2014 in young adults aged between 18 and 25 years old. There are also research findings showing that suicide and substance abuse are growing concerns in the university contexts (Becker et al. 2018; Knight et al. 2002). Besides personal and mental health issues, there are also research findings showing that university students become more egocentric and there is a drop in their empathy (Bourke and Mechler 2010; Konrath et al. 2011). The decline in social responsibility among university students is also a source of concern (Pryor et al. 2009).

With particular reference to Hong Kong, Shek (2010) highlighted several developmental issues among university students. These included stress and mental health issues, political apathy, and relatively poorer performance in psychosocial competencies when compared with students in mainland China. With reference to these issues, Shek (2010) raised the question of how we can nurture university students in a holistic manner. Shek and Wong (2011) also outlined the mental health and lifestyle issues of university students in the global contexts. In these two papers, the authors also argued that contemporary universities did not put enough focus on the

D. T. L. Shek (✉) · X. Zhu · D. Dou · M. Y. M. Law · L. Yu · C. M. S. Ma · L. Lin
Department of Applied Social Sciences, The Hong Kong Polytechnic University,
Hong Kong, People's Republic of China
e-mail: daniel.shek@polyu.edu.hk; xiaoqin.zhu@polyu.edu.hk; diya.dou@polyu.edu.hk;
ss.moon@polyu.edu.hk; lu.yu@polyu.edu.hk; cecilia.ma@polyu.edu.hk; jocelyn.lin@polyu.edu

© Springer Nature Switzerland AG 2020

G. H. Tonon (ed.), *Teaching Quality of Life in Different Domains*, Social
Indicators Research Series 79, https://doi.org/10.1007/978-3-030-21551-4_4

holistic development of university students. Similarly, Shek and Cheung (2013) further pointed out four developmental issues identified in university students. The first concern is related to unhealthy lifestyle and habits which included drinking problem, excessive use of Internet, use of online pornography, sleep problems, and interpersonal violence. The second concern is mental health issues which cover suicidal behavior, anxiety, depression, and stress faced by university students. The third concern is related to personal issues such as the lack of life goals and self-confidence as well as excessive materialism. The final issue is growing egocentrism and declining civic engagement in university students.

In the above-mentioned three papers, one key argument raised by the authors is that contemporary universities have failed to promote holistic development in university students. This deficiency is also clearly revealed by the remarks of Chickering (2010): higher education institutions have "generally ignored outcomes related to moral and ethical development as well as other dimensions of personal development" (p. 1) and colleges "failed to graduate citizens who can function at the levels of cognitive and moral, intellectual, and ethical development that our complex national and global problems require" (p. 3). With reference to the above background, two questions should be addressed. The first question is how we can promote the quality of life of university students so that they can become leaders of tomorrow. The second question concerns the means that can be used to promote quality of life in university students.

In this chapter, we introduce two credit-bearing subjects developed at The Hong Kong Polytechnic University (PolyU) that attempt to promote leadership qualities in university students via cultivating of their quality of life. The first subject is entitled "Tomorrow's Leaders" which was developed with reference to the positive youth development (PYD) approach. The basic philosophy of the subject is that intrapersonal and interpersonal competences are indispensable for becoming effective leaders. The second subject is entitled "Service Leadership" which was developed with reference to the Service Leadership and Management model (SLAM model) proposed by Chung (2011). According to the SLAM framework, an effective service leader should possess three attributes, including competence, character, and care, all of which can be regarded as indicators of well-being.

Leadership and Quality of Life

According to Felce and Perry (1995), quality of life is a multi-dimensional construct which includes physical well-being (e.g., health), material well-being (e.g., security), social well-being (e.g., interpersonal relationships), emotional well-being (e.g., self-esteem), as well as development and engagement in meaningful activities (e.g., competence/independence). Wallander et al. (2001) also argued that quality of life includes mental health, social health, social functioning, intimacy, and social functioning. In the literature on PYD, scholars used the 5Cs model to define adolescents' quality of life, whereby the Cs denote the concepts of connection, competence, confidence, character, and caring/compassion (Lerner et al. 2005). All these components of well-being are integral qualities for a healthy individual and leadership qualities as well.

Conceptually speaking, quality of life or well-being should be regarded as an integral part of leadership. Without good quality of life, a leader simply cannot function well. When one leads oneself (i.e., self-leadership), one has to possess a sense of purpose, resilience, and perseverance. When one leads others, one has to build relationships with others and resolve conflicts.

Different leadership models have emphasized the importance of quality of life or well-being as the basic attribute of effective leadership. For example, in spiritual leadership model (Fry 2003), it is argued that spiritual well-being (which includes hope, faith, altruistic love, and spiritual survival) is an intrinsic motivational force which propels effective leadership. In the servant leadership model (Greenleaf 1997), it is proposed that serving others (i.e., social well-being) is an important attribute of a good leader. Finally, in the 12 dimensions of leadership proposed by Chung and Elfassy (2016), several areas of well-being are proposed, including mental, emotional, spiritual, moral, and social well-being. Of course, whether we can promote university students' well-being via credit-bearing leadership subjects would be an important question to be considered. To answer this question, two credit-bearing leadership subjects are introduced in the sections below.

Tomorrow's Leaders

With rapid globalization and advances in technology, it is important for university administrators and teachers to re-think about how university students can lead in the rapidly changing world. With specific reference to Hong Kong, there is also an urgent need to develop holistic tomorrow's leaders who can lead in the service economy. What sorts of skills should tomorrow's leaders possess? For most people, they would argue that professional skills are important for leadership. While developing professional skills are important, people who advocate holistic development in young people think that university students would need more than just these skills. University graduates should also possess "soft skills" such as communication skills, collaboration skills, emotional competence, and sense of social responsibility. Interestingly, such an emphasis is consistent with the traditional Chinese view about ideal human development – "before one can bring peace to the world, one has to govern one's country. Before one can govern one's country, one has to put one's family in order. Before one can put one's family in order, one has to cultivate oneself" (The Great Learning).

To promote leadership qualities in university students, a three-credit subject entitled "Tomorrow's Leaders" has been developed and implemented at The Hong Kong Polytechnic University since 2012/2013 academic year. This subject adopted the PYD approach which upholds the thesis that both intrapersonal competences (such as resilience) and interpersonal competences (such as team building) are essential foundations of effective youth leadership. Besides cultivating leadership qualities of the students, the subject also attempts to promote well-being in university students. As a compulsory course, "Tomorrow's Leaders" has served more than 12,000 undergraduates since 2012.

Teaching Philosophy and Pedagogy

"Tomorrow's Leaders" is a credit-bearing subject which is based on the PYD approach (Shek 2013; Shek and Sun 2012b). The PYD approach focuses on the potentials and talents of young people instead of emphasizing problems and pathologies of youth development. It is argued that young people can thrive through being provided with suitable opportunities and support. Also, it is maintained that internal assets such as positive values and psychosocial competences (e.g., emotional competence, cognitive competence, and moral competence) are critical to the holistic development of university students. In Hong Kong, PYD constructs are utilized in the Project P.A.T.H.S. (Shek and Sun 2013a), such as resilience, self-efficacy, emotional competence, social competence, and spirituality. In some sense, "Tomorrow's Leaders" can be considered a "university version" of the Project P.A.T.H.S. which aims to promote holistic leadership development via cultivating intrapersonal and interpersonal skills in university students (Shek 2013).

Regarding curriculum development and pedagogy, we uphold three key beliefs. The first belief is that "every student has leadership potentials". Morbid emphasis on academic excellence is a basic feature of the Hong Kong education system, where good public examination result is commonly regarded as the hallmark of "successful" youth development. However, in "Tomorrow's Leaders", we strongly support the belief that every student has leadership potentials and should at least lead one's own life (i.e., self-leadership). This belief echoes the basic notion of the PYD approach which maintains that young people are "resources to be developed" rather than "problems to be solved".

The second belief is that we can nurture intrapersonal and interpersonal skills through credit-bearing subjects. Intrapersonal skills (e.g., emotional quotient) and interpersonal skills (e.g., conflict resolution) are fundamental to holistic student development. These skills are commonly regarded as "soft skills" or "21st century skills" which are strongly emphasized by employers in many employer surveys. Based on experience gained from Project P.A.T.H.S., a curricular-based PYD program which has benefited more than 600,000 man times (Shek and Sun 2013a), we believe curricular-based leadership programs and service-learning activities are powerful pedagogies which can be used to promote students' intrapersonal and interpersonal competences and social responsibility.

The third belief is that it is important to promote learning through experience, reflection, collaboration, and integration. Instead of using a didactic teaching approach, the subject adopts an experiential learning approach with the application of evidence-based pedagogies to facilitate the holistic development of the leadership qualities (particularly morality and integrity) among the students. Primarily, we believe that experiential learning is an important vehicle to help students understand themselves. As such, individual, group, and class experiential learning activities involving interactions among the students have been incorporated in the subject. In particular, we strongly emphasize students' reflective learning by encouraging them to deeply reflect on their own development and social responsibility in the learning process. In response to the research findings that students have become more egocentric, we highlight collaborative learning through group sharing, discussion, and presentation. As "Tomorrow's Leaders" is a credit-bearing subject, we also emphasize on academic integration with the personal lives of the students such as how to promote one's emotional quotient in daily life based on the theories and research findings.

Several special features are intrinsic to the classroom teaching of "Tomorrow's Leaders". These include: (a) high levels of teacher-student and student-student classroom interaction; (b) use of multiple teaching methods, including multimedia stimulation, discussion, sharing, presentation, role-plays, games, healthy competition, creative expression, and debates; (c) strong emphasis on student reflection and self-evaluation; and, (d) creation of an enjoyable classroom atmosphere that facilitates student learning and participation.

Student engagement is also a key focus in "Tomorrow's Leaders". We use several strategies to engage and inspire the students. First, students are engaged in group interaction through forming small groups in class. Second, new technology is used to facilitate student engagement. For example, students can share their opinions on the Internet instantly during class. Third, teachers are encouraged to share their views which would facilitate student reflection. Fourth, post-lecture evaluation that collects the feedback from students on each specific lecture also helps engage the students. Fifth, the adoption of the philosophy that "everyone can be a leader" promotes confidence and capability in the students.

We have encouraged teachers to document the curriculum of "Tomorrow's Leaders". For instance, Shek and Leung (2016b) outlined the topic on social competence. In the lecture, several topics are covered, including factors determining social competence and the outcomes of social competence, the association between social competence and leadership effectiveness, and hurdles on the development of social competence (e.g., egocentrism). Besides, ways to promote social competence and student feedback on the lecture were reported in the article. Another example is resilience as a quality of effective leadership (Shek and Leung 2016a). We define resilience and the related theories in the lecture. Besides, the link between resilience and leadership effectiveness as well as adolescent development is addressed. Finally, ways to promote resilience in university students are discussed.

Experiences in Students and Teachers

We believe that it is important to understand student experiences and outcomes through evaluation. Besides the routine e-evaluation conducted by the university, we have also conducted many evaluation studies for "Tomorrow's Leaders" to understand the experience of the students. Specifically, objective outcome evaluation (one-group pretest-posttest design and non-equivalent group design with an experimental group and control group), subjective outcome evaluation (assessing students' perceptions toward the subject teacher and benefits through the client satisfaction approach), process evaluation (assessment of the quality and adherence of subject implementation), and qualitative evaluation (individual reflection, interviews, and focus groups) have been carried out to investigate the effectiveness of the subject.

Objective Outcome Evaluation

We have used one-group pretest-posttest design to assess the impact of the subject using a validated instrument. For the pilot phase, the results revealed a significant increase in the scores in different domains, such as emotional competence and social competence. Based on the responses of 50 students to the Chinese Positive Youth Development Scale, Shek and Sun (2012c) found that students showed positive changes on subscale scores (such as emotional competence) and total score. Using a quasi-experimental design, Shek et al. (2013a) also found that the students in experimental group showed greater positive changes as compared to the students in control group on different measures of PYD. Shek (2013) summarized the findings in the pilot studies and concluded that "Tomorrow's Leaders" was able to promote the mental health of the students.

There were also findings suggesting that students changed in the positive direction in different measures for the full implementation phase. For example, Shek and Ma (2014) reported that in a sample of 1029 students, students showed positive changes on some measures of PYD and life satisfaction.

Subjective Outcome Evaluation

Subjective outcome evaluation data were collected after each lecture and upon the completion of the subject using validated instruments. Overall speaking, in the pilot and full implementation stages, the findings demonstrated that the students held positive views toward the subject and instructors. Moreover, students thought that the subject was beneficial to their overall development.

For the pilot stage, Shek and Sun (2013c) found that students regarded the subject as helpful to their resilience (97.9%), social competence (99.3%), and self-confidence (96.5%). Most important of all, over 97% of the students felt that the subject promoted their overall development. Similar findings were reported in another study of Shek and Yu (2014).

For the full implementation stage, according to the most updated findings based on the data collected in 2016/2017 academic year, most of the students expressed that the subject helped them to make moral decisions (88.66%), motivated them to perform lifelong learning to improve leadership qualities (85.61%), increased their capacity to practice ethical leadership (87.12%), and enabled them to understand (93.40%) and synthesize (92.99%) the attributes of effective leaders. Papers reporting these evaluation findings in details are under preparation.

Process Evaluation

Process evaluation was conducted using a validated instrument assessing the subject implementation quality and the extent to which the subject is delivered as designed. The related findings showed that the teachers basically followed the curriculum materials (i.e., high adherence) and the ratings on the subject implementation quality were high (Shek and Sun 2012a, b).

Qualitative Evaluation

Qualitative evaluation was conducted through written reflective journals and focus groups. In the pilot and full implementation stages, the findings informed that students held positive evaluations of the subject and instructors and they thought the subject benefited them in terms of promoting their leadership qualities (Shek and Sun 2012d; Shek et al. 2016a, e). Examples of students' reflective narratives are presented in the following section. Furthermore, teachers were also invited to share their own reflections, examples of which are outlined following by the students' reflections.

Reflection of Students

When we invited the students to reflect on the subject, they shared their experience on how the subject contributed to their holistic development. Some narratives are as follows:

It is a useful course for me to enhance my personal development, as it provided comprehensive topics about personal development and led me to have self-reflection. Some leadership skills also have been taught in the lesson in an interesting way.

I have developed self-reflection skills and acquired interpersonal skills which are very useful for my future development and growth. Finally, it is worth for me to take this course. I am confident that I would be a leader soon.

In the course of this subject, different activities, writings, and drawings enhanced my understanding of myself, including my strengths and weaknesses which helped me improve my interpersonal skills. The topics taught in this subject are important to our daily living. For instance, we need emotional competence when our feeling is fluctuating, we need resilience when we are in a deadlock.

For resilience, I've learnt that we can convert difficulties to opportunity. The course taught us positive thinking and encouraged me to deal with the difficulties. Now in my mind, difficulties just mean time to make decision and time to prove that I have the ability to solve problems. This concept is useful to give me power on dealing with the resilience in the rest of my life.

I liked the in-class activities, videos, and stories provided by the lecture. It got me involved in the class, and to cooperate with different people. When I attended other subjects, there was no chance to interact with people, and no chance to meet new friends. But in 'Tomorrow's Leaders' it has!

Another benefit I have gained from this subject is a better self-understanding. When learning the concept of personal qualities of effective leaders, the lecturer also encouraged us to think about ourselves. Therefore, I have learned to do the self-reflection. I think it helps me improve the self-awareness.

Reflection of Teachers

Besides students, we also attempt to understand the teaching experiences of teachers and how the subject influences their development. We have invited teachers to write reflections about their teaching and document such experiences in journal articles. Teachers also presented the evaluation findings on international conferences. Obviously, these strategies are empowering and rewarding for the teachers. A few examples are presented below:

In facing the growing trend of 'McDonaldization' and commercialization of university education, we sometimes may get misted over the missions and objectives of higher education. 'Tomorrow's Leaders', as a general education subject that emphasizes the intrapersonal and interpersonal qualities of the students, is a restatement of the importance of holistic development in university education. I am grateful to be one of the participants in the movement. (Leung 2016b, p. 227)

When conducting lectures in the past, I was confident that I was familiar with the theories being taught and was able to cite studies and figures that supported what I was teaching; to a great extent, I was convinced that I had the 'right' answers to many questions raised in class. Teaching TL is a different story; the subject is not about transferring truths to students, many of the discussions, for instance, on morality and integrity, and spirituality, do not require an absolute answer. I would share my views or what I would do under different circumstances with my students, but by no means were they considered as truths. My role, instead, was to act as a facilitator to help students find their own stance on these issues. (Leung 2016a, p. 217)

The experience in teaching 'Tomorrow's Leaders' has also changed me both as a teacher, and as a person … reflection on teaching the subject deepened my self-understanding and made me a more mature person. One insight I have gained is about my fear for interactive teaching. To conquer the fear, the first step may be to learn how to fully accept myself without any condition, i.e. I can make mistakes and this would not change the fact that I could still be a good person … Teaching the subject makes me further aware of the implication of scientific research to the society. By performing rigorously designed studies on important social issues, and disseminating the findings, we are able to educate the public, influence policy-making, and eventually make the world a better place. (Yu 2016, pp. 200–201)

Service Leadership

In the past several decades, the economic structure of Hong Kong has changed from a manufacturing economy to a service economy, with more than 90% of the GDP coming from service industries in the past decade. While manufacturing economy focuses on "doing things rights" (i.e., following procedures on the assembly lines), service economy emphasizes on "doing the right things" (i.e., making ethical decisions that benefit other people). In terms of requirements of effective leaders, Shek et al. (2015a) pointed out that direct leadership, task-orientation, and "doing" (e.g., functional skills) are emphasized in the manufacturing economy whereas empowerment, service-mindset, and "being" (e.g., character and care) are cherished under the service economy. With the new demands of service industries, higher education institutions should help their students to develop the basic attributes of effective service leaders. Unfortunately, Shek et al. (2013b) argued that higher education institutions in Hong Kong fail to nurture effective service leaders because care and moral character are often overlooked in university education. In particular, leadership programs normally focus on the cultivation of "doing" (i.e., skills) instead of the "being" (i.e., values and virtues) in students.

To promote the development of service leadership qualities in students, the Victor and William Fung Foundation provided financial support to eight government-funded universities in Hong Kong to develop service leadership education curriculum and materials. At PolyU, we have developed a credit-bearing subject named as "Service Leadership" based on the SLAM curriculum framework proposed by Po Chung, the Co-founder of DHL International (Asia Pacific). Chung (2011) defined service leadership as "satisfying needs by consistently providing quality personal service to everyone one comes into contact with, including one's self, others, groups, communities, systems, and environments". According to the SLAM model, leadership effectiveness (E) depends on three factors, including generic leadership competence (C), character (C) and the caring disposition of the leader (C) as perceived by others. In short, the SLAM model asserts that in addition to competences (i.e., doing), care, and moral character (i.e., being) are important qualities of an effective leader.

Development of Service Leadership Subjects

When we took up the project in 2012, Hong Kong still operated the 3-year undergraduate curriculum when we took up the project back in 2012. Therefore, a 2-credit "Service Leadership" subject involving 28 contact hours was initially developed and offered to students who enrolled in this previous 3-year undergraduate curriculum after taking the Advanced Level Examination in the 2012/2013 and 2013/2014 academic years. In this subject, the basic ideas of the Service Leadership Model are introduced. In particular, topics on generic leadership competence, character, and care were covered.

As the undergraduate education changed from a 3-year structure to a 4-year mode in 2012/2013 academic year, we developed another 3-credit "Service Leadership" subject with 39 contact hours for students taking the new 4-year curriculum for graduates of the Diploma of Secondary Education Examination. For this subject, we have added an additional component on the critical appraisal of the Service Leadership model and other major leadership models. This subject is opened to all the university students with an overarching goal to nurture effective service leaders.

This subject has several unique features. First, this subject intends to bring a paradigm shift in the students' mindset about leadership, particularly with reference to the notions that "leadership is a service" and "every student is (and can be) a leader". Second, instead of just focussing on the management skills (i.e., "doing"), students are invited to appreciate the importance of values and virtues (i.e., "being"). As such, this subject aims to help students reflect on and develop their competences (including intrapersonal and interpersonal competences), care (including listening, empathy and love), and character (including character strengths and Chinese virtues). Finally, this subject intends to cultivate an awareness of the importance of service leadership to the development and wellness of oneself, other people, and the society.

As far as the intended learning outcomes are concerned, after taking this subject, students are expected to be able to:

- Understand the major assertions, strengths, and weaknesses of contemporary models of leadership in the context of service economy;
- Acquire a basic understanding of attributes contributing to effective service leadership, including leadership competences, character, and care (i.e., 3Cs);

- Conduct personal reflections on the need and relevance of service leadership qualities to oneself; and
- Appreciate the value of the subject and the potential application of related knowledge to oneself.

Teaching Philosophy

We uphold several core beliefs when we designed and taught the "Service Leadership" subject. These include:

- Every student is (and can be) a leader. Teachers should encourage every student to develop his/her leadership qualities and appreciate the merits of every student. For Chinese students, they are usually timid, and they do not believe that they can be leaders. Therefore, adopting a humanistic orientation, we uphold the belief that every student has potentials and talents to be a leader, at least leading oneself.
- Self-understanding and self-reflection are very important for effective service leadership. Individual self-reflection exercises should be conducted, which allow students to enhance their self-understanding. This emphasis is important because without self-understanding and self-reflection, a person may have many blind spots on themselves.
- Experiential learning is an effective approach to enhance student learning. Experiential learning activities at individual, group, and class levels should be conducted, in which students can work individually or collaboratively to experience the knowledge covered in lectures. Instead of receiving "politically correct" answers from subject teachers, we believe that it is a better way for the students to find the answers by themselves. Therefore, activities were designed to elicit the experiences in students, which subsequently help them to reflect and eventually understand themselves better.
- Collaborative learning can help students develop competences, caring disposition, and moral character. Learning will be facilitated through group discussion, sharing, evaluation, and presentation. We believe that learning through a group would be beneficial because it helps to provide mutual support, care, and knowledge exchange amongst the group learners.
- Critical thinking is encouraged to deepen students' learning. As such, debates and critical appraisal on the SLAM framework and other leadership models are conducted, which allow students to think from multiple perspectives. Students are encouraged to recognize the strengths and weaknesses of different service leadership theories.
- Equal emphasis is placed on understanding the theoretical knowledge of service leadership and applying such knowledge in real life. We consider the application of knowledge acquired in the lectures an important element of service leadership education. Therefore, in-class activities and assignments are designed to help

students to apply such knowledge. Teachers should highlight the link between theoretical knowledge and students' daily lives as well as their future careers. Besides, students are encouraged to consciously apply the knowledge they learned from the subject in their lives and careers.

- Systematic evaluation utilizing different evaluation approaches is critical to understand the effectiveness of the subject. We adopt an evidence-based approach to understand students' changes after taking the subject as well as their subjective experiences and feelings during their study in the subject.

Teaching Methodology

The teaching/learning methodology includes lectures, experiential classroom activities, reflective exercises, a group project presentation, and an individual paper. Besides, this subject adopts a student-centered approach. Several strategies are used to enhance students' engagement.

- Formation of small groups: Students form groups at the beginning of the class. By doing this, we can promote collaborative learning through which students can have more opportunities to share and learn from each other.
- Student empowerment: The basic philosophy that "everyone is (and can be) a leader" promotes confidence and efficacy in the students. Teachers appreciate the participation, sharing, and cooperation (i.e., recognition for positive behavior) of every student.
- Creation of an enjoyable and inviting atmosphere: We consciously create an enjoyable and encouraging learning atmosphere in the classroom which would promote student involvement. For example, teachers interact with students in different ways, such as asking questions, which helps to engage the students (i.e., learning through engaging students).
- Teachers' disclosure: Teachers are encouraged to share their own experiences and opinions with students. It helps to build a trustful relationship between teachers and students, and also motivates the students to share their personal feelings and thoughts (i.e., facilitation of learning through trust).
- Use of multiple teaching methods: Apart from lecturing, multiple teaching methods including multimedia stimulation, group discussion, role-play, debate, drawing, and games are used in the class. These activities increase students' attentiveness, deepen their understanding of the knowledge, and stimulate their reflection (i.e., experiential learning).
- Emphasis on reflective exercises: We design worksheets, cases, group activities, and class discussion topics to facilitate individual and group reflection which can promote students' reflection on their own situations (i.e., reflective learning).

- Encouragement of practical application: Students are guided to understand how service leadership knowledge relates to their personal growth and career development. With an awareness of the link between service leadership qualities and personal development, students are more likely to participate in the class (i.e., learning with real-life application).
- Conscious use of different assessment methods to engage students in active learning: First, students' preparation for lectures and participation in class activities (e.g., completion of worksheets, voluntarily answering questions, and taking initiative to join group activities) will be assessed. Second, each group is required to do a group presentation, which enhances students' collaborative learning. Finally, students are invited to rate other group members' performance and contribution to the group presentation.

Outputs and Impacts

The two-credit subject was offered in 2012/2013 and 2013/2014 academic years to students under the 3-year undergraduate program. A total of 190 students took this subject. In 2014/2015 academic year, the "Service Leadership" subject was modified and enriched to be a three-credit General Education subject and has been offered to students under the 4-year undergraduate program. Since then, a total of 849 students completed this subject. Multiple evaluation studies have been conducted to understand the effectiveness of the subject.

Objective Outcome Evaluation

One-group pretest-posttest design was used to assess the outcome of the subject using a validated instrument. Generally speaking, students in the 3-year program and the 4-year program all showed significant increases in the scores of PYD, service leadership qualities and beliefs, and life satisfaction. For example, Shek et al. (2014b) examined changes in the students after taking the two-credit "Service Leadership" subject in 2012/2013 academic year, and found that students changed positively in character strengths, general PYD attributes, and service leadership qualities. In another evaluation study using a quasi-experimental design, Lin and Shek (2018) showed that students taking the three-credit "Service Leadership" subject in 2016/2017 academic year had significantly greater increases in life satisfaction, service leadership knowledge, and attitudes as compared to the students in control group who did not take the subject.

Subjective Outcome Evaluation

Students were invited to respond to a validated Subjective Outcome Evaluation questionnaire upon completion of the subject to express their views toward the subject, teacher(s), and benefits gained from the subject. The findings showed that students had positive views toward the three aspects under investigation. For instance, Shek et al. (2016c) reported that 91% of the students who enrolled in the two-credit subject offered in the second semester of 2013/2014 academic year liked the course very much, had a very positive evaluation of the subject teacher(s), and felt that the course enhanced their self-leadership.

Process Evaluation

Process evaluation was conducted, in which two raters observed and assessed the program implementation quality and program adherence. The findings showed that program adherence and the implementation quality of the subject were high (Shek et al. 2014a, 2016b).

Qualitative Evaluation

Qualitative evaluation was conducted using written reflective sheets and focus groups. In the studies adopting reflective sheets, students were invited to use a metaphor and three descriptors to express their experiences and feelings in learning the subject. The findings suggested that students had positive views toward the subject, instructor(s), and the benefits they gained from this subject (Shek et al. 2015b, 2016d, 2017). For example, among 463 descriptors and 152 metaphors used by 153 students, 446 (96.3%) descriptors and 151 (99.3%) metaphors were considered positive in nature (Shek et al. 2017).

Reflection of Students

Students shared their views toward the effectiveness of the subject in promoting their personal development in reflective writing and focus groups. Examples of their narratives are presented below:

> Service Leadership is an informative and inspirational subject which benefits my personal growth. Studying this subject helps me to connect my experiences with the theories and reminds me that I should pay more attention to what the expressed needs of the people around me or even the whole society are.

Table 4.1 Number of outputs related to Service Leadership course

Output type	Number
Books and special issues	9
Book chapters	54
Journal articles	49
Conference presentations	22
Conferences (organized by PolyU)	3
Total	137

My self-awareness was enhanced. Some concepts from this course were helpful. I learned something important about self-improvement in this course.

The knowledge that I have learned during the lessons did not directly contribute to my future career but changed my point of view towards things that happened around me as well as improved my attitude when facing problems and challenges in the future. More importantly, it taught me how to be an effective service leader for my own life, my career, and the whole society.

What I've learnt from the course can help me to perform better in my job as my job is related to service. It is like a light to guide me to become an effective staff.

To date, the evaluation findings have been published in refereed journals, a book series entitled "Quality of Life in Asia", and two special issues in "International Journal on Disability and Human Development". The achievement of the Service Leadership project will be also documented in a forthcoming special issue in "The International Journal of Adolescent Medicine and Health" edited by Shek, Chung, Lin, and Merrick.

In addition to evaluation findings, we also published papers and book chapters on curriculum development and related theoretical issues (e.g., Shek and Lin 2015; Shek and Yu 2015; Shek et al. 2013b). The number of different types of outputs related to the Service Leadership project is presented in Table 4.1.

Future Directions

Several future directions are noted regarding evaluation, teacher training, and program extension. Although multiple evaluation approaches were used, evaluation work can be enhanced in future. First, a quasi-experimental design with a control group will be conducted to replicate previous findings that students' positive changes are due to the subject. Second, a long-term follow-up study will be conducted to investigate the sustainability of the effectiveness. Finally, more attributes about service leadership will be assessed during the learning. Currently, our research team is conducting a 3-year study to develop assessment instruments of service leadership qualities, including knowledge scale, attitude scale, and behavior scale.

Besides, as the notion of service leadership is quite new, and an interactive teaching approach rather than a traditional didactic approach is used in the subject, the knowledge and qualities of teachers are very critical. To gain the knowledge of service leadership, teachers are required to attend a training program offered by Po Chung, who developed the SLAM framework of service leadership. For the training on teaching methodology, e-learning package that introduces the interactive teaching methods will also be developed.

Finally, we can extend the impact of the program. Actually, another service leadership-related subject using service learning pedagogy (i.e., "Service Leadership through Serving Children and Families with Special Needs") has been organized. Besides, the "Service Leadership" subject can benefit students from not only PolyU, but also other tertiary educational institutions in Hong Kong. In this case, we will deliver service leadership education in a condensed version such as a series of workshops to students from other tertiary education institutions. In addition, although SLAM framework was established under the socioeconomic background of Hong Kong, the notion of service leadership can also be applied to mainland China and other societies that need a postindustrial paradigm of leadership. Such application has been evident in the "Global Youth Leadership Program", which was co-organized by PolyU and Peking University, and "Silk Road Youth Leadership Program" which was jointly organized by PolyU, Peking University, and Xi'an Jiaotong University. For example, a service leadership summer school was offered to students from PolyU and Peking University in 2016, with 60 students involved. We will further deliver service leadership education to university students outside of Hong Kong.

Discussion

There is a noticeable need to promote holistic development and well-being in university students worldwide. As a timely response to this need, particularly in a Chinese context, two credit-bearing leadership subjects (i.e., "Tomorrow's Leaders" and "Service Leadership") have been well designed and successfully implemented at PolyU since 2012. The two subjects incorporate PYD approach and Service Leadership model respectively, uphold several key beliefs (e.g., every individual has potentials to be an effective leader), and adopt an experiential teaching and learning pedagogy. These unique features of the subjects establish a solid foundation for achieving the subject goals, which pertains to nurture qualified tomorrow's leaders who can meet the demands of growing service economies. As expected, multiple evaluation strategies have revealed that both subjects are well received by participating students and effectively in improving students' leadership attributes, promoting their whole-personal development, and increasing their quality of life. These findings suggest that it is a promising way to promote youth well-being and help them to develop a new set of leadership qualities demanded by the changing society through credit-bearing leadership courses.

Despite that the two leadership subjects are designed with respect to the context in Hong Kong, related experiences and insights presented in this chapter are applicable in other regions where educators and researchers may develop similar leadership training courses for university students and conduct evaluation studies as well. The importance of these two subjects can be shown by the fact that "Tomorrow's Leaders" was awarded the Silver Award (Ethical Leadership) in the QS Reimagine Education Awards 2017 and "Service Leadership" was awarded the Bronze Award (Ethical Leadership) in the QS Reimagine Education Awards 2016. In 2018, the teaching team for these two subjects were awarded the prestigious UGC Teaching Award in Hong Kong.

References

Becker, S. P., Holdaway, A. S., & Luebbe, A. M. (2018). Suicidal behaviors in college students: Frequency, sex differences, and mental health correlates including sluggish cognitive tempo. *Journal of Adolescent Health, 63*(2), 181–188. https://doi.org/10.1016/j.jadohealth.2018.02.013.

Bourke, B., & Mechler, H. S. (2010). A new me generation? The increasing self-interest among millennial college students. *Journal of College and Character, 11*(2), 1–9. https://doi.org/10.2202/1940-1639.1034.

Chickering, A. W. (2010). A retrospect on higher education's commitment to moral and civic education. *Journal of College and Character, 11*(3), 1–6. https://doi.org/10.2202/1940-1639.1723.

Chung, P. P. Y. (2011). *Service leadership definitions.* Retrieved from http://hki-slam.org/index.php?r=article&catid=1&aid=11#leadership

Chung, P. P. Y., & Elfassy, R. (2016). *The 12 dimensions of a service leader* (1st ed.). New York: Lexingford Publishing.

Felce, D., & Perry, J. (1995). Quality of life: Its definition and measurement. *Research in Developmental Disabilities, 16*(1), 51–74. https://doi.org/10.1016/0891-4222(94)00028-8.

Fry, L. W. (2003). Toward a theory of spiritual leadership. *The Leadership Quarterly, 14*(6), 693–727. https://doi.org/10.1016/j.leaqua.2003.09.001.

Greenleaf, R. K. (1997). The servant as a leader. In R. P. Vecchio (Ed.), *Leadership: Understanding the dynamics of power and influence in organizations* (pp. 429–438). Notre Dame: University of Notre Dame Press.

Knight, J. R., Wechsler, H., Kuo, M., Seibring, M., Weitzman, E. R., & Schuckit, M. A. (2002). Alcohol abuse and dependence among U.S. college students. *Journal of Studies on Alcohol, 63*(3), 263–270. https://doi.org/10.15288/jsa.2002.63.263.

Konrath, S. H., O'Brien, E. H., & Hsing, C. (2011). Changes in dispositional empathy in American college students over time: A meta-analysis. *Personality and Social Psychology Review, 15*(2), 180–198. https://doi.org/10.1177/1088868310377395.

Lerner, R. M., Lerner, J. V., Almerigi, J. B., Theokas, C., Phelps, E., Gestsdottir, S., et al. (2005). Positive youth development, participation in community youth development programs, and community contributions of fifth grade adolescents: Findings from the first wave of the 4-H Study of Positive Youth Development. *Journal of Early Adolescence, 25*(1), 17–71. https://doi.org/10.1177/0272431604272461.

Leung, H. (2016a). Levels of reflection on teaching a leadership and positive youth development subject. *International Journal on Disability and Human Development, 15*(2), 211–220. https://doi.org/10.1515/ijdhd-2016-0712.

Leung, J. T. Y. (2016b). Riding on a roller coaster: Personal reflections of teaching a subject on leadership and intrapersonal development. *International Journal on Disability and Human Development, 15*(2), 221–229. https://doi.org/10.1515/ijdhd-2016-0713.

Lin, L., & Shek, D. T. L. (2018). Does service leadership education contribute to student well-being? A quasi-experimental study based on Hong Kong university students. *Applied Research Quality of Life.* Advanced Online Publications. https://doi.org/10.1007/s11482-018-9644-x.

Mojtabai, R., Olfson, M., & Han, B. (2016). National trends in the prevalence and treatment of depression in adolescents and young adults. *Pediatrics, 138*(6), e20161878. https://doi.org/10.1542/peds.2016-1878.

Pryor, J. H., Hurtado, S., Deangelo, L., Blake, L. P., & Tran, S. (2009). *The American freshman: National norms fall 2009.* Los Angeles: Higher Education Research Institute, UCLA.

Shek, D. T. L. (2010). Nurturing holistic development of university students in Hong Kong: Where are we and where should we go? *The Scientific World Journal, 10*, 563–575. https://doi.org/10.1100/tsw.2010.62.

Shek, D. T. L. (2013). Promotion of holistic development in university students: A credit-bearing course on leadership and intrapersonal development. *Best Practices in Mental Health, 9*(1), 47–61.

Shek, D. T. L., & Cheung, B. P. M. (2013). Developmental issues of university students in Hong Kong. *International Journal of Adolescent Medicine and Health, 25*(4), 345–351. https://doi.org/10.1515/ijamh-2013-0032.

Shek, D. T. L., & Leung, H. (2016a). Resilience as a focus of a subject on leadership and intrapersonal development. *International Journal on Disability and Human Development, 15*(2), 149–155. https://doi.org/10.1515/ijdhd-2016-0704.

Shek, D. T. L., & Leung, J. T. Y. (2016b). Developing social competence in a subject on leadership and intrapersonal development. *International Journal on Disability and Human Development, 15*(2), 165–173. https://doi.org/10.1515/ijdhd-2016-0706.

Shek, D. T. L., & Lin, L. (2015). Core beliefs in the service leadership model proposed by the Hong Kong Institute of Service Leadership and Management. *International Journal on Disability and Human Development, 14*(3), 233–242. https://doi.org/10.1515/ijdhd-2015-0404.

Shek, D. T. L., & Ma, C. M. S. (2014). Do university students change after taking a subject on leadership and intrapersonal development? *International Journal on Disability and Human Development, 13*(4), 451–456. https://doi.org/10.1515/ijdhd-2014-0341.

Shek, D. T. L., & Sun, R. C. F. (2012a). Process evaluation of a positive youth development course in a university setting in Hong Kong. *International Journal on Disability and Human Development, 11*(3), 235–241. https://doi.org/10.1515/ijdhd-2012-0038.

Shek, D. T. L., & Sun, R. C. F. (2012b). Promoting leadership and intrapersonal competence in university students: What can we learn from Hong Kong? *International Journal on Disability and Human Development, 11*(3), 221–228. https://doi.org/10.1515/ijdhd-2012-0037.

Shek, D. T. L., & Sun, R. C. F. (2012c). Promoting psychosocial competencies in university students: Evaluation based on a one-group pre-test/post-test design. *International Journal on Disability and Human Development, 11*(3), 229–234. https://doi.org/10.1515/ijdhd-2012-0039.

Shek, D. T. L., & Sun, R. C. F. (2012d). Qualitative evaluation of a positive youth development course in a university setting in Hong Kong. *International Journal on Disability and Human Development, 11*(3), 243–248. https://doi.org/10.1515/ijdhd-2012-0040.

Shek, D. T. L., & Sun, R. C. F. (Eds.). (2013a). *Development and evaluation of positive adolescent training through Holistic Social Programs (P.A.T.H.S.).* Singapore: Springer.

Shek, D. T. L., & Sun, R. C. F. (2013b). Process evaluation of a leadership and intrapersonal development subject for university students. *International Journal on Disability and Human Development, 12*(2), 203–211. https://doi.org/10.1515/ijdhd-2013-0018.

Shek, D. T. L., & Sun, R. C. F. (2013c). Post-course subjective outcome evaluation of a course promoting leadership and intrapersonal development in university students in Hong Kong. *International Journal on Disability and Human Development, 12*(2), 193–201. https://doi.org/10.1515/ijdhd-2012-0136.

Shek, D. T. L., & Wong, K. K. (2011). Do adolescent developmental issues disappear overnight? Reflections about holistic development in university students. *The Scientific World Journal, 11*, 353–361. https://doi.org/10.1100/tsw.2011.5.

Shek, D. T. L., & Yu, L. (2014). Post-course subjective outcome evaluation of a subject on leadership and intrapersonal development for university students in Hong Kong. *International Journal on Disability and Human Development, 13*(4), 457–464. https://doi.org/10.1515/ijdhd-2014-0342.

Shek, D. T. L., & Yu, L. (2015). Character strengths and service leadership. *International Journal on Disability and Human Development, 14*(4), 299–307. https://doi.org/10.1515/ijdhd-2015-0451.

Shek, D. T. L., Sun, R. C. F., Tsien-Wong, T. B. K., Cheng, C. T., & Yan, H. R. (2013a). Objective outcome evaluation of a leadership and intrapersonal development subject for university students. *International Journal on Disability and Human Development, 12*(2), 221–227. https://doi.org/10.1515/ijdhd-2013-0020.

Shek, D. T. L., Yu, L., Ma, C. M. S., Sun, R. C. F., & Liu, T. T. (2013b). Development of a credit-bearing service leadership subject for university students in Hong Kong. *International Journal of Adolescent Medicine and Health, 25*(4), 353–361. https://doi.org/10.1515/ijamh-2013-0033.

Shek, D. T. L., Lin, L., Liu, T. T., & Law, M. Y. M. (2014a). Process evaluation of a pilot subject on service leadership for university students in Hong Kong. *International Journal on Disability and Human Development, 13*(4), 531–540. https://doi.org/10.1515/ijdhd-2014-0351.

Shek, D. T. L., Yu, L., & Ma, C. M. S. (2014b). The students were happy, but did they change positively? *International Journal on Disability and Human Development, 13*(4), 505–511. https://doi.org/10.1515/ijdhd-2014-0348.

Shek, D. T. L., Chung, P. P. Y., & Leung, H. (2015a). Manufacturing economy vs. service economy: Implications for service leadership. *International Journal on Disability and Human Development, 14*(3), 205–215. https://doi.org/10.1515/ijdhd-2015-0402.

Shek, D. T. L., Law, M. Y. M., & Liu, T. T. (2015b). Focus group evaluation of a service leadership subject in Hong Kong. *International Journal on Disability and Human Development, 14*(4), 371–376. https://doi.org/10.1515/ijdhd-2015-0458.

Shek, D. T. L., Fok, H. K., Leung, C. T. L., & Li, P. P. K. (2016a). Qualitative evaluation of a credit-bearing leadership subject in Hong Kong. *International Journal of Child Health and Human Development, 9*(2), 173–183.

Shek, D. T. L., Liang, J., & Law, M. Y. M. (2016b). Process evaluation of a university subject on service leadership in Hong Kong. *International Journal of Child and Adolescent Health, 9*(2), 253–261.

Shek, D. T. L., Liang, J., & Zhu, X. (2016c). Subjective outcome evaluation of a service leadership subject for university students in Hong Kong. *International Journal of Child Health and Human Development, 9*(2), 225–232.

Shek, D. T. L., Lin, L., & Xie, Q. (2016d). Service leadership education for university students in Hong Kong: A qualitative evaluation study. *International Journal of Child and Adolescent Health, 9*(2), 235–243.

Shek, D. T. L., Wu, F. K. Y., Leung, C. T. L., Fok, H. K., & Li, P. P. K. (2016e). Focus group evaluation of a subject on leadership and intrapersonal development in Hong Kong. *International Journal of Child Health and Human Development, 9*(2), 185–194.

Shek, D. T. L., Wu, J., Lin, L., & Pu, E. X. P. (2017). Qualitative evaluation of a service leadership subject in a Chinese context. *International Journal on Disability and Human Development, 16*(4), 433–441. https://doi.org/10.1515/ijdhd-2017-7012.

Wallander, J. L., Schmitt, M., & Koot, H. M. (2001). Quality of life measurement in children and adolescents: Issues, instruments and applications. *Journal of Clinical Psychology, 57*(4), 571–585. https://doi.org/10.1002/jclp.1029.

Yu, L. (2016). A teacher's reflection on teaching "Tomorrow's Leaders" in university students in Hong Kong. *International Journal on Disability and Human Development, 15*(2), 195–202. https://doi.org/10.1515/ijdhd-2016-0710.

Daniel T. L. Shek is Associate Vice-President, Chair Professor of Applied Social Sciences and Li and Fung Professor in Service Leadership Education at The Hong Kong Polytechnic University (PolyU). He is the Editor of the *Applied Research in Quality of Life*, ISQOLS-Springer.

Xiaoqin Zhu is Instructor at The Hong Kong Polytechnic University (PolyU).

Diya Dou is Instructor at The Hong Kong Polytechnic University (PolyU).

Moon Y. M. Law is a Teaching Fellow at The Hong Kong Polytechnic University (PolyU).

Lu Yu is Assistant Professor at The Hong Kong Polytechnic University (PolyU).

Cecilia M. S. Ma is Assistant Professor at The Hong Kong Polytechnic University (PolyU).

Li Lin is a Research Assistant Professor at The Hong Kong Polytechnic University (PolyU).

Chapter 5
Teaching Quality of Life and the Capability Approach

Paul Anand

Introduction

In this chapter, I want to consider some ways in which the capability approach (CA) might inform teaching quality of life. From almost a seedling complaint about utilitarian ethics in the early 1980s developed by Amartya Sen in his inspirational Oxford University lectures on welfare economics and seminars on economics and philosophy at All Souls College, the approach has made significant contributions to a range of disciplines from health through international development to social policy. It has helped to reinvigorate the social indicators movement and arguably also provided significant impetus for the rise of positive psychology though many of the early academic surveys focused on the foundational, philosophical issues and potential challenges for application and use. At this point in time, whilst the early conceptual and theoretical literature was both interesting and important, there is now scope to develop our thinking about the teaching of quality of life through a large body of empirical research that draws on CA.

Within graduate programs on international development for example, it is possible to conceive of modules that focus on quality of life, health, human development and many aspects of the sustainable development goals (SDGs) which relate direct to life quality and have arguably been inspired by the emphasis on multi-dimensionality and agency that CA encourages. In high income countries, quality of life teaching can feature in a range of social sciences from psychology

P. Anand (✉)
School of Philosophy Politics Economics Development and Geography,
The Open University, Milton Keynes, UK

Department of Social Policy and Intervention, Oxford University, Oxford, UK

Center for Philosophy of Natural and Social Sciences, London School of Economics,
London, UK
e-mail: paul.anand@open.ac.uk

© Springer Nature Switzerland AG 2020
G. H. Tonon (ed.), *Teaching Quality of Life in Different Domains*, Social
Indicators Research Series 79, https://doi.org/10.1007/978-3-030-21551-4_5

where it can be key focus through a range of other disciplines where it is often an issue to be taken account of at particular points. To (positive) psychology, CA contributes ideas of human flourishing and achievement which connect closely with pre-existing work on a range of psychological topics from flow (absorption) Csikszentmihalyi et al. (2014) to self-efficacy, Bandura (1982). But CA can and now has also been used to shed light on particular questions in a range of disciplines. Typically these applications draw on part of the CA approach and shed light on some aspect of quality of life in a particular context and it is natural to ask whether such applications help users to address or solve problems, or perhaps see them in a new light?

CA has been applied across a wide range of disciplines and to reflect the value of this in a teaching context I want to consider some of the applications that have emerged in the past decade or more. Any quality of life course that draws on CA will want to consider its theoretical foundations and so I prefix the survey of applications with a section that focuses on some key ideas by Sen (1985) and Nussbaum (2001). The chapter then identifies, in section "Some key theoretical themes", papers that apply and discuss CA in different areas with an emphasis either on empirical work and/or widely cited papers. For the most part, space only allows a brief mention of the paper but nearly all have been selected because they could be useful on graduate or higher level undergraduate courses. The following section then considers some early criticisms of the approach and suggests that discussions in teaching settings might lead students to conclude that most of the early objections to the approach have been addressed by its applications. One exception concerns some general ideas around objectivity which, I will suggest, might in some CA circles appear to have been misunderstood. A final section concludes.

The Contributions of Sen and Nussbaum

While there are a number good overviews of the approach (eg Qizilbash (1996) or Robeyns (2006)) in journal papers, it is often useful for students to consult original sources and Sen's (1985) account of the approach is a useful and authoritative starting point. The ideas in that monograph both identify previous theoretical difficulties and offer a constructive response to them. According to CA, quality of life has, at base, three aspects: the things we do or are, our experience of those actions and states, and the opportunities and constraints we face in life. All three aspects are widely recognised but often only objective actions and states are measured. This could be a starting point for teaching that explores what people do through time diaries for instance (eg see Kahneman et al. (2004)) or it might be interesting to consider which activities and states actually have an impact on subjective measures of experience. Perhaps most distinctive about this approach was the way it brought freedom and opportunity into research and discussions of quality of life.

To these definitional contributions, Sen adds an analysis of how quality of life is produced depending as it does both on the resources to which a person has access as well as their ability to convert those resources into activities, states or experiences. At this point, students might ask what are resources or 'conversion factors' which could be a good opportunity for students to consider their own views and answers to the question. Resources include income of course but they might also include social factors such as social capital. Conversion factors can be seen as a device by which the theory breaks with the concept of basic goods in Rawls. Instead of just giving everyone some quantum of basic goods, we need to allow for individual differences both in resources and in people's capacities to transform resources into valued activities or states. A final point to make concerns the emphasis on multi-dimensionality. Sen wanted to create a way of thinking about human wellbeing which did not simply reduce down to income and the fact that skills activities, and capabilities are all highly multi-dimensional is one way of doing this. Students could be encouraged to put these ideas together as Sen does into three fundamental relations: (1) activities/states depend on resources and conversion abilities, (2) happiness depends on activities and states experienced and (3) advantage or capabilities can be defined as the set of all activities/states a person could engage given their resource endowment and conversion abilities.

A second major contribution to the development of the approach can be found in a series of books and papers by political theorist Martha Nussbaum. Her approach is different to Sen's though there is a reading which sees it as complementary rather than alternative. Sen tells us formally that capabilities are multi-dimensional but we would like to know what specifically is the space of human wellbeing in which they operate. Nussbaum offers an answer to this question by providing a list of fundamental capabilities. These she claimed, were sufficiently important to quality of life, and perhaps implicitly often dependent on collective protection, that all democratic states should underwrite them. Her list covers: life, bodily health, bodily integrity, senses imagination and thought, emotions, practical reason, affiliation, other species, leisure, and control over the political and material environment. At the time there was much debate about whether there should or could be a single objective list given the cultural diversity within which democracies exist and this could give rise to useful and engaging classroom discussion.

The list could also make a useful basis for discussions about its contents (as well as the meaning of quality of life itself), the process by which it was constructed and claims made for its status. Is the list universally applicable around the world or even high income countries? Perhaps there are omissions? What would happen if one tried to make the list more detailed? Perhaps items on the list are not given the relative emphasis to which everyone agrees? In any case, taken together Sen and Nussbaum have provided a new conceptual framework for thinking about quality of life. On their foundations, thousands of papers have built though before moving on these applications, I want in the next section to highlight some key issues that have emerged from CA's approach to quality of life.

Some Key Theoretical Themes

The original core insights were distinctive in a number of ways as we have begun to see. Here are five.

(a) Individual differences

Perhaps most fundamentally, CA emphasises the need to be aware of individual differences, particularly in the ability of individuals to convert resources into desired activities or states. This provides an immediate connection both to a large body of research in psychology as well as advanced work in empirical economics on unobserved heterogeneity. The key point is not just that people have different preferences or values, but also that they have different social resources which help them transform financial resources into things that matter.

(b) Income is an input

A second point to highlight is that CA emphasises the fact that income and wealth are inputs into quality of life, and not to be confused with quality of life itself. Put this way, the point may seem obvious and it will generally be the case that there are positive relations between various aspects of quality of life and economic resources. However, correlation is only a measure of linear association and often relations to income are non-linear. Furthermore correlation does not imply causation and the connections between income and quality of life may need to allow for certain capabilities being predictors of future income, rather than the other way round. In any case, this emphasis is an important corrective to the theoretical and policy focus on income as the most important measurable variable when it comes to quality of life in many settings.

(c) The importance of agency

Early on in the development of the approach Sen drew attention to the concept of agency. The concept is widely used in philosophy and has also influenced the generation of measures and empirical work in international development. In these contexts, agency might be thought of as the power one has to bring about desired outcomes. Not only does it matter that individuals obtain the outcomes they need or desire, but individuals themselves and society at large, is often concerned that a person brings about those outcomes through their own actions.

(d) The value of public deliberation

Related to agency is the importance of public deliberation. It follows that if we value agency, in social decision-making problems we are likely to value processes that include meaningful deliberation and involvement. Whether this will be sufficient or effective are of course are open questions so the ideal need not be accepted uncritically even if the value of democratic processes for the promotion of quality of life remains one we believe important. CA tends to highlight the value of public deliberation and students might find this work can be supplemented by work from political science on its uses in practice or from community involvement studies in lower income countries.

(e) Subjective wellbeing depends on activities and states but is adaptable

A fifth and final point concerns questions about the extent to which the happiness or unhappiness that a state brings can be used a measure of value or importance. Perhaps outside economics this is not such a concern because subjective assessments of quality of life have always had varying degrees of use and application depending on the context (job satisfaction is a useful variable and arguably health satisfaction less so). In any case it is possible that a theoretical point has sometimes been confused or overstated. While the fact of adaptation mandates a need for caution about taking the absence of unhappiness as an assurance, that does not amount to support for the claim that all subjectively reported or evaluated data must disregarded as meaningless. From a scientific perspective, whether measures are informative or not depend particularly on the degree to which they are *reliable* and *valid* and from that perspective whether self-reported data is meaningful depends on the particular data measures employed and the data uses to which it is put. A blanket ban is not consistent with general practice in research methodology.

Beyond these five issues, it is worth recognising that a significant amount of CA research focusses on social justice. Social justice is implied by Nussbaum's approach but we might wonder whether this is so for the formal part of Sen's version which can be read as an abstract or general theory of quality of life and its production. Secondly, it is worth noting that several high level exercises have reported on the development of measures of economic and social progress that 'go beyond GDP'. The OECD backed report by Stiglitz et al. (2009) is the most prominent example and it provides both a good summary of problems as well as recommendations for future work on the development of non-financial measures of life quality. Thirdly, and perhaps least obviously, it should be recognised that there are significant affinities between the language of the capability approach, which has used terms such as human flourishing, and the emergence of the field of positive psychology particularly as articulated in *Flourish* by Seligman (2012) who claims that 'happiness is not enough'. Rather, his argument is that human flourishing depends on five 'pillars' which include 'positive emotion, engagement, meaning, achievement and social connections. This approach offers a potentially invaluable bridge between Sen's normatively driven concepts and empirical science though as yet it has to be said these strands of literature have developed somewhat independently and in isolation of each other. These ideas could be a minimum for students wanting to learn about CA as an approach to quality of life, and with them in place in should be possible to turn to applications.

Areas of Application

An early concern for CA researchers was to consider whether the approach might be made to work in practice – how it could be 'operationalised'. Centre stage of this debate has been the question whether human capabilities can be measured or not. Surely the list of things a person could do, given their resources and conversion abilities is infinite? Perhaps so but if we look at things from the sharp end first, we see that in fact household surveys, psychology researchers and economists all use some direct capability indicators and there is no reason why such indicators might not be extended to cover all the capabilities of interest. One way into this operationalisation literature can be found in Anand et al. (2009) which is one of the first papers to develop an extensive set of bespoke capability indicators.

Measurement Issues

Before getting on the main substantive areas of application, I want to discuss briefly the topic of measurement. This is a relatively technical area and there is certainly enough material for more than one session (depending on the background of students). In any case, I suspect many quality of life researchers and teachers would want to say something about this topic. While early doubts about the possibility of developing meaningful indicators of capabilities have probably been dispelled it is useful to rehearse the ways in which capability indicators are categorised and developed. Broadly speaking there are **explicit** approaches and **indirect** approaches to measurement. Explicit approaches ask respondents about the opportunities freedoms, constraints barriers and limiting factors that exist in their lives. They have been widespread in medical research for decades and can also be found in some national household surveys and international demographic surveys. Some direct capability indicators focus on what people are able to do on particular dimensions eg Anand et al. (2005, 2009, 2018), Al-Janabi et al. (2012), and Coast (2014). Another set focusses on the individual's level of agency – highlighting particular decision-making ability in particular areas of life and constraints on freedom of action deriving often from social relations. This work has been particularly influential in the development literature (see eg Kabeer (2018)) where decision-making inequalities can be a source of significant challenges to quality of life and is usefully reviewed in Alkire (2005).[1] There is in addition a series of papers that use techniques appropriate for situations where explicit indicators or measures do not exist. These latent variable methods can be very valuable for economists and a

---

[1] Care should be taken not to confuse this strand of work and thought with that on multi-dimensional poverty which at the time of writing focused more on available indicators which have been argued to be less explicitly related to capabilities. Basu (2016), Ferreira (2011), and Revallion (2011) are good accessible papers by leading economists that help students understand some of the challenges involved.

useful way into this literature is found in the pioneering work of Krisnakumar (2007). The relevant econometrics literature includes work by Andreassen and Di Tommaso (2018) for example and there is also an important body of work in economic theory which can be accessed through papers connected to the review by van Hees (2004). I make no attempt to discuss that literature here but do recommend it to those interested in these kinds of technical issues.

Health

There is a rich literature on health and CA which is likely to be of interest to many quality of life teachers both in and outside of medical training. Pereira (1993) is one of the earliest and offers a discussion of how CA can contribute to the understanding of health with some useful comparisons against alternative perspectives. Slightly earlier is the paper by Culyer (1989) which argues that CA could provide in health economics a non-welfarist approach and outlines again some of the conceptual reasons, in an accessible format, as to why this might be so. Anyone interested in the conceptual foundations of health might also wish to consult a subsequent follow-up by Brouwer et al. (2008) who discuss outcomes, sources of valuation, weighting of outcomes and interpersonal comparisons of wellbeing in the CA, again compared with the prevailing welfarist orthodoxy. Finally, in this foundational set, Prah Ruger (2006) uses CA to build a justification for the right to health drawing also on Aristotle's political theory as well as ideas about agreements which are incompletely theorised. This first set of papers help to set the stage for work that follows by outlining the rationale for moving beyond prevailing approaches to health particular within the health economics profession.

More empirically oriented applications of CA to quality of life issues followed on from this work first, notably, in the area of disability. A very widely quoted paper by Mitra (2006), for instance, shows how the approach can be used to analyse disability in terms of capabilities, potential and actual disability, as well as everyday functioning. And she also uses CA to highlight the fact that disabling factors derive not just from personal characteristics, but income and environment also. Shortly afterwards, Trani and Bakhshi (2008) report on a disability survey in Afghanistan that looks in considerable detail at the capability deprivations of those with a disability. The application of CA to quality of life with disability was perhaps an obvious target for researchers because of the emphasis on differential capacities and together this pair of papers could be used to make a strong case for the value of such applications.

Researchers have also sought to develop new CA-based instruments for measuring quality of life in health. Coast et al. (2008) for example developed an instrument known as the ICECAP which was originally designed around the needs of older patients and helps to identify the meeting of social health needs. Applied first in a clinical trial relating to community treatment orders for seriously ill patients, Simon et al. (2013) offer an alternative measure which has many more dimensions and can be traced back directly to Nussbaum's original list. Both papers help to illustrate how medical researchers use patient reported outcomes to operationalise capability assessment.

Other important works relating to health well worth considering for teaching include Ferrer et al. (2014) which uses CA to understand population access to health diet and physical activity, a book on social justice in health by Venkatapuram (2013), Wolff's (2009) philosophical discussions of disability, and Zaidi et al. (2017) on an European active aging index.

Childhood Education and Employment

Several applications of CA have been made to the closely related areas of education and childhood. Saito (2003) is one of the first to offer a sustained examination of how CA can be applied to children and argues for the need to develop *wisdom in the exercise* of capabilities. By contrast, one of the most widely cited empirical papers is Biggeri et al. (2006) who report an empirical analysis of the capabilities that matter to children developing a participatory method that emphases the contributions of children themselves. Many papers relevant to children focus on the contributions of education in some way. Tao (2013) for example, examines teacher under-performance by examining structural factors that constrain their behaviour while Murphy and Wolfenden (2013) draw on CA in their analysis of processes by which open educational resources were developed and adopted in the Teacher Education in Sub-saharan African (TESSA) programme. Finally, and reverting to two conceptual papers, students may be interested in Unterhalter's (2016) concept of creative negative capability which distinguishes between things that are measureable in education and those that are valuable but not measurable. In addition, Terzi (2005) offers a discussion of the 'dilemma of difference' in special needs education drawing particularly on a pamphlet by Mary Warnock. The problem follows from what Terzi describes as an unavoidable choice between categorisation for the identification of special needs and services and the opposing desire to be inclusive by treating all on an equal basis.

From childhood and education, it could be a natural step to look at work on transitions into and implications of CA for employment and related social and labour market policies. One recent review, Chiappero-Martinetti et al. (2015), discusses several research projects that connect CA to labour market policies and does so in a broader context of operationalising the approach. Several studies focus on activation policies including one by Dahmen (2014) in which he looks at the construction of employment identities recognising that how 'we conceptualise and realise who we are' is, like physical and social barriers and opportunities, a shaper of life quality. In a Sub-Sahara African context, Arubayi and Akobo (2018), respond to the view that education programs are failing youth transitions into the labour market by presenting research that identifies some of the additional factors and problems not envisaged by standard training programs. How quality of life relates to work is also an important sub-theme in CA, one that benefits from its multi-dimensional and agency emphases. Finally, students may appreciate studying a discussion paper by Sehnbruch (2004) in which she uses CA to look for evidence of, or risks to, decent work in the Chilean labour market. *Inter alia* the paper develops a new measure of employment quality, argues that CA provides a case for focussing on the freedom and wellbeing of workers in labour markets and suggests that employment quality be given greater emphasis in labour market policy.

Gender Agency and Empowerment

There is a significant literature on gender informed by CA which focuses mainly on issues particular to women. These are diverse and overlap inevitably with literatures other aspects of life quality but a useful recent and accessible paper that offers a route into this literature is Hanmer and Klugman (2016). The paper offers a review of the literature on women's agency from a theoretical and empirical perspective before reporting new analysis using the Demographic and Health Survey (DHS). It discusses econometric findings about women's agency in accessible fashion and reports inter alia that higher levels of education can be protective for women but only with male partners who also have secondary or higher levels of education. By contrast Unterhalter et al. (2013) look at empowerment, though issues of gender justice in schools. A key theoretical idea is that focussing just on differential access to education between boys and girls is not enough while novel data on reported obstacles provides useful additional insights about capabilities. Developed in a high income context though presumably with wider applications, Addabbo et al. (2010) use CA to develop a tool for auditing annual government budgets with respect to their impacts on multiple dimensions of women's quality of life. The paper has a particular focus on the ability to care (for oneself and for others) and again provides a nice illustration of how CA can be used to make theoretically informed contributions to policy debate. Finally, and returning again to a lower income country focus, a paper by Tiwari (2017) describes how connections between *social innovation* and capability expansion can be made. Drawing on current and historical case study research relating to women's self help groups, an m-finance project (M Pesa), and Gandhi's Indian Freedom Movement, the paper explains the nature of social innovations (as distinct from those that are purely market based) and argues for their potential to help address unmet aspirations as well as issues of equity and sustainability.

Design and Information Technology

While the design and information technologies are normally quite distant from the philosophical roots of CA, this subfield has generated some widely cited papers. Kleine (2010) for example addresses the paradox that information and communication technologies are widespread but have impacts difficult to identify. She develops a Choice Framework which relates structural factors and agency to development outcomes, provides a rich list of resources and uses the Framework to design ethnographic work on the impacts of telecentres in rural Chile. Her detailed discussion of implications for methodology/theory on the one hand, and development practitioners on the other could be valuable in many teaching settings. A second paper Oosterlaken (2009) is motivated by a paucity of research into 'the structures methods and objectives of social design'. She argues, inter alia, that the basic purpose of design is to expand what a person can do but that the working principles and discourse of designers focus on issues such as aesthetics or usability rather than the underling capabilities which good design is supposed to enhance. The paper includes a case-study of tricycles for the disabled in Ghana and a discussion of participatory design. The final paper in this trio, Swist and Collin (2017) considers three types of platforms that contribute the understanding of children's rights (based on a range of national indicators, specific issues and big data). They develop a 'networked' CA and apply to this to the Safe and Well online project that examined how social campaigns can foster safety and wellbeing in teenagers. A key finding was that the platforms have an orientation towards adult concerns and that greater involvement of the children who these platforms are intended to benefit is warranted.

Does Recent Research Rebut Early Concerns About CA as a Workable Approach to Quality of Life?

There are numerous theoretical, methodological issues and questions that could be considered. These were raised as the approach developed, many quite early on, and questioned whether the approach could be operationalised or whether it was a good way to think about quality of life. One of the themes that might be explored in a teaching session is the extent to which this now very rich framework and body of research provides a constructive opportunity for new work in old disciplines or to find new connections between them.

Measurability and Workability

As noted above, at the heart of doubts about CA lay concerns that capabilities are either difficult to measure or not often measured directly. We might still accept the second point when it comes to secondary data but point to many empirical studies both qualitative and quantitative that engage with or draw on the approach using direct indicators. All these data sources tap into capabilities in a direct albeit partial fashion. It could be argued that these measures operate in a similar way to income which is a partial indicator of quality of life most closely related to those aspects that depend on personal consumption but not non-market goods or goods provided by state. The diverse range of capability measures that have been used do not provide an explicit list of every possibility that a person but then neither does income. Rather they provide indicators of what is possible for a person with respect to a particular aspect of life, or so it could be argued. Rather than focus on early *a priori* of expressions of concern, students could be encouraged to engage with the positive examples of capability indicators that have been developed and draw conclusions based on these. Closely related is the problem of what Rawls called workability – for he was concerned whether the philosophically sophisticated approach could be operationalised in practice. The many qualitative applications combined with literatures on quantitative measures suggest that workability has been demonstrated in both qualitative and quantitative empirical work. Indeed it could be argued that while Rawls's own alternative was and is highly influential in theories of justice and political liberalism, it never established workability in the sense of becoming a foundation for empirical work.

Individualism and Under-Theorisation

A second critique that has emerged concerns the 'individualist' orientation of the approach. Many theories and accounts of quality of life do highlight the individual as the location for life quality while allowing a range of other factors as its source. But theories of quality of life (in a broad sense) range in their emphasis and purpose depending on whether they focus on what takes place at the location or what the sources might be. It could be interesting to explore with students whether in that context CA is a somewhat novel theory that emphasises neither the location nor the source per se but rather the bridging mechanisms between them. Several widely cited and student friendly papers now show how CA can connect to questions of collective action, Ibrahim (2006), Stewart (2005), Richardson (2007), and Tonon (2017). The approach according to this view can be seen as connecting up what happens at the individual level (studied by sociologists and psychologists for example) with external factors studied in social policy and economics. This bridging idea connects also with the criticism that the approach is under theorised. It could be argued that Sen's contribution was appropriately theorised as a general abstract theory (of the sort widespread in economics) and that subsequent applications and extensions are indeed essential for putting empirical flesh on these theoretical bones. One could argue that this generality is precisely what allows CA to make distinctive contributions to literatures on quality of life.

Staticness and Ambiguity

Sen's original account particularly has been critiqued for its static nature as well as for ambiguities in formulation. The static-ness of early work is easy to understand particularly given the fact his original equations did not mention time while Nussbaum's list also seems to envisage only limited evolution over time. That said in subsequent applications the dynamic possibilities of CA for empirical work are clear enough. Research on the development of children's non-cognitive skills and their impacts years later conducted by Heckman and colleagues provides an excellent example of how the time dimension can practically be brought into CA research. Elsewhere, work on empowerment which shows, for example, the impacts or otherwise of education clearly points to factors that could enhance agency. The human capital story which is predates CA is nevertheless an important aspect of it and invites researchers to consider not just averages but also heterogeneities. Recent experience might encourage the questions: can more human capital ever be unhelpful to an individual or is it now often wasteful to society and do improvements to education *always* enhance equity as many seem to suggest? Similarly, ambiguities in original discussions may not always carry over to empirical applications. Consider when measuring resources, a decision has to be made whether or not to include health status. A research might view having a healthy body as a valuable resource or see being able to live healthily as a capability indicator. Both the resource and the capability indicator interpretation make sense so any researcher has to make a decision about this and there is no obvious reason to think that all studies should make the same decision so long as they are clear about rationale. Discussing some of the decisions that researchers have made is likely to be a very useful exercise particularly in graduate level teaching related to quality of life where there is an emphasis on training for research.

Objectivity

Finally, it could be well be worth unpacking, what I see as a basic misunderstanding of standard research methods that arose in the CA though this misunderstanding may be fading over time as CA research develops as a body of empirical knowledge. It has been suggested that capabilities are objective and that the approach is not and should not use subjective data. If by subjective data is meant self-reported data used in demographic and household surveys, psychology experiments or clinical trials, then I would suggest that the prohibition is suspiciously broad. In fact one could go further and argue that it fails to acknowledge standard methodological practice in most health and social sciences. Whether data are acceptable from a scientific viewpoint is the key question and self-reports that are valid and reliable are accepted as meaningful. It might be interesting to consider whether some confusion has arisen from the term 'objective list' account applied to Nussbaum's list or Sen's concern about bias in self-reports due to 'adaptive preferences'. Students could for instance be encouraged to consider whether Sen's point was correct but over applied by others or whether an ethically objective list need have any implications at all for the epistemological status (methodological value) of self-reports.

Contributions to Quality of Life Pedagogy: Some Concluding Remarks

CA has a huge amount to contribute to teaching in the quality of life field. Connections to the pre-existing research on social indicators developed by sociologists in the 1970s are visible particularly though the rise of the UN's Human Development Index Anand and Sen (1994) or publications in *Social Indicators Research*. CA has given the latter research field a significant boost and both human development and the social indicators paradigms are likely to continue benefitting from mutual synergies over time. Relations to psychological research on quality of life have been much less evident despite the use of terms such as flourishing, a term favoured by Sen and adopted by Martin Seligman, one of the founder of positive psychology.[2] At the time of writing, there is evidence of growing literatures on CA and social justice, perhaps a reaction to persistent and increasing global inequalities. The approach, and its contributions to quality of life, have evolved along with the interests of those attracted to it, as well as its founders. In the appendix, I have suggested some possible titles for lectures of seminars based on some of the ideas here. Some of these topics might also include discussions of possible gaps in CA work. If running a class, on quality of life and CA, I might conclude with sessions on where the approach will go next. Obvious challenges or opportunities include sustainable development, the gig economy, non-cognitive skills and global warming as well as the ongoing interest in key areas some of which are reflected in the special interest group activities of the Human Development and Capability Association. Anyone teaching a course on quality of life or that includes a significant component of material on quality of life and freedom, opportunities or constraints, should find something of interest in CA.

---

[2] Though see for instance Hart (2016) on how aspirations matter for capabilities. Additional papers that merit consideration by teachers but are precluded from further discussion for reasons of space include Burchardt and Vizard (2011) on rights and consultation, Frediani (2010) on planning, Fukuda-Parr (2003) on gender, Alkire and Santos (2013) and Anand et al. (2019) on poverty.

Suggested Topics for 12 Lectures/Seminars on Quality of Life Through the Capability Approach

1. What is the Capability Approach and How Does it Conceive of Quality of Life
2. What are some of the Foundational and Application Problems that It Addresses
3. Some Measurement Issues
4. Applications in Health Care
5. Applications in Employment and Social Policy
6. Applications to Gender Minorities Agency and Inclusion
7. Applications in Design, ICT and Planning
8. Non-cognitive skills and other Psychological Issues in the Capability Approach
9. The Value and Importance of Engaging with Impacted Stakeholders
10. Applications to Poverty
11. Engaging with Sustainable Development and Social Justice
12. The CA paradigm and quality of life – challenges and synergies

References

Addabbo, T., Lanzi, D., & Picchio, A. (2010). Gender budgets. *Journal of Human Development and Capabilities, 11*(4), 479–501.

Al-Janabi, H., Flynn, T. N., & Coast, J. (2012). Development of a self-report measure of capability wellbeing for adults: The ICECAP-A. *Quality of Life Research, 21*(1), 167–176.

Alkire, S. (2005). Subjective quantitative studies of human agency. *Social Indicators Research, 74*(1), 217–260.

Alkire, S. (undated). *Measuring the freedom aspects of capabilities*, GEI Harvard University, http://citeseerx.ist.psu.edu/viewdoc/download?doi=10.1.1.516.7332&rep=rep1&type=pdf. Accessed 21 Feb 2019.

Alkire, S., & Santos, M. E. (2013). A multi-dimensional approach. *Social Indicators Research, 112*(2), 239–257.

Anand P., & Piketty T. (Eds.) (n.d.) Special issue in honour of Amartya Sen's 75th Birthday. *Journal of Public Economics, 95*(3–4).

Anand, P., & Roope, L. (2016). The development and happiness of very young children. *Social Choice and Welfare, 47*(4), 825–851.

Anand, S., & Sen, A. (1994). *Human development index: Methodology and measurement.* New York: Human Development Report Office.

Anand, P., Hunter, G., & Smith, R. (2005). Capabilities and well-being: Evidence based on the Sen–Nussbaum approach to welfare. *Social Indicators Research, 74*(1), 9–55.

Anand, P., Hunter, G., Carter, I., Dowding, K., Guala, F., & Van Hees, M. (2009). The development of capability indicators. *Journal of Human Development and Capabilities, 10*(1), 125–152.

Anand, P., Gray, A., Liberini, F., Roope, L., Smith, R., & Thomas, R. (2015). Wellbeing over 50. *The Journal of the Economics of Ageing, 6*, 68–78.

Anand, P., Saxena, S., Gonzalez R., Dang H. (2018). Can women's self help groups contribute to sustainable development: Evidence of capability changes from Nothern India, Discussion paper available from authors.

Anand, P., Jones, S., Donoghue, M., Teitler, J. (2019). Non-monetary poverty and deprivation: A capability approach, Discussion paper available from authors.

Andreassen, L., & Di Tommaso, M. L. (2018). Estimating capabilities with random scale models: women's freedom of movement. *Social Choice and Welfare, 50*(4), 625–661.

Arubayi, D. O., & Akobo, L. A. (2018). The capability approach and national development in Nigeria: Towards a youth transition model. *Human Resource Development International, 21*(5), 463–492.

Bandura, A. (1982). Self-efficacy mechanism in human agency. *American Psychologist, 37*(2), 122.

Biggeri, M., Libanora, R., Mariani, S., & Menchini, L. (2006). Children conceptualizing their capabilities: Results of a survey conducted during the first children's world congress on child labour. *Journal of Human Development, 7*(1), 59–83.

Brouwer, W. B. F., Culyer, A. J., van Exel, N. J. A., & Rutten, F. F. H. (2008). Welfarism vs. extra-welfarism. *Journal of Health Economics, 27*(2), 325–338.

Burchardt, T., & Vizard, P. (2011). 'Operationalising' the capability approach as a basis for equality and human rights monitoring in twenty-first-century Britain. *Journal of Human Development and Capabilities, 12*(1), 91–119.

Carter, I. (2011). Respect and the basis of equality. *Ethics, 121*(3), 538–571.

Chiappero-Martinetti, E., Egdell, V., Hollywood, E., & McQuaid, R. (2015). Operationalisation of the capability approach. In *Facing trajectories from school to work* (pp. 115–139). Cham: Springer.

Coast, J. (2014). Strategies for the economic evaluation of end-of-life care: Making a case for the capability approach. *Expert Review of Pharmacoeconomics & Outcomes Research, 14*(4), 473–482.

Coast, J., Flynn, T. N., Natarajan, L., Sproston, K., Lewis, J., Louviere, J. J., & Peters, T. J. (2008). Valuing the ICECAP capability index for older people. *Social Science & Medicine, 67*(5), 874–882.

Csikszentmihalyi, M., Abuhamdeh, S., & Nakamura, J. (2014). Flow. In *Flow and the foundations of positive psychology*. Dordrecht: Springer.

Culyer, A. J. (1989). The normative economics of health care finance and provision. *Oxford Review of Economic Policy, 5*(1), 34–58.

Cunha, F., & Heckman, J. (2007). The technology of skill formation. *American Economic Review, 97*(2), 31–47.

Dahmen, S. (2014). The capability approach and sociological conceptions of human agency: An empirical assessment on the basis of an analysis of activation policies. *Social Work and Society-International Online Journal, 12*(2), 1–14. https://www.socwork.net/sws/article/view/404.

Duckworth, A. L., & Quinn, P. D. (2009). Development and validation of the Short Grit Scale (GRIT–S). *Journal of Personality Assessment, 91*(2), 166–174.

Ferreira, E. H. G. (2011). Poverty is multi-dimensional, but what are we going to do about it? *Journal of Economic Inequality, 9*(3), 493–495.

Ferrer, R. L., Cruz, I., Burge, S., Bayles, B., & Castilla, M. I. (2014). Measuring capability for healthy diet and physical activity. *The Annals of Family Medicine, 12*(1), 46–56.

Frediani, A. A. (2010). Sen's capability approach as a framework to the practice of development.

Fukuda-Parr, S. (2003). The human development paradigm: Operationalizing Sen's ideas on capabilities. *Feminist Economics, 9*(2–3), 301–317.

Hanmer, L., & Klugman, J. (2016). Exploring women's agency and empowerment in developing countries. *Feminist Economics, 22*(1), 237–263.

Hart, C. S. (2016). How do aspirations matter? *Journal of Human Development and Capabilities, 17*(3), 324–341.

Heckman, J. J. (2006). Skill formation and the economics of investing in disadvantaged children. *Science, 312*(5782), 1900–1902.

Hobson, B. (2011). The agency gap in work-life balance. *Social Politics, 18*(2), 147–167.

Ibrahim, S. S. (2006). From individual to collective capabilities. *Journal of Human Development, 7*(3), 397–416.

Kabeer, N. (2018). *Gender livelihood, capabilities and women's economic empowerment*. London: GAGE program office, ODI.

Kahneman, D., Krueger, A. B., Schkade, D. A., Schwarz, N., & Stone, A. A. (2004). A survey method for characterizing daily life experience: The day reconstruction method. *Science, 306*(5702), 1776–1780.

Kanbur, R. (n.d.) Capability, opportunity, outcome and equality. Working Paper 2016–05. Ithaca: Charles H. Dyson School of Applied Economics and Management Cornell University.

Kleine, D. (2010). ICT4WHAT? – using the choice framework to operationalise the capability approach to development. *Journal of International Development, 22*, 647–692.

Krishnakumar, J. (2007). Going beyond functionings to capabilities: An econometric model to explain and estimate capabilities. *Journal of Human Development, 8*(1), 39–63.

Mitra, S. (2006). The capability approach and disability. *Journal of disability policy studies, 16*(4), 236–247.

Murphy, P., & Wolfenden, F. (2013). Developing a pedagogy of mutuality in a capability approach: Teachers' experiences of using the open educational resources (OER) of the teacher education in sub-Saharan Africa (TESSA) programme. *International Journal of Educational Development, 33*(3), 263–271.

Nussbaum, M. C. (2001). *Women and human development: The capabilities approach* (Vol. 3). Cambridge, UK: Cambridge University Press.

Oosterlaken, I. (2009). Design for development. *Design Issues, 25*(4), 91–102.

Pereira, J. (1993). What does equity in health mean? *Journal of Social Policy, 22*(1), 19–48.

Qizilbash, M. (1996). Capabilities, well-being and human development: A survey. *The Journal of Development Studies, 33*(2), 143–162.

Revallion, M. (2011). Mashup indices of development. *The World Bank Research Observer, 27*, 1–32.

Richardson, H. (2007). The social background of capabilities for freedoms. *Journal of Human Development and Capabilities, 8*(3), 389–414.

Robeyns, I. (2006). The capability approach in practice. *Journal of Political Philosophy, 14*(3), 351–376.

Ruger, J. P. (2006). Toward a theory of a right to health: Capability and incompletely theorized agreements. *Yale J Law Humanit, 18*(2), 3.

Saito, M. (2003). Amartya Sen's capability approach to education: A critical exploration. *Journal of Philosophy of Education, 37*(1), 17–33.

Sehnbruch, K. (2004). *From the quantity to the quality of employment*. Berkeley: Center for Latin American Studies, U of California. Paper No 9.

Seligman, M. E. (2012). *Flourish: A visionary new understanding of happiness and well-being*. New York: Simon and Schuster.

Sen, A. K. (1985). Commodities and capabilities. Currently available *OUP Catalogue*.

Simon, J., Anand, P., Gray, A., Rugkåsa, J., Yeeles, K., & Burns, T. (2013). Operationalising the capability approach for outcome measurement in mental health research. *Social Science & Medicine, 98*, 187–196.

Stewart, F. (2005). Groups and capabilities. *Journal of Human Development, 6*(2), 185–204.

Stiglitz, J. Sen, A. & Fitoussi, J.P. (2009). *The measurement of economic performance and social progress revisited: Reflections and overview*. France. HAL.ffhal-01069384f. https://hal-scienc-espo.archives-ouvertes.fr/file/index/docid/1069384/filename/wp2009-33.pdf.

Sugden, R. (1993). Welfare resources and capabilities. *Journal of Economic Literature, 31*(4), 1947–1962.

Swist, T., & Collin, P. (2017). Platforms, data and children's rights. *New Media and Society, 19*(5), 671–685.

Tao, S. (2013). Why are teachers absent? Utilising the capability approach and critical realism to explain teacher performance in Tanzania. *International Journal of Educational Development, 33*(1), 2–14.

Terzi, L. (2005). Beyond the dilemma of difference: The capability approach to disability and special educational needs. *Journal of Philosophy of Education, 39*(3), 443–459.

Tiwari, M. (2017). Exploring the role of the capability approach in social innovation. *Journal of Human Development and Capabilities, 20*, 1–16.

Tonon, G. (2012). Quality of life in Argentina. In K. Land, A. Michalos, & M. Sirgy (Eds.), *Handbook of social indicators and quality of life research*. Dordrecht: Springer.

Tonon, G. (2017). Communities and capabilities. *Journal of Human Development and Capabilities, 19*(2), 121–125.

Trani, J.-F., & Bakhshi, P. (2008). Challenges for assessing disability prevalence: The case of Afghanistan. *Alter, 2*(1), 44–64.

Trani, J. F., Bakhshi, P., Bellanca, N., Biggeri, M., & Marchetta, F. (2011). Disabilities through the capability approach lens: Implications for public policies. *Alter, 5*(3), 143–157.

Unterhalter, E., Heslop, J., & Mamedu, A. (2013). Girls claiming education rights. *International Journal of Education Development, 33*, 566–575.

Unterhalter, E. (2016). Negative capability? Measuring the unmeasurable in education. *Comparative Education, 53*(1), 1–16.

Van Hees, M. (2004). Freedom of choice and diversity of options: Some difficulties. *Social Choice and Welfare, 22*(1), 253–266.

Venkatapuram, S. (2013). *Health justice: An argument from the capabilities approach*. Malden: Wiley.

Walker, M. (2003). Framing social justice in education: What does the 'capabilities' approach offer? *British Journal of Educational Studies, 51*(2), 168–187.

Wolff, J. (2009). Cognitive disability in a society of equals. *Metaphilosophy, 40*(3–4), 402–415.

Zaidi, A., Gasior, K., Zolyomi, E., Schmidt, A., Rodrigues, R., & Marin, B. (2017). Measuring active and healthy ageing in Europe. *Journal of European Social Policy, 27*(2), 138–157.

Paul Anand   is Professor of Economics at The Open University and a Research Associate at the Centre for Philosophy of Natural and Social Science at the London School of Economics at the Department for Social Policy and Intervention Oxford University, UK. He has published widely on the operationalization of the capability approach and been principal investigator on grants from the Arts and Humanities Research Board and the Leverhulme Trust on the topic. He holds a DPhil from the University of Oxford, is author of *Happiness Explained* (OUP) and lives in Oxford.

Chapter 6
Teaching Quality of Life in Political Science

Takashi Inoguchi

People's Satisfaction with Daily Life (Inoguchi et al. 2014)

Aside from political leaders' popularity rates and the stock exchange index of business firms, ordinary people are highly interested in aspects of daily life, such as housing, income, health, family, food, human relations and work. Cross-national opinion polls on daily life satisfaction were carried out in Japan, South Korea, Thailand, Hong Kong, Macao, the Philippines, India, Myanmar, Taiwan, China, Malaysia, and Pakistan in the fall of 2013 and winter 2014. The percentage difference index (PDI) is formulated as the sum of two positive responses (satisfied and somewhat satisfied) minus the sum of two negative responses (dissatisfied and somewhat dissatisfied). Percent difference indices are given according to society and daily life aspects. For our analysis to go beneath national average and to g o beyond national borders, two lines of analyses are carried out. First, the distance between the level of satisfaction of the top and bottom quartiles is given for each society and according to each of the daily life aspects. Second, the regional sum of satisfaction of the top quartiles and bottom quartiles are shown crossed by daily life aspects. Two key threads stand out from these comparisons. First, social relations (family and human relations) stand out as most satisfied aspects of life in most of 12 societies. Second, the need to go beneath national averages and beyond national borders in analyzing cross-national surveys is confirmed. The compatibility and validity of cross-national surveys with varying sampling method and survey mode are briefly discussed at the end.

T. Inoguchi (✉)
Institute of Asian Cultures, J.F. Oberlin University, Machida, Japan

University of Tokyo, Tokyo, Japan
e-mail: inoguchi@ioc.u-tokyo.ac.jp

© Springer Nature Switzerland AG 2020   99
G. H. Tonon (ed.), *Teaching Quality of Life in Different Domains*, Social
Indicators Research Series 79, https://doi.org/10.1007/978-3-030-21551-4_6

Cicero famously noted that *cedant arma togae* (that the military yield to civilizations). This cross-national survey was carried out by following this dictum. *Togae* in Latin means the daily press (togas) of Roman citizens. *Togae* are a symbol of daily life. This survey goes deeper into seven aspects of daily life, as follows: housing, incomed, health, family, food, human relations, and work, to see how satisfied or dissatisfied ordinary people are (cf. Inoguchi and Fujii 2013; Iwai et al. 2009, 2011, 2013).

In an era of deep and wide globalization, one cannot afford to be disinterested in the gaps and differences within a society. Comparing national averages of satisfaction with health, for instance, is not enough. One must go beyond averages. One of the ways to go beyond national averages is, for instance, to take the two quartiles at the top 25% quartiles and the bottom 25% quartiles for health satisfaction gives a profile "beneath" the national average. For instance, the ANT (Asian National Total) for health is the sum of BNA (Beneath National Average) of satisfaction with health in the 12 societies. One then compares ANT for health, income, family, etc. By way of factor analysis (via varimax rotation), these profiles are drawn in two dimensional forms country by country. Thus ANT profiles for daily life aspects both within a nation and across nations gives a picture of whether these gaps within a nation are large or small. Both profiles portrayed by averages and profiled by BNA are drawn in Table 6.1.

Observing across societies, it is most striking how ubiquitous and solid the importance of human relations, food, and family satisfaction are (Fig. 6.1). Human relations are secondary in terms of social relations. The family equates with primary social relations. Food demonstrates materialist survival in Asia. Seen in this way, it is most striking, how pronounced the weight of social relations is. According to the formulations of Maslow 1943, and Inglehart 1977, human survival motivates materialist satisfaction such that this comes top, followed by social relations. They may be underestimating the critical importance of social relations in Asia.

As far as satisfaction with daily life aspects is concerned, social relations are ranked higher. This point is further strengthened by the fact that the across-nation tendency shows that secondary grouped (human relations) are ranked higher than primary groups (family). It is most important to note the fact that gaps in satisfaction level region-wide between the top quartiles and the bottom quartiles are greater in (1) income, (2) housing, (3) or, and (4) health, in that order. The tide of globalization makes the world both flattened (Friedman 2006) and diversified (Stiglitz 2012). Across societies, some low-income levels in the developing world tend to go up while some low-income levels in the developed world tend to go down. Within each country, the gaps between low-level income earners and high-income level people tend to widen.

The increasing gaps of daily life aspect-satisfaction are moderated by other factors. Health, for instance, has been improving in each country and thus gaps between top and bottom quartiles moderated, as are work satisfaction gaps. It is because market adjustment takes time and labor contractual adjustment takes more time. Housing is more directly affected by market mechanisms as well as income.

Table 6.1 Difference level top quartiles and bottom quartiles in term of each satisfaction aspect

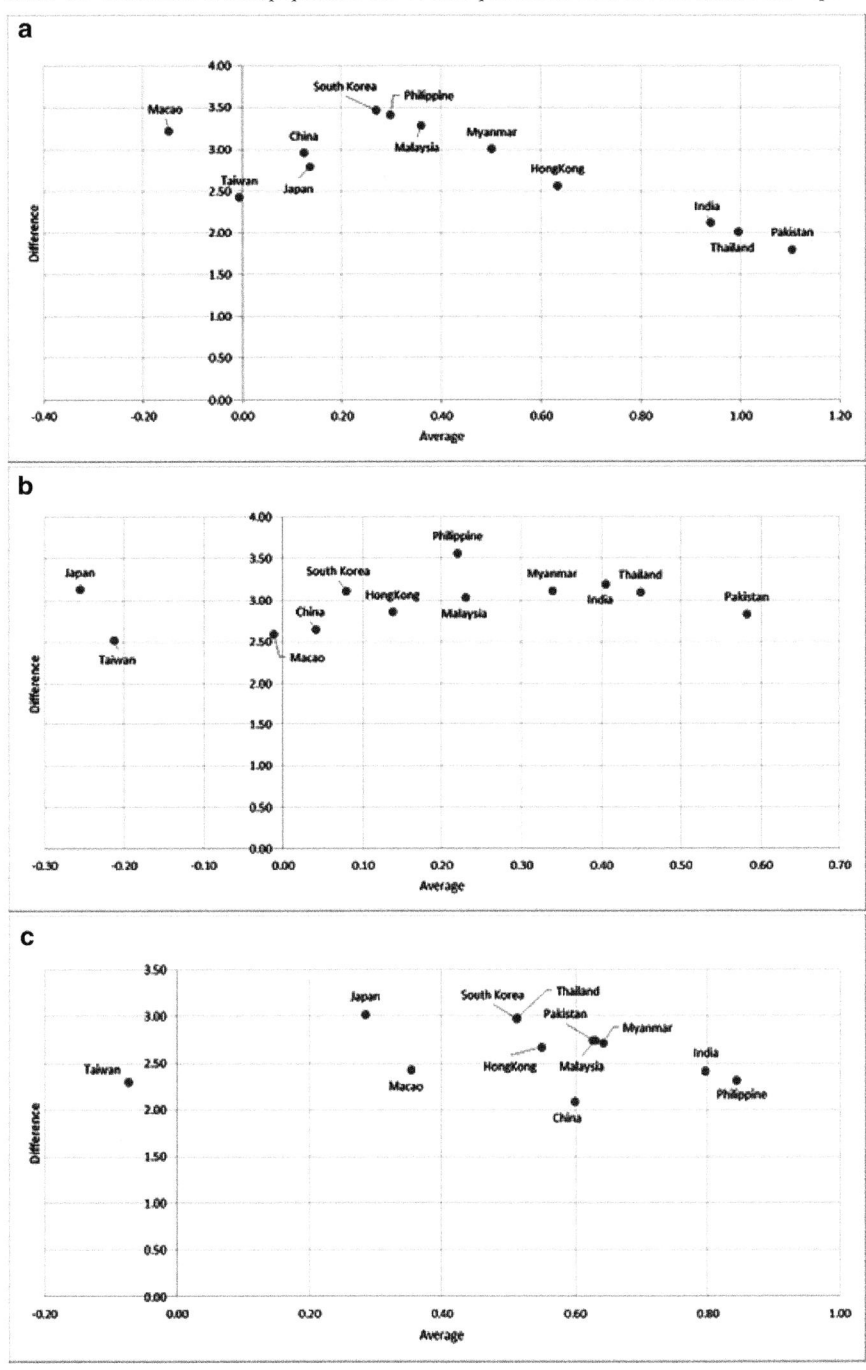

(continued)

Table 6.1 (continued)

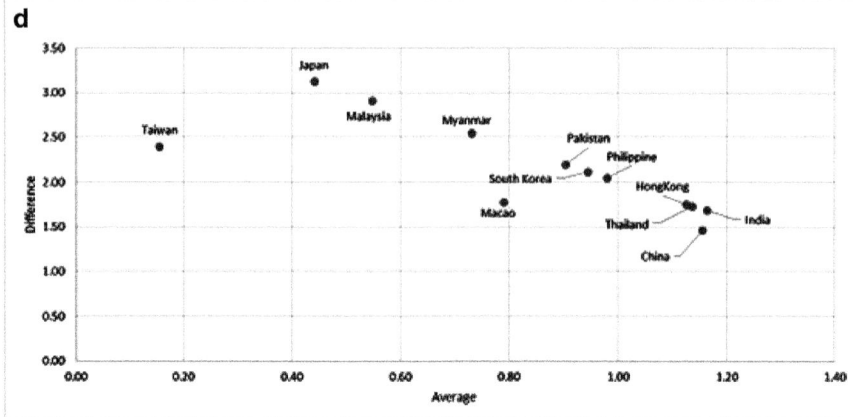

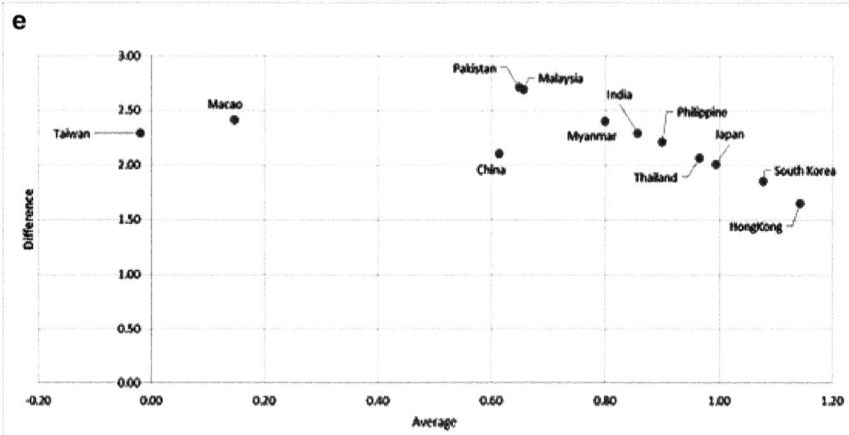

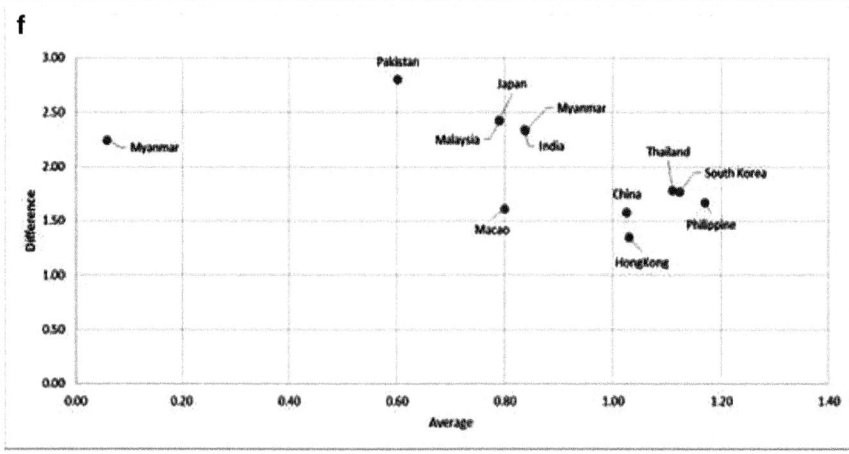

(continued)

Table 6.1 (continued)

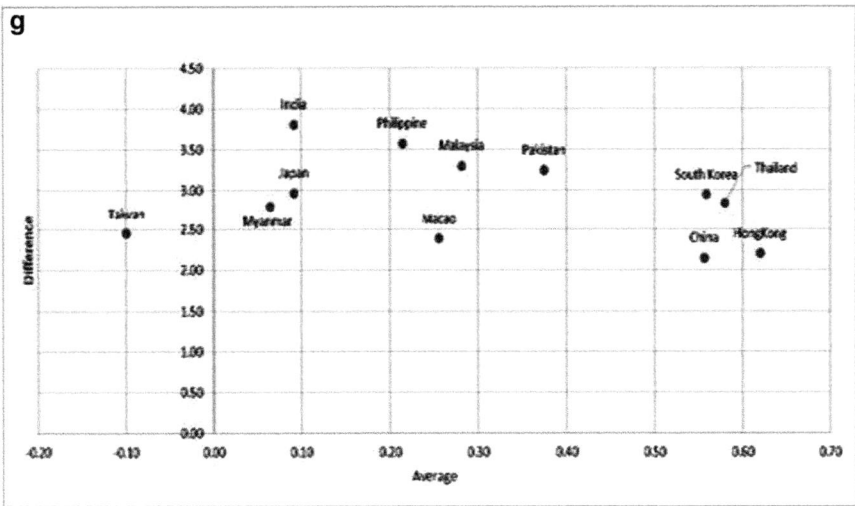

(a) Difference level top quartiles and bottom quartiles in terms of housing satisfaction (b) Difference level top quartiles and bottom quartiles in terms of income satisfaction (c) Difference level top quartiles and bottom quartiles in terms of health satisfaction (d) Difference level top quartiles and bottom quartiles in terms of family satisfaction (e) Difference level top quartiles and bottom quartiles in terms of food satisfaction (f) Difference level top quartiles and bottom quartiles in terms of human relations satisfaction (g) Difference level top quartiles and bottom quartiles in terms of work satisfaction

To sum up, two threads come out. The first striking finding is that social relations gives a very high level of satisfaction in most of the 12 societies. Important to note here is that the finding stands out irrespective of the difference in the per capita national income level in the 12 societies. The second striking finding is that the level of satisfaction with daily life aspects differs within each society and across societies. In an era of globalization, going beneath national averages and beyond national borders should be the spirit of cross-national surveys. One methodological caution is important. Given the varying sampling method and survey mode among the 12 pollings, the problem of comparability ad validity should be thoroughly discussed. This was prompted by the consideration of giving utmost freedom to each polling leader who was inescapably constrained by such factors as finance, time, and personnel. Our hunch so far is that as long as we stick to the principle of not pooling multi-society data into one basket for executing factor analysis or logit regression analysis, we should be able to come up with fairly broad comparisons.

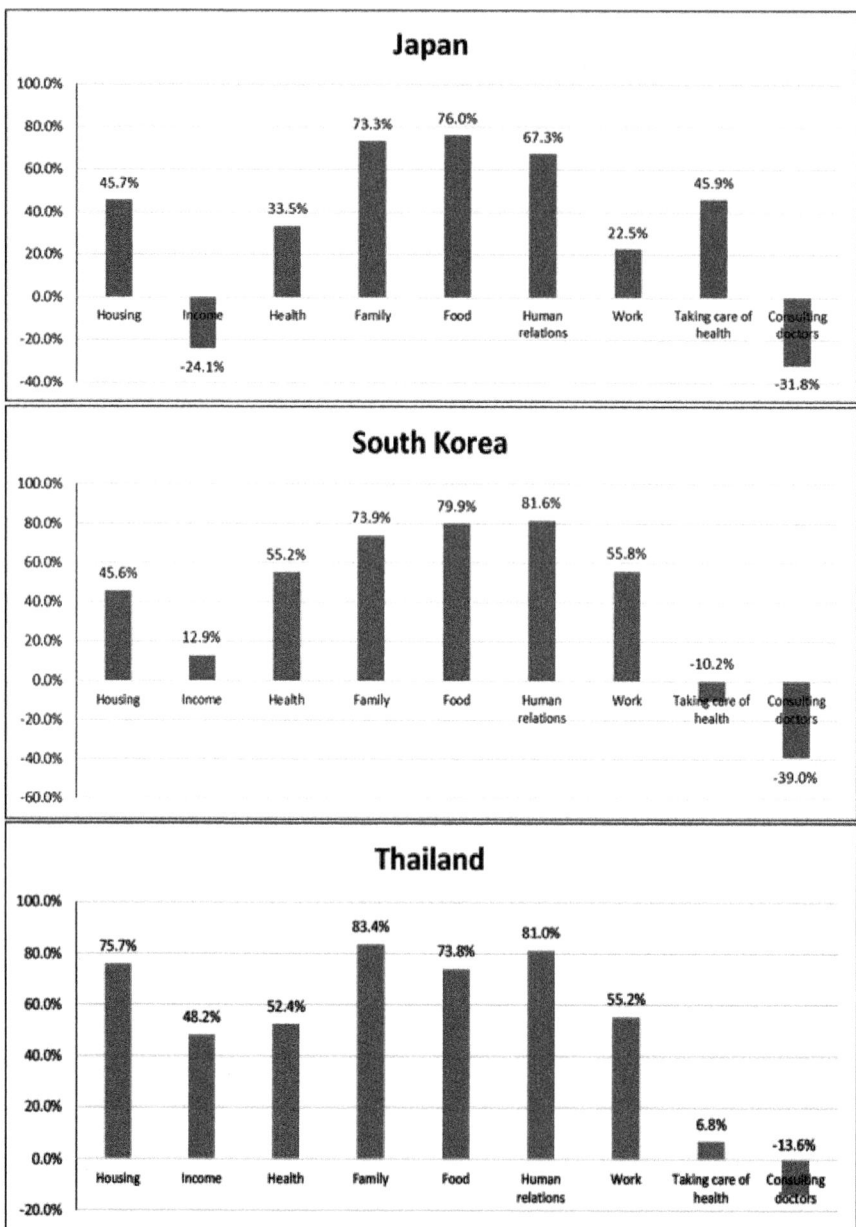

Fig. 6.1 Satisfaction with Daily Life Aspects in terms of Percent Difference Index (PDI):PDI = (satisfied + somewhat satisfied) – (dissatisfied + somewhat dissatisfied) in Each Society

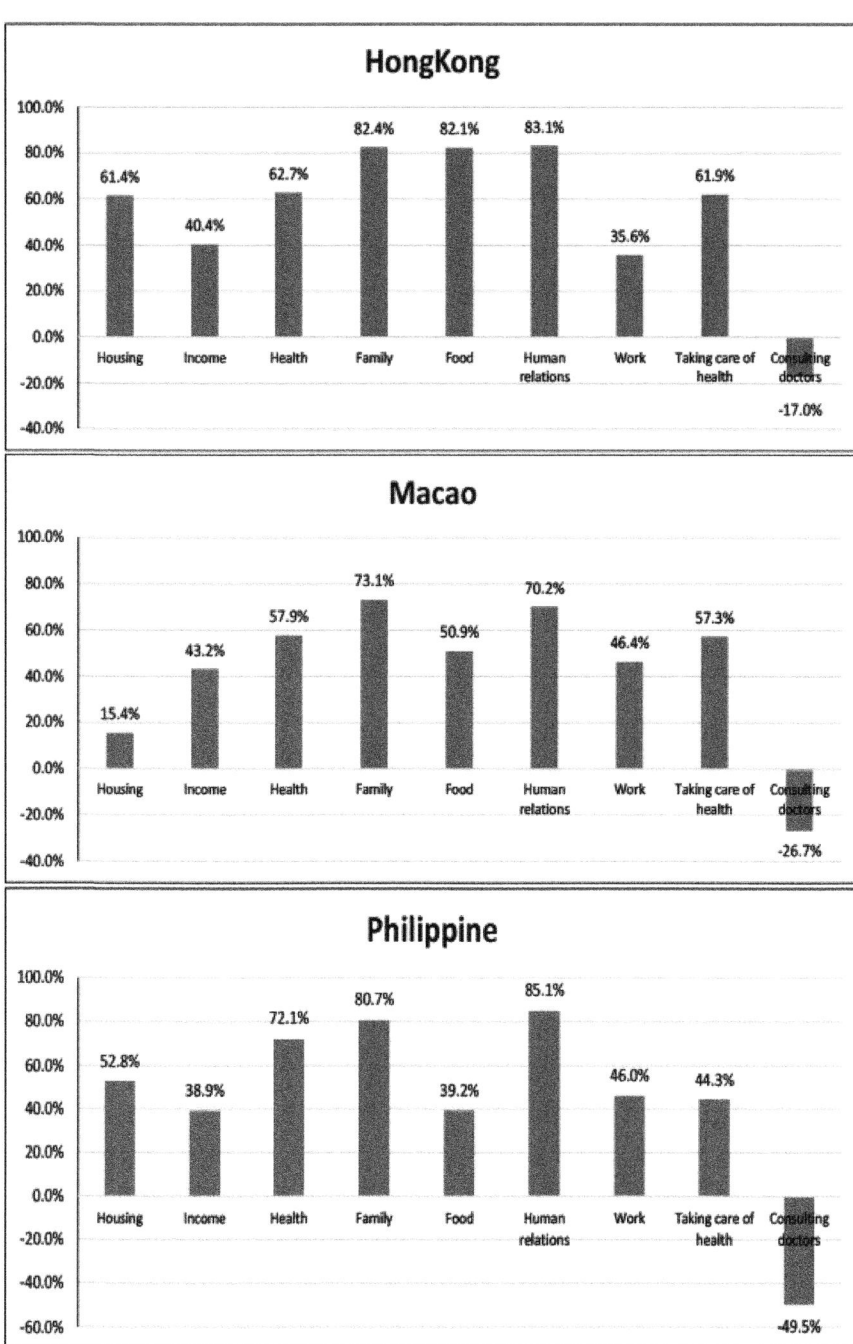

Fig. 6.1 (continued)

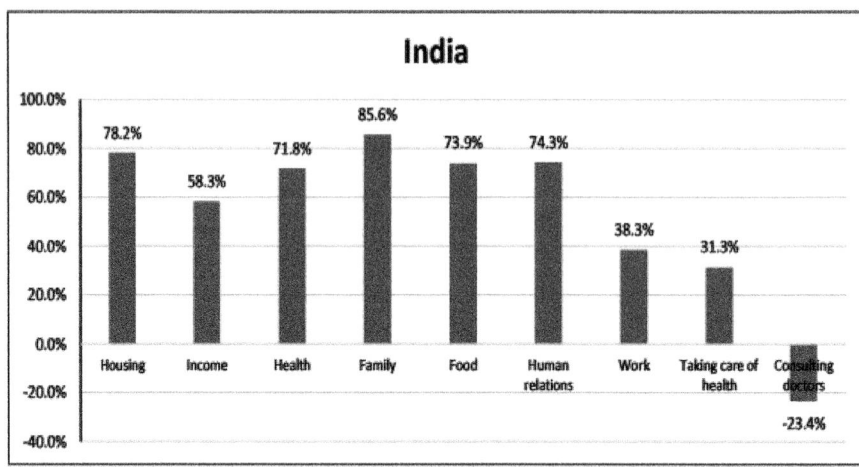

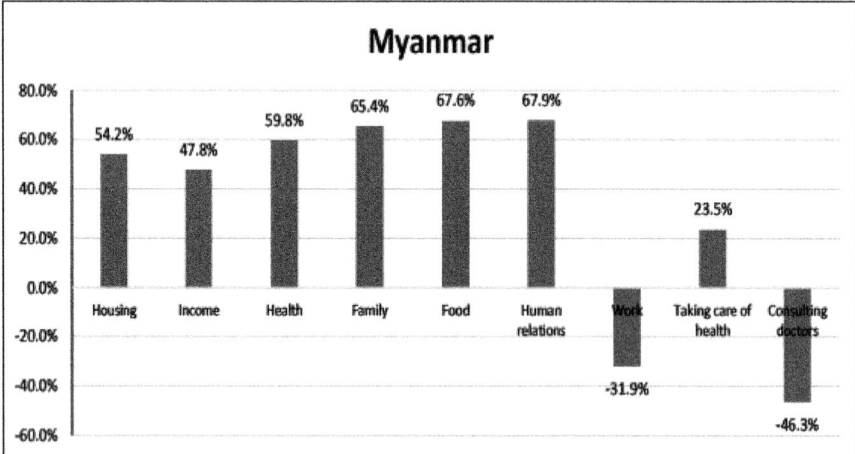

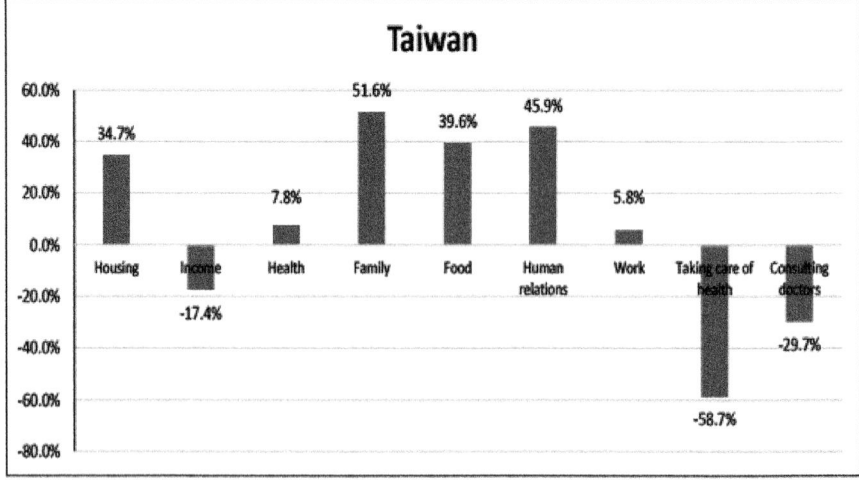

Fig. 6.1 (continued)

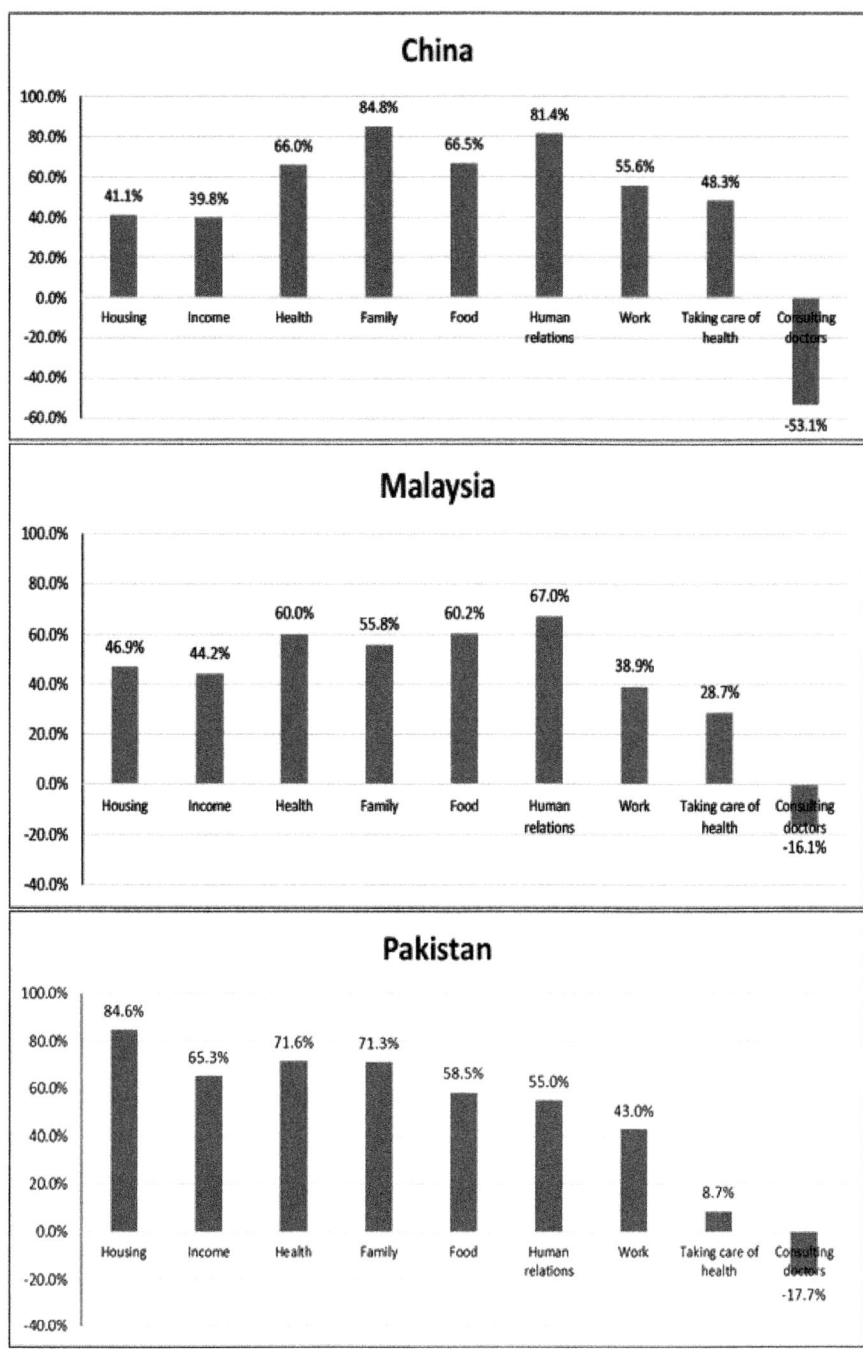

Fig. 6.1 (continued)

People's Approval of Government Conducts
in Economic Policy

Popularity rating of the government has been one of the key indicators both the government and people watch just like the stock exchange index of business and the foreign exchange rates in currency. The Japanese government established the monthly polls on this in 1955 when the Japanese economy had been registering the accelerated annual growth rates after steadily recovering from ruins and ashes of the war defeat. When watching quality of life, it is important to comprehend both the cycles of economic change and the cycle of people's mood change. In democracy and non-democracy alike both are two key indicators of quality of life.

There are soft times and hard in running the economy. Taking Japan, let us say that 1960–1976 are soft times whereas 2006–2018 are hard times. In the former the economy registered fairy steady upward movement albeit the oil crisis of 1973 hitting Japan hard. The world economy was on the whole on the moderated upswings of the US-led liberal international order. In the latter period the economy experienced hard times: the great depression took place in 2008 in the United States triggering the great depression the world over. To add salt to the wounds, the Great Japan earthquake took place in 2011, devastating northeast Japan and ruining the Pacific coasts by tsunami and causing the Fukushima No. 1 nuclear power plant meltdown. The recovery process was long.

The spirit of the government in running economic policy at soft times may be phrased as "Surfing over economic waves" (Inoguchi 1979). When the economy was on the whole on the steady upward swings, what the government does is to let the economy take care of itself while the government focused on carrying out auxiliary tasks for the positive growth rates to continue. As a contrast, the spirit of the government in running economic policy at hard times may be phrased as "Skirting tax hikes." It is natural for the government to raise taxes when the economy registers virtually zero growth annually. To make things worse, demographic contraction has been on the way and government social policy expenditure needs keep on the steady rise. In other words, the percentage of younger population has shrunk steadily whereas the percentage of older population has expanded dramatically.

"Surfing over economic waves" and "skirting tax hikes" are both my own characterization of Japanese government's economic management in the third quarter of the last century and the first quarter of this century respectively. In the conventional parlance of the discipline of political economy, the flavor of human control of economic policy is pronounced. Hence the ideological or partisan difference of economic policy target often comes to the fore. For instance, high income strata tend to favor anti-inflation policy whereas low income strata tend to favor anti-unemployment policy in the third quarter of the last century. In a similar vein, in the first quarter of this century high income strata tend to favor low corporate tax whereas low income strata tend to favor income-gap-reducing policy. The mainstream political economic literature of government economic policy making in the third quarter of the last century tends to highlight ideological and partisan origin in Western democracy.

In Japan economic policy making in the third quarter of the last century is shouldered by national bureaucracy, which abhors partisan colors and parliament-based politicians' intervention. Hence surfing over economic waves is an apt characterization. Japanese national bureaucracy preferred its neutrality from political partisan forces and the cabinet led by prime minister preferred its basic harmony with national bureaucracy. With the catch-all center-right party long keeping power except 1991–1994 when this catch-all center-right party lost power.

"Skirting tax hike" is the spirit of economic policy in the first quarter of this century (Inoguchi 2010, 2012). The tide of globalization has been accelerating since the last quarter of the last century world-wide. Not only economic interdependence but vulnerability have become a key feature of the globalized economy. Hence to Japan a series of vulnerability have manifested themselves in 1991 (Japanese bubbled economy burst out), in 1997–1998 (the Asian financial crisis assaulted Asia, especially Thailand, South Korea, and Indonesia which surrendered their power to the IMF about foreign exchange control), in 2008–2009 (Lehman Brothers-triggered Great Depression permeated the world over). The last of which hit Japan hard as well. The economy did not grow much with the deflationary trend continuing and thus registering barely below 1% annual economic growth rate. If consumption tax hike were to be carried out, the popularity rate f or prime minister is bound to go down. In 1990 prime minister Kiich Miyazawa raised consumption tax and he and his Liberal Democratic Party lost power. In 2012 Yoshihiko Noda of the Democratic Party of Japan raised consumption tax and he and his Democratic Party lost power. Shinzo Abe succeeding him continuously dodged or delayed timing of tax hike twice despite his promise. Instead he declared Abenomics whereby very loose monetary policy of printing Japanese yen notes massively was introduced and instituted. Deflationary economy continues and commodity prices do not go up much. Business firms abhor risk-taking entrepreneurial decisions on new investment for R & D and abroad. Consumers do not spend much. Annual economic growth rate keeps highly dependent on foreign exports, which in turn are increasingly vulnerable to US-triggered massive protectionism. To add salt to wounds, the need to spend massive expenditure on pension, medical care, education keeps on the alarmingly steady rise. "Skirting tax hike" has been the guiding spirit of the day while very loose monetary policy of printing Japanese yen notes massively has got Japanese citizens to approve government economic policy with citizens' satisfaction registered 74.0%, the highest for the past two decades.

People, Propensity to Nurture Certain Self of Norms and Values (QOL Runs in Harmony of Culture)

Barrington Moore (1966) argues that the solid bourgeois class leads democracy and that agriculture being commercialized in capitalism is a key to divergent paths on which major societies chose their respective regimes in the twentieth century: Britain and France to democracy, Germany and Japan to fascism, Russia and China to communism. Underlying his argument is the strong adherence to the modernity scroll. Schmuel Eisenstadt makes a strong but balanced argument on multiple modernities in which the Europo-centric notion of modernization is patently wrong by citing many historical advanced societies. Alexander Woodside gives a strong argument and rich historical examples on multiple modernities focusing on China, Vietnam and Korea in all of which the three criteria of modernity did exist since long ago and the negative consequences of modernity plagued them for long and were maintained in their predicament in their nineteenth and twentieth centuries. Such predicament may be manifested in those moral virtues preached by parents to children.

The AsiaBarometer survey 2006 question 44 asks the following question in respondents in East Asia: Vietnam, Taiwan, Singapore, R. Korea, Japan, Hong Kong, China.

Here is a list of qualities that children can be encouraged to learn at home. Please select two you consider to be most important.

1. *independence*
2. *diligence*
3. *honesty*
4. *sincerity*
5. *mindfulness*
6. *humbleness*
7. *religiosity*
8. *patience*
9. *competitiveness*
10. *respect for senior persons*
11. *deference for teachers*
12. *don't know*

Sample sizes are 2000 for China, 1000 for Hong Kong, 1003 for Japan, 1000 for R. Korea, 1038 for Singapore, 1006 for Taiwan, 1000 for Vietnam. (taken from Takashi Inoguchi, "Post-Modernity and Multiple Modernities as Discourse of Quality of Life", presented at the 10th International ISQOLS conference, Bangkok, December 9–11) (Fig. 6.2).

A glance at responses by country and by quality enables us to find three propositions: (1) Even within East Asia, the clear differentiation is registered with regard to how parents inculcate values and virtues among children in family; (2) the Continental or Confucian or Chinese civilization versus the maritime or Buddhist or Japanese civilization; (3) in the former the troika of virtues, independence, diligence and honesty, is more or less uniformly stressed in continental societies of East Asia; (4) Japan, representing the maritime East Asia, mindfulness is singularly stressed in Japan and Japan only.

The contrast between continental and maritime Asia has been propounded by anthropologists and geographers in explaining group organizations, family, society, and the state (cf. Robert D. Kaplan, Tadao Umesao, James C. Scott). This section contrast continental and maritime East Asian societies in terms of moral virtues parents wish their children to inculcate.

AsiaBarometer 2006 Q44 country:
Here is a list of qualities that children can be encouraged to learn at home. Please select two you consider to be most important.

1. Independence

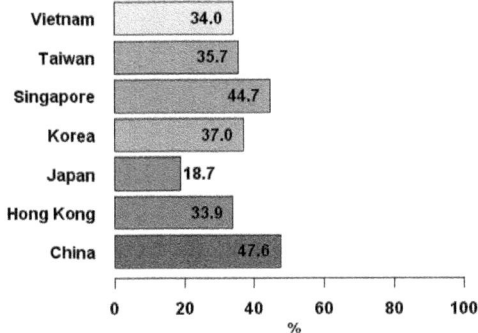

Inoguchi, Takashi et al., AsiaBarometer Survey Data 2006 [computer file], AsiaBarometer Project (www.asiabarometer.org)

2. Diligence

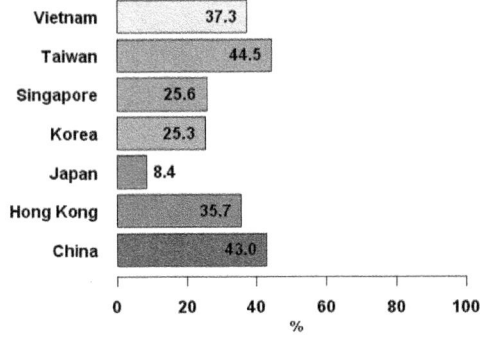

Inoguchi, Takashi et al., AsiaBarometer Survey Data 2006 [computer file], AsiaBarometer Project (www.asiabarometer.org)

3. Honesty

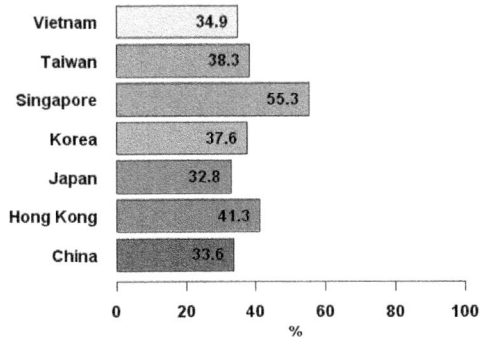

Inoguchi, Takashi et al., AsiaBarometer Survey Data 2006 [computer file], AsiaBarometer Project (www.asiabarometer.org)

Fig. 6.2   Moral virtues preached to children by parents in family

4. Sincerity

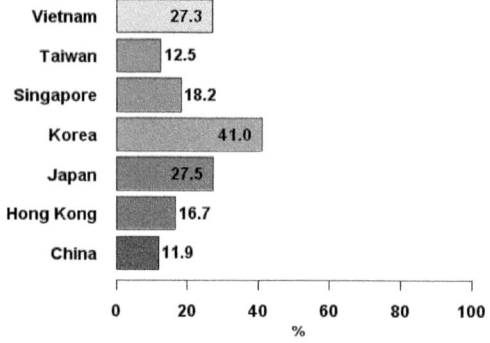

5. Mindfulness

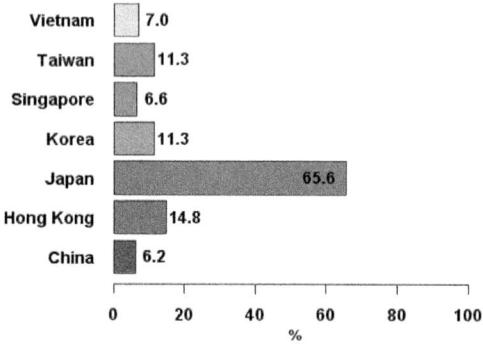

6. Humbleness

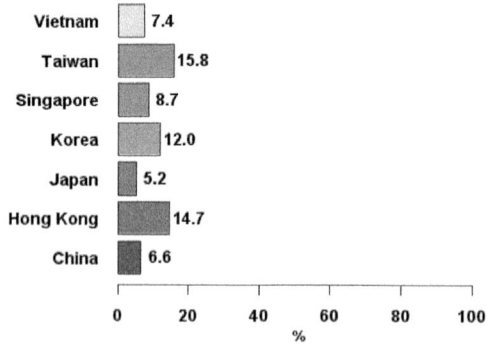

Fig. 6.2 (continued)

7. Religiosity

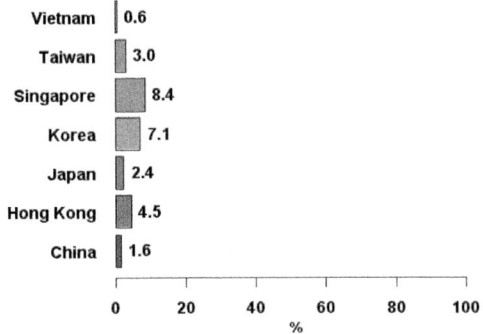

Inoguchi, Takashi et al., AsiaBarometer Survey Data 2006 [computer file], AsiaBarometer Project (www.asiabarometer.org)

8. Patience

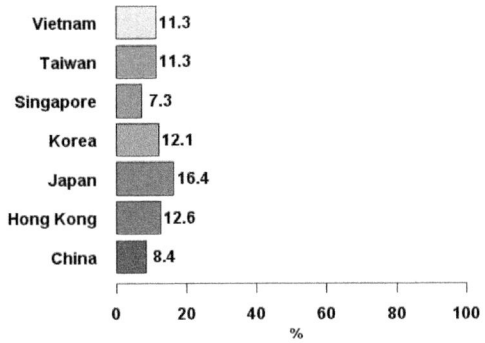

Inoguchi, Takashi et al., AsiaBarometer Survey Data 2006 [computer file], AsiaBarometer Project (www.asiabarometer.org)

9. Competitiveness

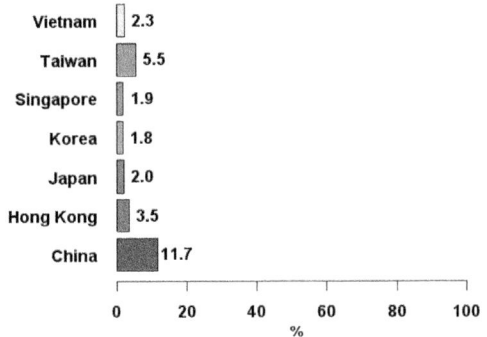

Inoguchi, Takashi et al., AsiaBarometer Survey Data 2006 [computer file], AsiaBarometer Project (www.asiabarometer.org)

Fig. 6.2 (continued)

10. Respect for senior persons

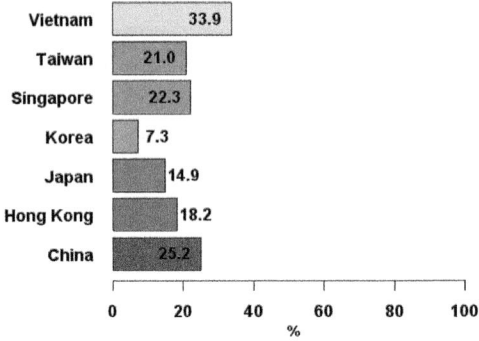

Inoguchi, Takashi et al., AsiaBarometer Survey Data 2006 [computer file], AsiaBarometer Project (www.asiabarometer.org)

11. Deference for teachers

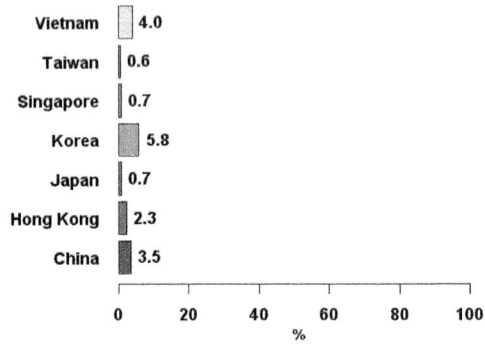

Inoguchi, Takashi et al., AsiaBarometer Survey Data 2006 [computer file], AsiaBarometer Project (www.asiabarometer.org)

12. Don't know

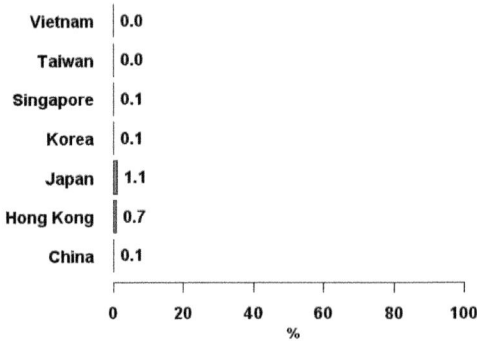

Inoguchi, Takashi et al., AsiaBarometer Survey Data 2006 [computer file], AsiaBarometer Project (www.asiabarometer.org)

Fig. 6.2 (continued)

AsiaBarometer 2006 Q44 country:
Here is a list of qualities that children can be encouraged to learn at home. Please select two you consider to be most important.

China

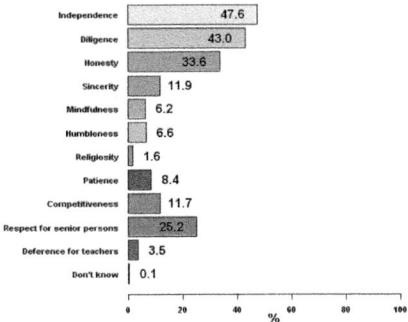

Inoguchi, Takashi et al., AsiaBarometer Survey Data 2006 [computer file], AsiaBarometer Project (www.asiabarometer.org)

Hong Kong

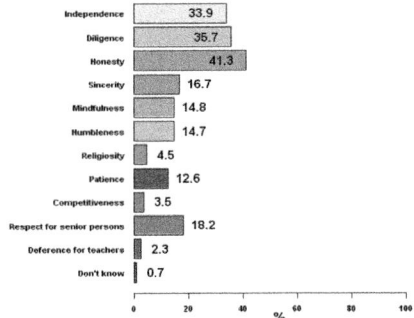

Inoguchi, Takashi et al., AsiaBarometer Survey Data 2006 [computer file], AsiaBarometer Project (www.asiabarometer.org)

Japan

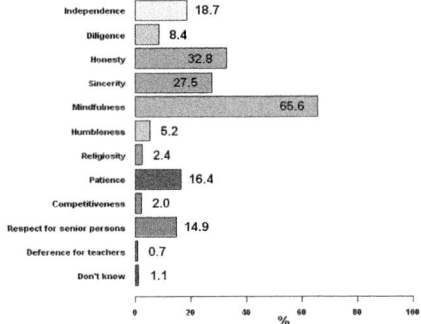

Inoguchi, Takashi et al., AsiaBarometer Survey Data 2006 [computer file], AsiaBarometer Project (www.asiabarometer.org)

Fig. 6.2 (continued)

Korea

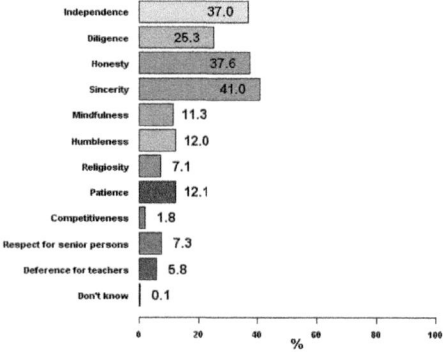

Singapore

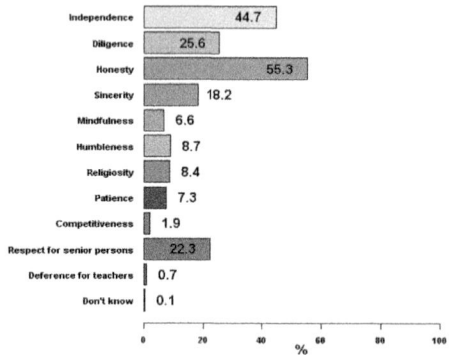

Taiwan

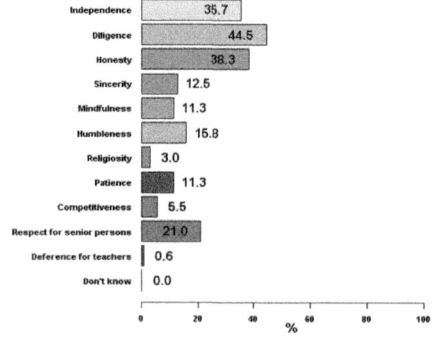

Fig. 6.2 (continued)

Vietnam

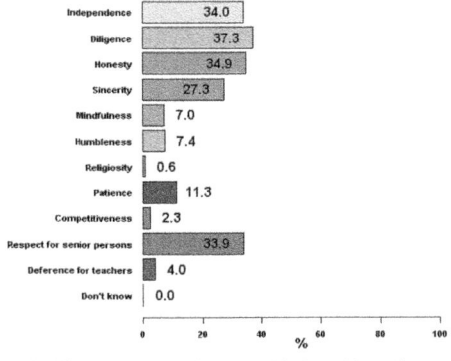

Fig. 6.2 (continued)

QOL and Confidence in Institutions

(taken from Takashi Inoguchi and Yasuharu Tokuda, eds., *Trust with Asian Characteristics*, Springer, 2017, pp. 169–175)

Confidence in institutions constitutes an important part of quality of life. For instance, if confidence in mass media is exceedingly low, one is placed at a loss to get reliable news on what happens in the world in relation to daily life. If confidence in police is very low, one needs to take care of oneself when a theft takes away one's huge amount of savings kept at home. If confidence in civil service extremely low, one needs to take care of oneself when the amount of one's pension seems to be miscalculated.

The Asia-Europe Survey (2000) directed by Takashi Inoguchi with Grant from the Ministry of Education (project number 11102000) carried out 16 country surveys on confidence in institutions, eight in Asia and eight in Europe (Inoguchi and Tokuda 2017. Cf. Blondel and Inoguchi 2006; Inoguchi and Blondel 2008; Inoguchi and Marsh 2008). The Asia-Europe Survey, focusing on democracy, was carried out in Japan, South Korea, Taiwan, Singapore, Malaysia, Indonesia, Thailand, and the Philippines in Asia whereas in Europe the United Kingdom, Ireland, France, Germany, Sweden, Italy, Spain, Portugal, and Greece. The list of institutions asked responses about confidence is as follows:

1. parliament
2. political parties
3. (elected) government
4. law and the courts
5. leaders

6. police
7. civil service
8. military
9. big business
10. mass media

Two tables are shown here with regard to Asian confidence in institutions and European confidence in institutions. Two important observations are made first (Tables 6.2 and 6.3).

1. People have higher confidence in such professional institutions that are not necessarily governed by democratic principle. They are the military, the police, the civil service, and the courts.
2. People have lower confidence in such democratic institutions as political parties, parliament, elected government, and political leaders.

Important to note in relation to the above two observations is that these two observations are made irrespective of being fully democratic or not. The principle of selection in such professional institutions like the military, the police, the civil service and the courts is some combination of meritocratic, technocratic and bureaucratic, but not necessarily democratic rules. The picture is not very different between Asian and European societies. The major difference between Asian and European patterns is that in Asian democracies the highest confidence people have tends to be with the military and the civil service whereas in European democracies people tend to have confidence in the military and the police.

How to explain the difference of confidence in institutions with regard to non-professionally recruited institutions such as parliament, political parties, (elected) government, leaders? For instance, confidence in political parties in Europe is often regarded as being very low. If you take a look at Whiteley (2011), you may be convinced of this low confidence in political parties. (Paul Whitely published the article, "Is the Party Over? The Decline of Party Activism and Membership across the Democratic World," *Party Politics*, 17(1), pp. 21–44) I would add two more reasons to Whiteley (2011): the introduction of one unified currency by the Maastricht Treaty (2000) to the European Union's selective members and the consequent consolidation of many institutional mechanisms of the European Union short of many aspects of national economic policy which national political parties used to make use of to navigate national economic futures and people's lives. In other words, national economic life is more strongly in charge of the European Union (the European Commission, the European Council and their offshoots).

In Asia, Northeastern Asian democracies, Japan, South Korea, and Taiwan, are "disaffected democracies" (Putnam and Farr 2000) with confidence in political institutions tend to be very low. Singapore and Malaysia are authoritarian states where confidence in political institutions was relatively high. Thailand, the Philippines and Indonesia were intermittently stumbling Third-wave democracies (with the first wave being southern Europe in the 1970s and the second wave being East Asia in the 1980s).

Table 6.2 Asian confidence in institutions

%	Japan	South Korea	Taiwan	Singapore	Malaysia	Indonesia	Thailand	Philippines
80–90				Police courts govt civil service military leaders			Military	
70–80				Parliament business parties media		Civil service		Media
60–70					Gov't courts military leaders civil service	Military media gov't parliament	Business civil service media	
50–60	Military courts police civil service	Military	Civil service		Police parliament media business parties	Police	Courts	Military civil service gov't courts
40–50		Media	Military leaders gov't business			Leaders unties	Police	Parliament police
30–40		Police courts civil service	Police media courts			Courts business	Leaders parliament	Leaders business parties
20–30	Business media parliament	Gov't	Parties				Gov't parties	
10–20	Gov't parties leaders	Business	Parliament					
0–10		Leaders parties parliament						

Source: Nippon Research Center. *The Asia-Europe Survey*. Tokyo: Nippon Research Center for the project on democracy and political cultures in Asia and Europe, led by Takashi Inoguchi, funded by a grant from the Ministry of Education. Culture. Sports. Science and Technology, for the period between 1999–2003 (Project number 11102000)

Table 6.3 European confidence in institutions

%	UK	Ireland	France	Germany	Sweden	Italy	Spain	Portugal	Greece
80–90									
70–80	Military		Business civil service					Military	Military
60–70	Police	Police military	Police military	Police		Police business		Media civil service business police	
50–60		Civil service courts	Media		Police courts	Military	Police parliament		
40–50	Courts business civil service	Media	Courts parliament gov't	Courts military	Business	Media	Military courts gov't media civil service	Parliament gov't courts	Police courts
50–40	Parliament	Business gov't parliament		Parliament business leaders	Military parliament civil service		Parties leaden business	Leaders	Gov't business
20–30	Media gov't	Leaders parties	Leaders	Gov't civil service media	Media gov't leaders	Civil service courts gov't parliament	Parties	Media parliament civil service	
10–20	Leader parties		Parties	Parties	Parties	Leader parties			Leader parties
0–10									

Source: Nippon Research Center. *The Asia–Europe Survey.* Tokyo: Nippon Research Center for the project on democracy and political cultures in Asia and Europe, led by Takashi Inoguchi funded by a grant from the Ministry of education. Culture, Sports, Science and Technology, for the period between 1999–2003 (Project number 11102000)

Looked at this way, confidence in institutions is a concept not easy to handle. One needs to use it with history, geography, culture and contexts carefully examined.

QOL-Based Typology of Asian Societies

(taken from Takashi Inoguchi, Hong Kong ISQOLS annual meeting, PPT Materials)

Life satisfaction is based on the text to which societies construct themselves. To gauge quality of life, life satisfaction is one of its good indicators because life consists of fairly mundane and concrete things like a workplace life domain, an aspect of nuclear family life, and an urban middle class life style. Life satisfaction can be contrasted to happiness. If one asks how happy are you, responses differ tremendously. Leo Tolstoy says that all happy families resemble one another; every unhappy family is unhappy in its own way. He is wrong! Every happy family too is happy in its own way. Gauging happiness indicators must surpass difficulties of inevitable variations of responses because happiness is a difficult word to use and more importantly to respond to.

Thus I would like to propose the 16 item list of life satisfaction to gauge the aggregate indicators of a society:

1. housing
2. standard of living
3. household income
4. health
5. education
6. job
7. friendships
8. marriage
9. neighbors
10. family life
11. leisure
12. spiritual life
13. public safety
14. conditions of the environment
15. social welfare system
16. democratic system

With the question "how satisfied are you about each of the sixteen items of life domains, life aspects or life styles?", I attempt to sort out the types of Asian societies. It may be called a QOL-based typology of Asian societies.

One of the complaints often heard of typologies propounded about Asian societies is that depending on the academic discipline the question is fairly predetermined and the answer is fairly predetermined. Why? If an anthropologist proposes a typology of Asian societies, the question is often related to a nuclear family or an extended family, a matrimonial family or a patrimonial family. If it is categorized a nuclear family dominant, then the answer can be that a society heavy with a nuclear family tends to produce political instability because ideas and emotions are not very likely to be inherited through families and generations. If a geologist and a geographer proposes a typology of Asian societies, the question is often related to a temperate society, a dry weather society and a humid weather society or a vertically pronounced society with many mountains and a horizontally pronounced society with endless plains after plains. The answer can be that the combination of dry weather and high plateaus and mountains produces a fragmented society and an autocratic political regime. If a philosopher proposes a typology of Asian societies, the question is often related to the extent of freedom enjoyed by people at the grass roots level. The answer can be that the freedom enjoyed by one person, by a small number of elites or by a large member of a society determine the types of a society, i.e., autocracy, oligarchy or democracy.

These and many others are a dominant way of typologizing Asian societies. I am not entirely happy about it although by sharpening conceptualization and deepening analysis it has widened and enriched our knowledge of Asian societies. Because it is driven disciplinary biases and foci and because it is not necessarily evidence based in the narrow sense of solidly empirical and systematic. No less important is that many typologies adopt the top down approach, not the bottom up approach. I like the bottom up approach here because a society consists of how satisfied they are with which life domains, aspects and styles.

The AsiaBarometer survey carried out in 2003–2008 covers 32 societies in Asia (29) and its vicinities (the US, Russia and Australia) with the national random sampling method and face-to-face interviewing mode (Inoguchi and Fujii 2013; Inoguchi and Tokuda 2017). It contains the question which asked the 16 items of life satisfaction. All the responses to the question on life satisfaction were factor-analyzed by each of the 28 Asian societies. Therefore 28 factor analysis results were produced. One of them, Turkmenistan, was not examined by factor analysis for reasons of data irregularities.

The method used is factor analysis with varimax rotation. Three key dimensions are:

1. materialism or survival (denoting A or a, with capitalized A meaning first dimension).
2. post-materialism or social life (denoting B or b, with capitalized B first dimension).
3. public sector dominance or power (denoting C or c, with capitalized C meaning first dimension).

The order of associated eigen values or weight of explanatory power varies from society to society. This variety of order means the types of societies. For Asia, the combination of three dimensions yield six types. One of which places the society of post-materialism first, followed by public sector dominance, and lastly materialism, in other words, such a prioritizing society does not exist in any of the 28 Asian societies.

Six types are:

1. Abc: Japan, Afghanistan, Indonesia, Tajikistan, Uzbekistan, and Taiwan
2. Acb: Bangladesh, Cambodia, China, Laos, Mongol, Myanmar, India, Nepal, and South Korea
3. Bac: Hong Kong, Vietnam, Thailand, Kyrgyzstan, and Malaysia
4. Bca: not found among the 28 Asian societies
5. Cab: Pakistan, Brunei, Bhutan, the Philippines, Kazakhstan, and the Maldives
6. Cba: Singapore and Sri Lanka

How should I label each type of Asian societies? Abc is a "normal type" in Ronald Inglehart's research (1997), materialism versus post-materialism. In other words, human beings strive for survival. After attaining enough for survival, they can then afford social life, whether this means a further accumulation of wealth or political influence or pursuit of other goals like honor. What lacks in Inglehart's paradigm is limited attention to the public sector. In human societies, this is natural. The difference is large or small or effective or ineffective. Abc type societies consist of those societies where power is essentially decentralized. In other words, in Asian cases, democratic societies, which are designed to curtail power dominance and authoritarian societies which are less than effective for reasons of multiethnic fragmentation, foreign military influence, people-alienating dictatorial exercise of power, and poor communications and transportation infrastructure.

Acb reflects the strong influence of the public sector as perceived by people at the grassroot level of life when compared to Abc societies. Former British colonial influence on bureaucratic and military institutions are strong in India, Bangladesh, Myanmar and Nepal (albeit Nepal keeping independence). Communist party-run societies like China and Laos, ex-communist societies like Cambodia and Mongolia, and former Japanese colonial and present Confucian bureaucratic influence like South Korea are included.

Bac includes those societies where ethnic diversities like in Kyrgyzstan, Thailand and Malaysia and hegemonic coalitions like Vietnam (northern Vietnam over southern) and Hong Kong (two systems in one country scheme) enable people to invigorate social life, including connections, position seeking, and wealth accumulation.

Bca societies prioritize in descending order social life, power and survival.

Bca is not found among 28 Asian societies.

Cab is a society where the public sector is dominant whether it is the military and police, the trenched hereditary political elites, or the rentier elite class of foreign investment in natural resources.

Cba is a society where the public sector is dominant whether it is because of government actively pursuing and implementing policies on housing, pension, and medical insurance and/or the military and police are dominant.

I know that the labeling of each type of Asian societies would help readers to comprehend the virtue of the QOL-based typology of societies, especially in Asian societies. This exercise is not attempted here. It is sufficient for me to be able to show that the wholesome nature of society can be reflected in such indicators of the QOL-based typology of Asian societies without damaging the basis of individual satisfaction and dissatisfaction of daily life in society at the grassroot level.

Applying Quality of Life Studies in Sustainable Developmental Goals (Health, Education and Income in East Asia)

One of my purposes of proposing a QOL-based typology of Asian societies is this: a concept and an associated indicator must be of use in practice. In this case, as one of the proponents of multiple modernities, I am of the view that a QOL-based typology of Asian societies does not lead readers and practitioners to rank societies according to one criterion. Rather the multidimensional understanding of societies is what we need. I have made it clear that societies contain three key dimensions, survival, social life, and public sector dominance. Typology of societies makes it precise about the weight of such key dimensions, society by society. By knowing such differentiated weights of key dimensions one can go forward to think about public policy to achieve certain goals, say, sustainable developmental goals. In other words, a QOL-based typology of Asian societies helps to contextualize a certain public policy goal and approach in a certain society. Here I take us three of such goals: health, education, and income.

Health

One of the pronounced diseases that plague a large number of people in East Asia which has achieved very dynamic economic development is cancer. Economic development brings about household income. The increase in household income has changed their food intake pattern from rice-and vegetables-focused to flower, milk and animal meat-focused. This change has been very pronounced in East Asia. One of the earliest manifestations of the suspected relationship between animal-protein-focused food intake and the increase of cancer is Okinawa people. Okinawa was occupied and administered by the United States after 1945 till 1972. War-devastated Okinawa received the large amount of food assistance from the United States g overnment. Although calorie intake has increased dramatically, the death of cancer has also increased in number. Mainlander Japanese followed the path of Okinawa in this respect. The death causes of cancer has become No 1 ahead of heart disease, brain disease, neumonia. Although Japanese longevity is one of the longest in the world, those afflicted by cancer do not necessarily enjoy healthy longevity.

China has experienced 30 year-long double digit economic development per annum since the 1990's. Even shortly after the 1949 revolution, animal-protein intake increased steadily. Thus prime minister Zhou Enlai, himself afflicted by cancer ordered to carry out a large scale of food study in China involving 0.9 billion Chinese subjects in 1973–1974. Prof Colin Campbell of Cornell University further carried out a solid and through study on Chinese food, habit, and death (Campbell and Campbell II 2016). In spring 2018 I had an occasion on which eight Japanese and one Chinese dined together in a restaurant. The eight Japanese ordered beef steak while one Chinese ordered Atlantic salmon. This episode might as well inform of the fairly wide spread awareness of the Chinese of the creeping cancer disease.

Then what can QOL studies do within the SDGs movement? My answer is: to carry out Colin's China study on food, habit and death across East Asia. After examining the societal type (Abs, Acb, Bac, Bca, Cab, or Cba), thus exploring which kind of public policy can be effective, health enhancing policy package should be drawn.

Education

The number of universities and colleges in Japan is 800. Before 1945 it used to be ten or so imperial universities, some two dozen or so vocational higher schools and 40 odd normal higher schools. The United States ordered the Japanese government to have at least one national university in each of the 49 prefectures and normal and vocational higher schools were trans formed to colleges and universities. During the high economic development period of the 1950s through 1980s colleges and universities mushroomed with 80% being private universities. The expansion of manufacturing and service sector personnel needs matched the expansion of universities.

Prof Henry Rosovsky, Dean of Harvard College, once contrasted education in Japan and the United States. Japanese education is best in primary education whereas U.S. education is the best in graduate school. Modernization in Japan was driven by the compulsory education for 6 years old pupils through 15 years old with solid literacy, arithmetic, and social knowledge, which were indispensable to all out modernization. Higher education was also stressed to man national bureaucracy. For that purpose, ten or so imperial universities were set up. Imperial universities produced bureaucrats in law, finance, civil engineering, construction, transportation, electric communication, agriculture, pharmaceutics etc. Imperial universities produced academics to reproduce bureaucratic rats and academics. Hence literature, history, philosophy, foreign languages were also emphasized. Most important however, is that the size of professors was extremely small and that the size of student body at imperial universities was far more extremely small. In the United States, primary education is weak. Good education is privately financed in elite privileged schools. With lower literacy rate prevailing, primary education cannot be very effective. Higher education is not the goal of attaining the status and requirement to become bureaucrats or doctors but the starting point for those ambitious students to explore power and prosperity in the next stages of life. At Harvard Nobel laureates can converse on the same elevator of one of the buildings. In Japan, Nobel laureates are accumulated number two since 1945 after the United States. At the University of Tokyo, many graduates-laureates have got those works done while they were in the United States.

Then what can the QOL-based typology of societies do in relation to level up education in Japan and East Asia? My answer is: Given the global demand for receive higher education in non-Western world of higher income and academic level, why not grade up graduate education in English solely because English is the language universally used in non-Western students. Then we have to examine which type of society fits Japan and East Asia well and explore the kind of public policy package is created in sync of society type.

Income

East Asia is one of the regions in the world, which has experienced solid economic development besides North America and Western Europe in the last century and early this century. In other words, income level is high on average in the non-Western world. The task confronting East Asia is how to solidify income level on the basis of domestic market demand and how to amplify global income level by taking initiatives to make norms, rules and regulations of global economic and trading activities. Multilateral treaties and accords are such things. Where there is no world assembly, it is the task of multilateral agreements that can work. Multilateral treaties are quasi-legislation in the sense that they become laws which regulate those sign and ratify and which become symbols of solidarity to move together toward dreams and goals. East Asia is one of the regions which register the fairly solid supporters of such multilateralism besides Northwestern European states and their vicinities (Inoguchi and Le 2019).

Then what can the QOL-based types of societies do to facilitate for East Asian starts to play such roles? My answer is: Identifying domestic impediments against such multilateral initiatives toward global income equity, the package of public policy should be designed and implemented.

Conclusion with a Syllabus

Quality of life cannot be gauged without the cognitivism that human life is bound to be affected by politics. In other words, quality of life cannot be understood without the awareness that politics, large or small, has something to do with politics. Hence the rationale of teaching quality of life studies and politics.

Syllabus: Quality of Life Studies and Politics
1. Introduction: Definition of QOL and Its Scope
2. People's Satisfaction with Daily Life
3. People's Propensity to Nurture Children Values and Norms
4. QOL and Confidence in Institutions
5. QOL-Based Societal Profiling or Typology of Asian Societies
6. Applying QOL Studies in Sustainable Development Goals (SDGs)

References

Blondel, J., & Inoguchi, T. (2006). *Political cultures in Asia and Europe*. London: Routledge.

Campbell, C., & Campbell, T., II. (2016). *The China study: Revised and expanded edition: The most comprehensive study of nutrition ever conducted and the startling implications for diet, weight loss, and long-term health*. Dallas: BenBella Books.

Friedman, T. L. (2006). *The world is flat [Updated and expanded]: A brief history of the twenty-first century*. Farrar Straus & Giroux. Expanded, Updated Edn.

Inglehart, R. (1977). *The silent revolution*. Princeton: Princeton University Press.

Inoguchi, T. (1979). *Political surfing over economic waves: A simple model of the Japanese political economic system in comparative perspective*. Presented at the world congress of the international political science association, Moscow, 1979. 8.12–18.

Inoguchi, T. (2010). *Post-modernity and multiple modernities as discourse of quality of life*. Presented at the inaugural meeting of the Asian social research association, November 4–5, 2010, Tokyo, Japan.

Inoguchi, T. (2012). Voters swing, and swing away soon. *Asian Survey, 53*(1), 184–197.

Inoguchi, T., & Blondel, J. (2008). *Citizens and the state: Attitudes in Western Europe and East and Southeast Asia*. London: Routledge.

Inoguchi, T., & Fujii, S. (2013). *The quality of life in Asia: A comparison of quality of life in Asia*. Dordrecht: Springer.

Inoguchi, T., & Le, L. T. Q. (2019). *The development of global legislative politics: Rousseau and Locke Writ Global*. Springer. (Forthcoming).

Inoguchi, T., & Marsh, I. (Eds.). (2008). *Globalization, public opinion and the state: Western Europe and East and Southeast Asia*. London: Routledge.

Inoguchi, T., & Tokuda, Y. (Eds.). (2017). *Trust with Asian characteristics: Interpersonal and institutional* (pp. 169–175). Dordrecht: Springer.

Inoguchi, T., et al. (2014). Daily life satisfaction in Asia: A cross-national survey in twelve societies. *Asian Journal for Public Opinion Research, 1*(3), 153–202.

Iwai, N., et al. (2009). *East Asian views of family in graphs*. Kyoto: Nakanishiya shuppan.

Iwai, N., et al. (2011). *East Asian cultures and values in graphs*. Kyoto: Nakanishiya shuppan.

Iwai, N., et al. (2013). *East Asian health and society in graphs*. Kyoto: Nakanishiya shuppan.

Maslow, A. (1943). A theory of human motivation. *Psychological Review, 40*(4), 370–396.

Putnam, R., & Farr, S. (2000). *Disaffected democracies: What's troubling the trilateral countries?* Princeton: Princeton University Press.

Stiglitz, J. (2012). *The price of inequality: How today's divided society endangers our future*. New York: W. H. Norton.

Whiteley, P. (2011). Is the party over? The decline of party activism and membership across the democratic world. *Party Politics, 17*(1), 21–44.

Chapter 7
Developing Quality-of-Life Pedagogy in Marketing Courses: A Structured Approach

Don R. Rahtz, M. Joseph Sirgy, Stephan Grzeskowiak, and Dong-Jin Lee

Introduction

This chapter explores how the concept of Quality of Life (QOL) has been an integral part of marketing from its earliest days as a discipline of study. In the very beginning of marketing, the discipline was concerned with delivering a variety of goods to consumers to enhance their quality of life. A broad system of elements was constructed to effectively create and deliver those goods. This system included such things as (1) creating needed goods for individuals and households, (2) the distribution architecture and vessels/vehicles that deliver the desired goods, (3) the valuation of these various goods by setting prices, and (4) informing the target consumers as to the availability and use of these goods designed to "make their lives better." Over the years, marketing evolved into a much more managerially-focused discipline that lost focus of its macro mission, namely "to make consumer's lives, their greater communities, and societies better."

In this chapter we explore how those in the marketing discipline can further develop a viable pedagogy that applies QOL theories, tools, and concepts when teaching marketing. In doing so, we seek to disseminate a perspective to the next

D. R. Rahtz (✉)
College of William and Mary, Williamsburg, VA, USA
e-mail: Don.Rahtz@mason.wm.edu

M. J. Sirgy
Virginia Polytechnic Institute & State University, Blacksburg, VA, USA
e-mail: sirgy@vt.edu

S. Grzeskowiak
NEOMA Business School, Mont-Saint-Aignan, France
e-mail: research@grzeskowiak.ch

D.-J. Lee
Yonsei University, Seoul, South Korea
e-mail: Djlee81@yonsei.ac.kr

© Springer Nature Switzerland AG 2020
G. H. Tonon (ed.), *Teaching Quality of Life in Different Domains*, Social
Indicators Research Series 79, https://doi.org/10.1007/978-3-030-21551-4_7

generation of marketers that again focuses on "making consumers lives better" through the marketing of goods. It is these next-generation marketers who will need to better engage with a global consumer market that is faced with a variety of challenges—those that are inherently linked with issues of QOL.

A Little History

Recently Witkowski and Jones (2016) examined the historical journey of marketing. In their piece they look back to both the roots and the application of this thing we call "marketing." They also examined where the teaching of marketing methods began and how it has evolved as both a discipline in both application and teaching. The first textbook that was published on the system of marketing was in 1917 by Ralph Starr Butler. Powers (2015) examined the publication and its impact going forward in the discipline. Benton (1987) recounts Butler's providing a name for the discipline that came to be known as marketing. He cites Bartels (1976, p. 24).

> ...the subject matter that I intended to treat was to include a study of everything that the promoter of a product has to do prior to his actual use of salesmen and of advertising. A name was needed for this field of business activity ... I finally decided on the phrase "marketing methods." (Ralph Starr Butler 1911)

This definition leads to the understanding that producing goods that people need required a system of activities to move those goods from point of product development to consumer acquisition and use of those goods. Benton (1987) provides an excellent examination of the journey forward from the 1911 articulation by Butler. He introduces the reader to an economist, Weld, who in 1913 taught a course on how farm products are "marketed" through what was referred to "distributive industries" (p. 421). He asserts that this was the first time "Marketing" appeared in the title of an academic course.

While the source of the following quote has been attributed by some to a story in *Brownel's* (1916) *Dairy Farmer*, it has also been at times attributed to Charles Palin, regarded as many as the founding father of market research. Either way, the thought from 1916 shows recognition that the road to the modern "Marketing Concept" started long ago.

> We may talk as long as we please about manufacturers, wholesalers, and retailers. But in the last analysis, the consumer is king. The whim of the consumer makes and unmakes the manufacturers, the jobbers, and the retailers. Whoever wins the confidence of the consumer wins the day; and whoever loses it, is lost (p. 7).

Anyone who has studied marketing will recognize the arrival of the consumer focus in the marketing of goods and services, the cornerstone of the marketing concept. In 1957, two pieces were published that highlighted the need for the marketing field to recognize that understanding and satisfying the consumer were the key to a successful business endeavor. Borch (1957) and McKitterick (1957) both articulated the ideas that marketing needed such a "philosophy" to support the construction of a *system* to focus on the desires and needs of these markets. Benton (1987) notes that it was recognizing the need for a clear intent for managers to bring about "consumer sovereignty" through customer satisfaction that led Phillip Kotler (modern dean of the marketing discipline) and others to clearly advocate the link between a company's commitment to this sovereignty and long-term success.

Marketing over the years has evolved into both macro and micro-marketing sub-disciplines (Shapiro 2008a, b). This division has led to a divergence in both philosophical and practical views what "marketing" is. It can be argued that macromarketing, with its concern for the interactions between markets, marketing, and society is clearly connected to this idea of Quality of Life (QOL) due to its recognition of the entire system that delivers QOL to the society. George Fisk, one of the founding fathers of macromarketing within the discipline, in one of his many presentations, noted that "The role of macromarketing is to save the world" (Fisk 2001).

As mentioned in the opening paragraph, QOL connections to micromarketing, however, have not been clearly recognized and have been met with some resistance by those who adhere to the more narrow managerial view of marketing. This resistance is, in the view of many, based on a combination of both cultural and structural elements in the discipline itself. In other words, the widespread acceptance of the micromarketing view across both academe and business has created an environment where there is hesitancy to embrace the broader systemic, yet unfamiliar and possibly disruptive, adjustment view to a system that appears to be working "just fine." Due to this broader discipline structural and cultural resistance, macromarketing scholars such as Benton (1985), Shapiro (2008a, b), Shultz (2007), and Radford et al. (2015) have noted that this resistance has placed marcomarketing at a disadvantage in the discipline. The authors note that these structural and cultural aspects are wide and far reaching. Examples include limited curriculum space in university programs of study, availability of and ranking of mainstream marketing research outlets, and the demand from the private sector for managerial-focused tools from marketing scholars.

An historical examination of the evolution of marketing, however, finds common ground for both the macro and micro camps for embracing the "philosophy" of a significant role for a QOL perspective in the marketing discipline. It is proposed here that this role, especially in today's world, is relevant both conceptually and methodologically. There is a clear value in the understanding and the application of the QOL perspective for practitioners in the marketplace. If so, this, in turn, gives marketing educators a strong impetus to recognize the need to develop pedagogy for teaching QOL theory and methods. This also drives the need to create QOL applications to illustrate to both students and practitioners how to leverage their use in the marketplace.

The lynch pin of the philosophy that brings unity to embrace the QOL perspective in both the macromarketing systems view and the micromarketing managerial view is the philosophy that has dominated the mainstream marketing discipline for years, namely the *Marketing Concept*. The purported importance of "consumer sovereignty" in regards to achieving "profit through long-term consumer satisfaction" points to any number of areas where QOL concepts and measures can make significant contributions to the discipline. It is important, again, to illuminate the importance that the early ideas in marketing were driven by "consumer sovereignty." The obvious connection between consumer sovereignty and consumer well-being is a logical place to begin our examination of how practitioners can incorporate a QOL perspective in their marketing research, strategies, and tactics.

Quality of Life (QOL) Marketing and Consumer Well-Being

Enhancing consumer well-being is an important goal for marketing. Quality of Life (QOL) marketing is defined as marketing practice designed to enhance the well-being of customers while preserving the well-being of the firm's other stakeholders. QOL marketing is based on ethical marketing philosophy involving two dimensions: enhancement of consumer well-being (beneficence) and preservation of other stakeholders (non-maleficence) (Lee and Sirgy 2004; Sirgy 1996, 2001; Sirgy and Lee 1996, 2008; Sirgy et al. 2012). The key prescription stemming from this literature is: *QOL marketing should result in increased customer trust and commitment, company goodwill, consumer well-being, and other benefits to society at large.*

The Consumer Well-Being (CWB) construct is an excellent, wide reaching construct that provides a theoretical foundation to guide marketing research, strategy, and tactics. That is, CWB can be operationalized and applied in a host of settings for strategic planning and executions and the subsequent measurement of marketing performance. With that in mind, the purpose of the next sections is to explore specific guidelines on how to develop beneficent QOL marketing strategies while minimizing any damage done to any of the firm's stakeholders. We will address the beneficence dimension of QOL marketing and present specific strategic guidelines that marketers can use in designing and implementing QOL marketing strategies that lead to enhancement of consumer well-being. We will also address how QOL strategies are equally based on the non-maleficence dimension—"thou shall do no harm."

So how do we define CWB? One good definition is a definition based on the consumption life cycle (Sirgy and Lee 2008). That is, CWB is a state of objective and subjective well-being[1] involved in the various stages of the consumption life cycle in relation to a particular consumer good. The consumption life cycle refers to consumer experiences with various types of marketplace stages starting from the stage of purchasing the product to the last stage involving product disposal. Specifically, the stages of the consumption life cycle are: product acquisition (purchase), preparation (assembly), consumption (use), ownership (possession), maintenance (repair), and disposal (selling, trade-in, or junking of the product). See Table 7.1 for a more detailed definition of consumer well-being based on the dis-

---

[1] *Subjective* consumer well-being refers to positive feelings the consumer may have in a manner that contributes to his or her quality of life (i.e., life satisfaction). In contrast, *objective* consumer well-being refers to expert assessments regarding consumers' costs and benefits as well as safety assessments—consumer safety, public safety, and safety to the environment (Sirgy and Lee 2008).

Table 7.1 A conceptualization of consumer well-being based on the consumption life cycle

Consumption life cycle	Consumer well-being captured in terms of consumer satisfaction in relation to a particular stage of the consumption life cycle	Consumer well-being captured in terms of experts assessment in relation to a particular stage of the consumption life cycle
Stage 1: Product acquisition	Consumer satisfaction with the manner leading to product acquisition (i.e., shopping)	Experts' assessment that
		The product is high quality and the price is fair and affordable, and
		The purchase experience is safe to the purchasers, the sales person/facility, the general public, and the environment
Stage 2: Product preparation	Consumer satisfaction with the preparation or assembly of the product	Experts' assessment that the product is
		Easy (or convenient) and
		Safe to prepare or assemble to the preparer, the general public, and the environment
Stage 3: Product consumption	Consumer satisfaction with the consumption or use of the product	Experts' assessment that the consumption of the product is
		Significantly beneficial to consumers and
		Safe to consumers, the general public, and the environment
Stage 4: Product ownership	Consumer satisfaction with the ownership of the product	Experts' assessment that the ownership of the product
		Has appreciable value and
		Is safe to the owners, the general public, and the environment
Stage 5: Product maintenance	Consumer satisfaction with product maintenance and repair	Experts' assessment that the maintenance of the product is
		Easy (or convenient),
		Not costly (affordable), and
		Safe to the repair person/facility, the general public, and the environment
Stage 6: Product disposal	Consumer satisfaction with product disposal (or trade-in or re-selling)	Experts' assessment that the disposal of the product is
		Easy (or convenient),
		Not costly (affordable), and
		Safe to the disposal person/facility, the general public, and the environment

Source: Adapted from Sirgy and Lee (2008)

tinction of subjective and objective consumer well-being and the various stages of the consumption life cycle.

Making Marketing Decisions Guided by the Concept of Well-Being

The American Marketing Association in their 2013 definition taken from their website defines Marketing as:

> ...... the activity, set of institutions, and processes for creating, communicating, delivering, and exchanging offerings that have value for customers, clients, partners, and society at large.

We again see the focus on "consumer." This most recent definition has added the society element. This is consistent with a broader QOL perspective. Well-being marketing is addressed as a higher-level ethical business philosophy. Sirgy and Lee (2008) were able to articulate this philosophy by contrasting well-being marketing with traditional marketing, what they call "transactional marketing." The ethics supporting transaction marketing is based on the concept of consumer sovereignty of business ethics. Although consumer sovereignty is considered to be an ethical concept, it falls short in contrast to the ethics of well-being marketing. Well-being marketing is grounded on business ethics concepts of duty of beneficence and non-maleficence. Well-being marketing is more ethical than transactional marketing in serving the business community, consumers at large, and society overall.

Specifically, transactional marketing is guided by neo-classical economic theory. Marketers focus on maximizing sales and profit by recruiting more and more customers to purchase the firm's product. Transactional marketing is justified, ethically speaking, by the notion that high levels of product sales signify that the firm serves society by marketing a product that consumers need or want. Hence, a firm meeting market demand for consumer goods is a firm that serves society well. Making more sales leads to financial profitability. Profitability translates into more jobs and economic security for the firm's employees. Society also benefits through taxation. That is, the more the firm sells, the more it is taxed, the more the tax revenues are used by government to provide public services that benefit society at large. The prosperity cycle feeds on itself. The more people are employed, the more tax revenues are generated through personal income taxation, which also serves society at large. Competition is good; it benefits society. Competition among firms is the motivating force that drives firms to develop higher quality products and selling them at lower prices. This motivational force translates into higher levels of innovation and efficiency. The drive to do better than the competition prompts a business enterprise to innovate and develop new and better quality products, and market those products at lower prices. When consumers purchase high quality products at low prices, they reward firms that are innovative and efficient. Thus, firms that are able to meet market demand for better products at lower prices are rewarded financially, and those that cannot compete are punished. Hence, consumer sovereignty is an ethical concept reflecting the fact that when consumers vote with their pocketbooks they serve society at large by rewarding good business and weeding out bad business. When consumers shop around they end up buying those products that are highest in quality at the lowest price. However, for consumers to exercise their sovereignty they have to be informed about the product's quality and price. Much of today's business laws (e.g., anti-trust laws, consumer protection laws) are designed to increase consumer sovereignty by making consumers better informed about their market choices. However, in spite of consumer sovereignty, market inefficiencies do occur in the form of sales that have little to do with market demand or consumers making wise decisions to purchase the highest quality products at lowest prices. Many firms survive and prosper not because they market higher quality products at lower prices but because they have *countervailing power*. Large firms overwhelm their competitors through massive marketing communications campaigns. They control the channels of distribution restricting consumer access to competitor brands.

In contrast, the business philosophy underlying well-being marketing is based on the concept of "societal marketing" (Kotler 1979). This concept refers to integrated marketing activity aimed at generating consumer satisfaction and long-run consumer well-being. Kotler (1987) made an attempt to couch the concept of societal marketing in a historical context. He made the argument that marketing thought evolved in three stages. The first stage is essentially based on the *marketing concept*. The marketing concept emerged when firms abandoned the product/sales orientation of marketing—marketing comes in at a later stage of the product commercialization cycle to focus on selling an existing product; that is, marketing has very little to do with the inception and design of the product. The product/sales orientation gave way to the marketing orientation (i.e., the marketing concept). The marketing concept focuses on wants of target consumers and is used to guide product, price, place, and promotion strategies and tactics. Then came *humanistic marketing* as the second stage of marketing evolution. This concept refers to the notion that marketers consider both consumer wants and consumer interests. Humanistic marketers focus on making "better" goods and services after which they educate consumers about the benefits of the new and improved products. Humanistic marketing was then followed by *societal marketing*. This concept addressed the shortcoming of humanistic marketing in that some marketing practices may serve consumer wants and interests but yet hurt society's interests.

Guided by the societal marketing concept, Sirgy and Lee (2008) have developed the concept of *well-being marketing* and defined as a business philosophy that guides the development, pricing, promotion, and distribution of consumer goods and services to individuals and families for the purpose of enhancing consumer well-being at a profit (in the long run) in a manner that does not adversely affect the public, including the environment. Thus, marketers focus not only on meeting consumption demand of target consumers safely (and in ways to enhance their quality of their life) but also do so in ways to avoid any adverse impact on other stakeholder groups such as employees, distributors, suppliers, stockholders, etc. (Sirgy 2001). This conceptualization of well-being marketing is grounded on two principles based on duty ethics, namely beneficence and non-maleficence (e.g., Beauchamp 1999). The principle of *beneficence* argues that one ought to promote good or "beneficence." In contrast, the principle of *non-maleficence* refers to injunction not to inflict harm on others. As such, well-being marketing should be viewed on a higher ethical plane than transactional marketing. Well-being marketing takes into accounts the well-being of both consumers and society at large. In the next section of the chapter, we analyze how the concepts of well-being marketing is used to guide marketing decision-making and pedagogy. We will contrast marketing decision-making guided by well-being marketing with decision-making guided by transactional marketing.

Teaching QOL in Relation to the Product Element of the Marketing Mix

In keeping with our use of the Marketing Mix to frame our discussion, the American Marketing Association's definition taken from their website defines Product as:

> ... a bundle of attributes (features, functions, benefits, and uses) capable of exchange or use; usually a mix of tangible and intangible forms. Thus, a product may be an idea, a physical entity (a good), or a service, or any combination of the three. It exists for the purpose of exchange in the satisfaction of individual and organizational objectives. ... While the term "products and services" is occasionally used, product is a term that encompasses both goods and services.

Sirgy and Lee (2008) argued that transactional marketers make product decisions (product design, packaging, labeling, branding, warrantee, technical assistance, etc.) by focusing on short-term profitability—maximize sales and reduce costs. As such, product strategy and tactics are guided by an understanding of consumers' purchase expectations. The product, the package, the warranty, etc. are all designed to meet consumers' purchase expectations. The goal is a product mix resulting in consumers' preference and choice of the firm's brand over competitor brands. In contrast, product decisions, guided by well-being marketing, focus on developing products that are significantly beneficial to consumers with little or no adverse effects on consumers as well as other stakeholders (employees, the local community, the environment, and the general public). Furthermore, product decisions guided by well-being marketing focuses on maximizing consumer satisfaction across all six stages of the consumption life cycle (product acquisition, preparation, consumption, possession, maintenance, and disposal) with minimum negative externalities. Let us explore these in some detail (see Table 7.2).

With respect to product decisions related to *product purchase*, a transaction-oriented firm would design the product in units most attractive to target consumers, making the transaction easy and convenient. In contrast, well-being-oriented firms would make a concerted effort to ensure that product design is not only guided by customer satisfaction and loyalty goals but also by safety concerns—safe to consumers, the general public, and the environment. With respect to *product preparation*, transaction marketers attempt to maximize sales by ensuring that the product

Table 7.2 Making marketing decisions guided by transaction versus well-being concepts

Marketing decisions	In telation to:	Transactional marketing	Well-being marketing
Product decisions (product design, packaging, warranty, etc.)	Product acquisition, ownership, preparation, consumption, maintenance, and disposal	Consumer purchase expectations (purchase criteria)	Customer satisfaction, trust, and commitment
			Safety concerns
Place decisions (breadth of channel, channel members, etc.)	Product acquisition, ownership, preparation, consumption, maintenance, and disposal	Customer access and convenience	Customer satisfaction, trust, and commitment
			Safety concerns
			Access to customers most likely to benefit from the product (inclusivity)
Promotion decisions (e.g., message and media decisions)	Product acquisition, ownership, preparation, consumption, maintenance, and disposal	Brand awareness, beliefs, preference, purchase	Customer satisfaction, trust, and commitment
			Safety concerns
			Use of the product to maximize consumer well-being
Pricing decisions (pricing of product, accessories, warranty, retail, etc.)	Product acquisition, ownership, preparation, consumption, maintenance, and disposal	Costs, profit, what the market can bear, competition	Customer perceived value
			Expert assessment of value
			Costs related to possible environmental remediation

Source: Adapted from Sirgy and Lee (2008)

can be *easily* assembled or prepared for consumption. Furthermore, to ensure that the product is not returned, many transaction-oriented firms make a concerted effort to provide technical assistance to customers to assist with product assembly. Well-being marketers would design the product in such a way to avoid the possibility of customer injury while assembling the product and to ensure safety to others as well as the environment. Well-being marketers would also make every attempt possible to make the preparation experience fun, exciting, and meaningful to their consumers. Doing so should significantly increase consumer satisfaction with product preparation. With respect to *product consumption*, a transaction-oriented firm designs a product to meet consumer purchase expectations. Once the product is designed guided by purchase expectations, the transaction marketer promotes the product to tout those benefits. Doing so enhances the marketability of the product. In contrast, well-being marketers design a product by taking into account both pre-purchase expectation and post-purchase perceptions of product performance. That is, the well-being marketer is also guided by safety concerns during consumption and a consumption experience that is most meaningful and enriching. With respect to *product ownership*, many transaction-oriented firms design their products with product obsolescence in mind. In other words, durability is not a major concern, unless market research shows that target consumers use criteria such as durability in purchase decision-making. If so, a transaction marketing firm would design the product in such a way to convince consumers that their brand is better than competitor brands on durability. Well-being marketing would design the product to make its durable irrespective of whether consumers consider durability as a significant criterion in their purchase decision-making. Well-being marketers place high priority on safety concerns as well as customer satisfaction, trust, and customer loyalty. In other words, well-being firms design a product to ensure that there are no safety issues associated with product ownership—safety to the owners and their families, safety to the local community, the environment, and the general public. Furthermore, the well-being firm would design the product in such a way that its ownership becomes a part of an overall constellation of goods and services signifying a lifestyle. As such, ownership of the product is likely to be most satisfying to the consumer. With respect to *product maintenance*, many transaction-oriented firms provide their customers a product warranty to help the customer when the product needs servicing or repair. Consumers expect a good warranty and, as such, warranty is treated as a significant criterion in purchase decision-making. In contrast, well-being marketing firms do the same to increase brand loyalty and enhance the chances of repeat business, but they do so by focusing on preventative maintenance too. Well-being firms are also very conscientious about safety concerns. The maintenance warranty offered by the firm is safe-proof. That is, the maintenance program ensures that no aspect of maintenance is likely to jeopardize the safety of customers, employees, the environment, as well as the general public. In addition to the safe-proof maintenance program, well-being firms would not hesitate to recall their products when evidence arises concerning lack of safety. Finally, with respect to *product disposal*, transaction-oriented firms are likely to use environmentally-friendly product ingredients and/or packaging only if consumer research uncovers that consumers do indeed consider environmental-friendly dimensions of the product in purchase decision-making. In contrast, well-being firms are motivated by corporate social responsibility and environmental stewardship. The product is designed in ways to ensure that disposal would not contribute to environmental degradation. Table 7.3 provides a categorization of several studies examining how various aspects of the "Product" have been examined by researchers recently. Table 7.4 below offers some suggestions for classroom discussions that would help the student understand how QOL concepts and measures can be applied successfully in today's world.

Teaching QOL in Relation to the Place Element of the Marketing Mix

The American Marketing Association definition taken from their website defines Distribution as:

> … the act of marketing and carrying products to consumers. It is also used to describe the extent of market coverage for a given product. … In the 4Ps, distribution is represented by place or placement.

Table 7.3 Issues related to product decisions and references of interest

Issues related to:	References of interest
Product development	Tourism programs to support QOL of local residents of host communities (Konu 2015; Nguyen et al. 2014)
	Ecosystem surveying (Maynard et al. 2010)
	Assessing new product processes (Salari and Bhuiyan 2018)
Product usage and production	Design and usage of products (Cooper 2005)
	Consumer goods and QOL valuations (Sirgy and Lee 2008)
	Palliative health care (Wong et al. 2018)
	Linking QOL to consumer behavior (Loo et al. 2016)
	The silver lining of luxury consumption (Hudders and Pandelaere 2012)
	Materialism and consumption behavior (Kasser and Sheldon 2000)
	Compulsive buying (Ridway et al. 2008)
	The buying impulse (Rook 1987)
	Impulse buying and variety seeking (Sharma et al. 2010)
Ethical issues	QOL and marketing (Constantinescu 2011)
	Design of sustainable products (Sotamaa 2009)
	Branding and consumption (Olbrich et al. 2016)
	Sustainable consumption (Sandeen 2009)

Table 7.4 QOL discussion questions related to the product element of the marketing mix

Topic	QOL discussion questions
Product development	How can marketers use QOL perspective and measures to optimize product development processes?
	Should marketers use such things as sustainability as a necessary deliverable before moving to market?
	How does consumer well-being fit into a product development process for consumer product companies? For B2B companies?
Product usage and production	Do companies have a duty to produce only goods they know will lead to a positive QOL impact?
	Should materials that cause significant environmental damage (like plastics) be banned or phased out quickly?
Ethical issues	The demand for products from the consumer market can be quite strong. Sometimes these products are either unhealthy or cause long-term negative impacts on consumers, environment. Should those products be produced and be allowed to be produced and sold by the public policy officials?

Marketing distribution (or the Place element of the marketing mix) includes the study of the structure, functions, interactions, and activities of marketing channels. Students learn how to analyze and develop integrated physical distribution and logistics systems for the firm. A course on Marketing Channels explores the relationships among manufacturers, wholesalers and distributors, and retailers.

Distribution decisions guided by a well-being philosophy are very different from distribution decisions guided by transactional marketing (Sirgy and Lee 2008; see

Table 7.2). A firm oriented towards transactional marketing makes distribution decisions guided sales, market share, and profitability objectives. The channel is designed with those financial goals in mind—the type of channel and channel members that provide consumers access and convenience in purchasing are likely to meet financial objectives. In contrast, well-being marketers make distribution decisions guided by both financial and societal goals. The well-being firm considers safety (safety to consumers, other publics, and the environment) and the extent to which the channel can effectively reach target consumers—those likely to benefit from the product the most.

Let us now focus on how the channel goals may differ in relation to various stages of the consumption life-cycle. With respect *to product purchase*, transaction firms tend to aim at cost reduction in customer service, offering assortments with high-margin or high repurchase-rate products, and tend to develop channel structures that drive high sales volumes. These goals may not only impact retail intermediaries, but can also be achieved with electronic marketing channels or direct sales intermediaries to ensure maximum sales, market share, and profit. In contrast, well-being firms are likely to identify intermediaries based on business philosophy, reputation for ethical conduct and social responsibility, customer satisfaction ratings, and value propositions (assortment). The channel goal would be to focus on long-term customer benefits. They create a shopping environment that empowers consumers in their shopping decisions, calibrates consumer spending with expected product benefits, pre-selects assortments of high value, and perhaps customize products to better suite individual needs. With respect to *product preparation,* transaction firms may pay attention to customer concerns about product preparation only to the extent that customers express these concerns as purchasing criteria. Transaction firms stock and/or order inventory of parts, tools, manuals, assembly instructions necessary to prepare or assemble the product successfully. They may also develop training programs to help distributors with product installation. In contrast, well-being firms may focus on helping consumers to integrate new products into their lives. This could be an installation service, but maybe it means that consumers would be coached into using the product in a way that yields maximum QOL benefits. One example is the involvement of new customers into experience sharing platforms that allow consumers to learn from other product users. It could also mean showing consumers how the new product can improve various life domains. By making these linkages with various life domains, well-being firms can improve consumers' lifestyle. Compared to marketing channels for transaction firms, the well-being focus are likely to require marketing channels that allow consumers to participate in the value creation process. With respect to *product consumption*, most transaction firms train their channel members on how to demonstrate the use of the product to customers by adhering to the legal requirements of the transaction contract or warranty, especially if customers expect such demonstration at the point of purchase. Well-being firms go beyond transaction firms in that they train their channel members not only on how to demonstrate the use of the product but also how to use the product responsibly—safely for the consumer and with no negative impact on the general public and the environment. With respect to *product ownership*, transaction firms select channel members who can provide lease versus buy options to customers. Providing options to own or lease facilitates product sales. In contrast, well-being firms not only provide lease versus buy options but also train retailers to help their customers understand the differential benefits of these options, ultimately to protect the investment value of the product. Well-being firms may also aim at reducing materialistic product ownership and its negative impact on consumer well-being. For example, marketing channels could be designed to reduce the number of products consumers own (or replace) in a specific product category and rather focus on preserving performance and value of already owned products. This shift of channel goals requires a new skill set across all channel members. In relation to *product maintenance*, transaction firms make replacement parts available at their channel members to honor the warranty, and of course make a profit. Well-being firms go further by helping educate and train customers on how to maintain the product themselves to save money. Finally with respect to *product disposal*, many transaction firms typically develop programs to encourage customers to trade-in their old product for a newer model. Of course, the objective is to drum up sales. Well-being firms assist their distributors develop product trade-in/disposal programs that encourage customers to turn in their old products for proper and environmentally-friendly disposal. Compared to transactional channels with predominantly downward channel-flows, such trade-in programs are likely to require channel flows that move up the channel as well as the integration of new types of intermediaries. See Table 7.2.

From a teaching perspective, it is instructive to recognize QOL impact as key competitive advantage and therefore a reason for channel redesign. The instructor may identify a case example and ask students to set distribution objectives related to QOL. Once these objectives have been defined the instructor may identify one or two objectives as focal for specifying distribution tasks. This exercise tends to generate a heterogeneous mix of distribution tasks if assigned in the context of small group work. The results should be shared and discussed with the whole class. Table 7.5 provides a categorization of several studies examining how various aspects of distribution have been examined by researchers recently. Table 7.6 provides examples of QOL discussion questions related to distribution.

Teaching QOL in Relation to the Promotion Element of the Marketing Mix

In keeping with our use of the marketing mix to frame our discussion, the American Marketing Association definition taken from their website defines Promotion as follows:

Promotion: An advertising or marketing campaign is a set of coordinated, specific activities that are based on a common theme and are designed to promote a product, service or business through different advertising media.

Table 7.5 Issues related to place decisions and references of interest

Issues related to:	References of interest
Growing power of distributors	Category killers (Spector 2005)
	Distributor market orientation (Siguaw et al. 1998)
	Distributor power (Butaney and Wortzel 1988)
Need for cost reduction and growth	Distribution cost reduction (Spence 1986)
	Cost reduction and customer satisfaction (Rust et al. 2002)
	Distributor market development (Siguaw et al. 1998)
Electronic marketing channels	Non-store retailing (Korgaonkar 1984)
	Inter-channel competition and conflict (Webb and Hogan 2002)
	Mass-customization (Pine and Davis 1993)
Marketing channels for services	Customer co-creation (Vargo et al. 2008)
	Channel relationship type (Cannon and Perreault 1999)

Table 7.6 QOL discussion questions related to the place element of the marketing mix

Topic	QOL discussion questions
Growing power of distributors	Are channel intermediaries a gatekeeper for consumers' QOL?
	How can category killers define the QOL impact of products?
	Retailers have shifted from selling products for manufacturers to buying products for their customers
	How can they make the next shift towards assuring the delivery of QOL?
Need for cost reduction and growth	Distribution has been discovered as another source for potential cost reduction
	Does cost reduction in marketing channels jeopardize the delivery of QOL?
	How can a focus on QOL in marketing channels contribute to increasing market share or market development?
Electronic marketing channels	Which aspects of a QOL strategy can non-store retailing meaningfully address?
	How does inter-type competition challenge QOL distribution goals?
	Can QOL be mass-customized?
Marketing channels for services	How can marketing channels be designed to allow customer co-creation of QOL?
	What types of relationships need to be formed across marketing channel members to generate QOL know-how at different channel levels?

IMC: Integrated marketing communication (IMC) is a cohesive combination of marketing communications activities, techniques, and media designed to deliver a coordinated message to a target market with a powerful or synergistic effect, while achieving a common objective or set of objectives.

The Promotion element in the marketing mix has been referred to by a number of different names depending on schools and departments. In the 1980s, there was the rise of IMC courses that drove the discourse on Promotion. IMC, in some ways, was a simple repackaging of the mix of previous combined incarnations of Advertising, Promotions, and Sales and Personal Selling. The discipline's naming of the various elements should not cause confusion; however, as the "Promotion" encompasses the contacts and communications with the consumers and businesses with whom the company or commercial entity is engaged. In today's world, those contact points are substantial and complex. The twentieth century world in which Ralph Starr Butler existed has become the firm's constant contact with consumers, either directly or indirectly. Many of the issues in QOL these days seem to emanate from our use of media, social media in particular.

Promotion decisions guided by a well-being philosophy are recognizably different from decisions guided by a transactional marketing orientation (Sirgy and Lee 2008; see Table 7.2). A transaction firm makes promotion decisions guided by goals such as creating brand awareness, informing prospective customers about the brand's benefits, generating brand preference and purchase. With a different twist, well-being marketing firms do the same but pursue additional goals of informing customers of benefits likely to lead to customer satisfaction, trust, and commitment, and product safety.

Specifically, let us break the distinction between transactional and well-being marketing by stage of the consumption life cycle. Consider promotion decisions in regards to *product purchase*. Transaction firms tend to develop their marketing communications campaign to generate maximal sales through a hierarchy of effects: brand awareness → brand beliefs → brand preference → brand choice and purchase. Well-being firms pursue the additional goal of generating high levels of customer satisfaction, loyalty, and safety (to consumers, general public, and the environment). Well-being companies are more willing to share information about their product's potential hazards. With respect to *product preparation*, transaction-oriented firms tend to focus on educating and training customers how to assemble or prepare the product for consumption. In addition to what transaction firms do, well-being marketing firms do more. They inform customers about the availability and cost of installation services from selected retail outlets, and they inform customers about the availability of replacement parts and tools needed for product assembly or preparation. They also educate customers how to assemble or prepare the product in a manner safe to themselves, the general public, and the environment. In relation to *product consumption*, transaction firms inform their customers about the use of the product in a manner to influence brand choice and purchase. Well-being firms go one step further by informing their customers how to effectively use the product in ways to meet customers' expectations and make the consumption experience most satisfying. Furthermore, the emphasis is on establishing and maintain trust and customer loyalty. And of course, safety in use (safety to the consumers, the general public, and the environment) is an imperative. With respect to *product ownership*, transaction firms typically inform their consumers about incentive programs to trade-in their current product for a new model, ultimately to drum up sales. Well-being firms go the extra mile by informing customers about any financing deals to ensure customer retention. They make an effort to educate their customers on how to retain the product safely (safe to the consumer, safe to the general public, and safe to the environment). With respect to *product maintenance*, transaction firms do very little in terms of communicating to customers much about product maintenance. There is no financial, short-term return in doing so. In contrast, well-being firms are motivated to foster customer goodwill, customer satisfaction/trust/commitment. They do so by informing their customers about how to service the product to enhance its reliability and durability. They also instruct customers on how to do their own repairs safely—to ensure their own safety, bystanders and others, as well as the environment. Finally, with respect to *product disposal*, transaction firms usually say very little in regards to disposal issues. However, there are instances in which manufacturers have a financial, short-term stake in product disposal such as trade-in programs. Here, the transaction firm informs customers of the availability of any trade-in programs and the market value of the trade-ins. In contrast, the goal of well-being firms is to generate customer satisfaction/trust/commitment. And of course a major goal of well-being firms is to inform their customers about how to dispose the product safely, safely to the customers and their families, safely in relation to the general public and the environment. See Table 7.2.

The communication landscape is intertwined with a digital world of brand advocates, influencers, and brand communities that exist in both the cyber and real world. How marketers manage the ever evolving and complex web of information flow can be a formidable and daunting task, to say the least. Privacy, security, and mental health are all personal well-being issues related to this "P." Are consumers being exploited, bullied, and even spied upon as part of product promotional campaign? These are clear QOL issues and have become part of both the discussion in both the private and public sectors. In Table 7.6, we provide examples of QOL discussion topics under four broad categories that reflect the common managerial splits within the Promotion area—advertising, personal selling, promotions, and digital and social media. In exploring these four areas of Promotion, students can expand their learning horizon by discussing many of the social, ethical, and health policy concerns. If you examine Table 7.6, you will see that the QOL issues in Promotion are widespread and reflect a real plethora of important issues. The development and use of QOL concepts in many of these areas are crucial for both public policy and marketing practitioners. In regards to Advertising, we find advertising being accused of a variety of social ills and harmful promises. At the same time, we know that we need advertising to gather a great deal of positive information. Of interest too, is the increasing use of QOL concepts being used in the Personal Selling component of Promotion. Wellness and well-being of the salesforce and job performance are critical issues in today's environment. Promotional programs are sometimes thought to entice consumers to make choices that are counter to long-term consumer well-being. At the same time, promotions can give incentives to consumers to be much more likely to be involved with QOL-enhancing activities such as gym memberships. Finally, there are many QOL studies and applications related to Digital and Social Media. Today's world is "totally connected"; public policy and marketers

Table 7.7 Issues related to promotion decisions and references of interest

Issues related to:	References of interest
Advertising	Negative impact of mass media on consumer well-being (Lowery and Sloane 2014)
	Negative impacts on societal well-being (Vokey et al. 2013)
	Quality of life and obesity (Segar et al. 2012)
	Misleading and unsubstantiated advertising (Stewart and Neumann 2002)
	Persuasive advertising and materialism (Sandhu 2015)
Personal selling	Implement indicators of QOL in aspects of sales force performance and well-being (Kantak et al. 1992)
	Measures regarding wellness lifestyles (Porter et al. 2008)
	Measures of workplace isolation and job performance from a QOL perspective (Mulki et al. 2008)
	Measures and methods for monitoring and preventing job burnout (Shepard et al. 2011)
	Job and life satisfaction (Kantak et al. 1992)
Promotions	Develop socially responsible promotional programs that reduce unethical and harmful marketing practices (Parker and Pettijohn 2003)
Digital and social media	Impacts and issues regarding the use of digital platforms and social media to influence individuals and society (Sashi 2012)
	Subjective well-being assessments (Chen et al. 2017)
	Social media use and health impacts (Foerster and Roosli 2017; Jiang 2017; Weinstein 2018)

should employ QOL concepts and measures to maintain and monitor the consumer well-being. This is especially true among the youth market.

Table 7.7 provides examples of studies linking Promotion with QOL. From a teaching perspective, one can argue that students in the class should be exposed to some of the QOL issues discussed above. Discussion of these issues can help students better evaluate marketing performance. Table 7.8 below offers some suggestions for classroom discussions that should help the student understand how QOL concepts and measures can be applied successfully the Promotion area of the Marketing Mix.

Teaching QOL in Relation to the Price Element of the Marketing Mix

The typical Pricing course introduces the management of the firm's pricing function as part of the marketing mix. This includes the management of the firm's pricing function within the entire system that delivers the product to the ultimate consumer. In other words, the pricing and valuation of a product needs to also consider channel partners within the broader system of manufacturers, wholesalers and distributors, and retailers when employed.

Table 7.8 QOL discussion questions related to the promotion element of the marketing mix

Topic	QOL discussion questions
Advertising	How can advertising depictions impact the well-being of the target markets that the ads are directed to?
	How can advertising create negative personal well-being perceptions by overpromising results and creating unrealistic expectations of beauty etc.?
Personal selling	Have unreasonable demands for performance created significant threats to sales people regarding health and overall well-being?
Promotions	Do promotions aimed at various health practitioners and others create unrealistic demands that lead to unethical outcomes?
Digital and social media	How have digital platforms and social media impacted our marketing in society in positive ways? In negative ways?

Sirgy and Lee (2008) argued that a transaction firm typically makes pricing decisions guided by factors such as cost-plus (plus a margin to achieve a desired profit level), what the market can bear, and competition. In contrast, well-being firms are guided by customer perceptions of value, experts' assessment of product value, price affordability, and cost of safety and remediation. A well-being firm tries to balance societal goals with the firm's financial goals. Specifically, with respect to the *purchase* stage of the consumption life cycle, well-being firms are guided by other factors in addition to cost, profitability goals, what the market can bear, and competition. They may use both subjective and objective assessments in determining value (e.g., *Consumer Reports* value ratings). Well-being marketers also take into account price affordability. Making the price affordable increases the likelihood in placing the product with as many consumers who need the product as much as possible. Well-being firms are also safety-conscious in their pricing decisions. If their product is determined to degrade the environment in certain ways, then the cost of environmental restoration has to be included in the price of the product. The same factors (customer perceived value, objective value, price affordability, and safety/remedial costs) are equally involved in pricing decisions involved in product preparation, use, ownership, maintenance, and disposal. Specifically, in *product preparation*, well-being marketers price parts and tools necessary to prepare or assemble the product or for providing technical assistance (in the form of customer service) to assist customers in the product assembly or preparation. With respect to *product consumption*, there are many consumer products in which consumers not only pay for the purchase of the product but also every time the product is used (e.g., wired telephone, cellular telephone, Internet access, satellite television, and cable television). With respect to *product ownership*, many firms help consumers assume ownership of high-ticket items (e.g., automobiles). Well-being marketers' pricing of credit ought to be guided by customer perceived value, experts' assessment of value, consumer affordance, and other costs related to safety. With respect to *product maintenance*, many consumer goods companies offer repair services from the manufacturing site. Well-being firms strive to price repair services affordably. With respect to *product disposal*, transaction firms price their products without taking into account environmental concerns. Well-being firm do. See Table 7.2.

Table 7.9 Issues related to price decisions and references of interest

Issues related to:	References of interest
Price setting	How much should medical care cost? (Padua and Padua 2016)
	Drug pricing (Karpman and Höglund 2017)
	Mortgages and insurance (Ashton and Hudson 2017)
	Consumer wine purchasing (Barber 2012)
	Health insurance (O'Conner 2018)
Value	Energy consumption (Press and Arnould 2009)
	Value of health (Garrison 2009)
	Hedonic pricing in real estate (Lu 2018)
Ethical issues	Constructed value of health (Brown 2011)
	Access to stores and the pricing of goods (Kyureghain and Nayga 2013)
	Alcohol consumption (Kozak 2013)
	How much is a life worth? (Brock 2006)
	Ethical choices in society (Olson et al. 2016)

In Table 7.9, we discuss pricing issues in the context of a wide group of market settings under three broad categories, namely (1) price setting, (2) value, and (3) ethics. If you examine Table 7.9, you will see that the QOL issues are extremely widespread and reach across all strata of our society. In regards to price setting, there have been a whole host of pricing studies that explore a broad mix of consumer social issues in relationship to QOL. From a teaching perspective, pricing lends itself to a potentially rich discussion around the ideas of consumer "valuation" of products. As with the previous examples of elements of the marketing mix, using studies of QOL-focused pricing topics can be most impactful. For example, if the students in the class are exposed to these issues, they might well have personal experience from their own extended family or friends who have faced similar situations. For example, how much should they pay for insurance as a family member ages? The importance of fitting pricing-related discussions into a QOL perspective can be highlighted by the instructor to show the wide applicability of QOL in pricing assessments. The example applications provided here cross a number of public and private sectors and are selected to help students consider QOL aspects in evaluating marketing performance. Table 7.10 below offers some suggestions for classroom discussions that should help the student better understand how QOL concepts can be applied successfully in a pricing context.

Developing Pedagogy and Building Applications for Integrating a QOL Perspective Into Coursework

The previous section has laid out a number of ways in which the concept of well-being marketing can be discussed and applied in the practice of marketing. This final section of the chapter seeks to provide a brief summary of the issues related to

Table 7.10 QOL discussion questions related to the price element of the marketing mix

Topic	QOL discussion questions
Price setting	How can marketers make sure they set a price consistent with the desires of consumers in target markets?
	The pricing of drugs for maintaining health or even life is fraught with peril. How would you price a "life-saving" drug?
	Are services and products subject to the same issues in price-setting?
Values	Valuation in consumer goods is quite variable based on any number of issues
	Choose one luxury brand versus staple types of goods. How do you quantify value as it relates to QOL?
Ethical issues	Should rich and poor be allowed to have access to medicines and products that extend life?

teaching QOL in marketing and provide suggestions on how those in marketing education can think about building a variety of applications into a marketing course framework. Shapiro (2012) and Radford et al. (2015) have noted the business school accrediting organization (AACSB) has set QOL-related topics such as sustainability and ethics, as topical priorities. This call crosses a variety of borders, both international and disciplinary studies. Pantelic, Akal, and Zehetner (2016) has advocated engaging students regarding these issues in the classroom. They argue that students are the future decision makers in regard to sustainable business practices. Consequently, students should be involved now and primed to make informed decisions in critical discussions regarding these issues in the future.

As it turns out though, currently very few of the top schools have these topical courses in their curriculum. In other words, it seems that the managerial focus of micromarketing has refused to yield curriculum space in programs. In addition, the paucity of these types of courses might also be the victim of an external market driven by program content and time demands. These external demands also have led to the stream lining of programs built on specific marketing "skill sets," such as data analytics and a continuing demand for degree programs (especially at the graduate level) whose hour requirements have been reduced to allow for quicker completion of degrees.

As noted at the very beginning of this chapter, marketing has historically been linked to the idea of consumer well-being and delivering goods and services that, by definition, is designed to enhance consumers' lives and contribute positive to society at large. That should also be viewed within the context of long-term environmental sustainability.

A number of authors from the marketing education field have provided suggestions on how to create better learning experiences in the classroom for teaching not only QOL-focused content, but a myriad of other marketing-related content. For example, several macromarketing scholars have offered a variety of suggestions to demonstrate and highlight aspects of well-being marketing to practitioners and students alike. For example, Shapiro (2008a, b, 2012) suggested the development of online course offerings that would then be posted online to allow free access to any interested parties with internet availability. There are also suggestions by Radford et al. (2015) for a variety of experiential learning projects (see Elam and Spotts 2004) that can be used to help frame the complex and constantly evolving markets and their relationships with consumers and society.

Macromarketers are being joined in their advocacy with marketing education scholars for broader stakeholder-focused/long-term goals and measures in the marketing curriculum. Lee and Benza (2015) have offered a good summary of the need to expand our traditional managerial focus into the field of Design Logic. They present a template for the development and application in a graduate course. Taylor and Judson (2014) have provided an excellent exploration concerning the need for marketing education to evolve the current curriculum (which is currently based on the short-term managerial view) into a more societal, sustainable, and QOL curriculum. The article offers a set of 28 propositions regarding the need for marketing education to not only be addressing the traditional short-term marketization teaching structure but to also embrace a more enlightened long-term view that includes such QOL elements such as "eudaimonic happiness" and other measures such as "flourishing." Readers of this chapter are urged to spend the time to read the Taylor and Judson (2014) piece in its entirety.

Next Steps

In this chapter we made an attempt to provide a quick look at how educators in the marketing discipline can better identify and use well-being concepts and measures in the teaching of marketing. The chapter touched upon a variety of tools to help educators understand how well-being marketing can be a useful tool for decision making by marketers in both strategic and tactical situations. As noted in various places in this chapter, marketing education has historically been focused on the micro/managerial perspective in both theory and application. This more narrow focus has produced students who often cannot see the systemic nature of marketing in the greater systems of consumers, markets, and society. In a time when business needs to reach across a wide variety of academic and public policy domains, we find ourselves stymied by an outdated system of "silos" within academe. These silos limit professors, researchers, and our students in thinking to be innovative and forward looking in confronting marketing problems in an ever-changing world. It is up to us all to engage the leadership at both the local, national, and global levels to be cognizant of the value and contribution to the long-term well-being of the discipline itself and its interface with society. Only then will we be able to effectively continue our quest to "make consumer's lives better" and strive to meet George Fisk's challenge to "Save the world."

References

American Marketing Association. *Common language marketing dictionary.* http://marketing-dictionary.org/. Accessed Oct 2018.

Ashton, J. K., & Hudson, R. S. (2017). The price, quality and distribution of mortgage payment protection insurance: A hedonic pricing approach. *British Accounting Review, 49*(2), 242–255.

Barber, N. (2012). Consumers' intention to purchase environmentally friendly wines: A segmentation approach. *International Journal of Hospitality & Tourism Administration, 13*(1), 26–47.

Bartels, R. (1976). *The history of marketing thought* (2nd ed.). Columbus: Grid, Inc.

Beauchamp, T. L. (1999). Ethical theory and bioethics. In L. Beauchamp & L. Walters (Eds.), *Contemporary issues in bioethics* (3rd ed.). Belmont: Wadsworth Publishing Company.

Benton, R. (1985). Micro bias and macro prejudice in the teaching of marketing. *Journal of Macromarketing, 5*(2), 43–38.

Benton, R. (1987). The practical domain of marketing: The notion of a 'free' enterprise market economy as a guise for institutionalized marketing power. *The American Journal of Economics and Sociology, 46*(4), 415–430.

Borch, F. J. (1957). The marketing philosophy as a way of business life. In *The marketing concept: Its meaning to management* (Marketing series no. 99) (pp. 3–5). New York: American Management Association. (Reprinted in Classics in Marketing edited by C. Glenn Walters and Donald Robin. Santa Monica, CA: Goodyear Publishing Company, 1978, pp. 385–96).

Brock, D. W. (2006). How much is more life worth? *Hastings Center Report, 36*(3), 17–19.

Brown, P. R. (2011). The dark side of hope and trust: Constructed expectations and the value-for-money regulation of new medicines. *Health Sociology Review, 20*(4), 410–422.

Brownel, G. H. (1916) *Brownel's dairy farmer.* Vol. 7.

Butaney, G., & Wortzel, L. H. (1988). Distributor power versus manufacturer power: The customer role. *The Journal of Marketing, 52*, 52–63.

Cannon, J. P., & Perreault, W. D., Jr. (1999). Buyer-seller relationships in business markets. *Journal of Marketing Research, XXXVI,* 439–460.

Chen, L., Gong, T., Kosinski, M., Stillwell, D., & Davidson, R. L. (2017). Building a profile of subjective well-being for social media users. *PLoS One, 12*(11), 1–15.

Constantinescu, M. (2011). The relationship between quality of life and marketing ethics. *Romanian Journal of Marketing, 6*(3), 41–44.

Cooper, R. (2005). Ethics and altruism: What constitutes socially responsible design? *Design Management Review, 16*(3), 10–18.

Elam, E. L. R., & Spotts, H. (2004). Achieving marketing curriculum integration: A live case study approach. *Journal of Marketing Education, 26*(1), 50–65.

Fisk, G. (2001). "Reflections of George Fisk" (from plenary session presentation at the 2001 Macromarketing Conference). *Journal of Macromarketing, 21*(2), 121–122.

Foerster, M., & Röösli, M. (2017). A latent class analysis on adolescents media use and associations with health related quality of life. *Computers in Human Behavior, 71*, 266–274.

Garrison, L. P., Jr. (2009). Editorial: On the benefits of modeling using QALYs for societal resource allocation: The model is the message. *Value in Health, 12*, S36–S37.

Hudders, L., & Pandelaere, M. (2012). The silver lining of materialism: The impact of luxury consumption on subjective well-being. *Journal of Happiness Studies, 13*(3), 411–437.

Jiang, S. (2017). The role of social media use in improving cancer survivors' emotional well-being: A moderated mediation study. *Journal of Cancer Survivorship, 11*(3), 386–392.

Kantak, D. M., Futrell, C. M., & Sager, J. K. (1992). Job satisfaction and life satisfaction in a sales force. *Journal of Personal Selling & Sales Management, 12*(1), 1–18.

Karpman, D., & Höglund, P. (2017). Orphan drug policies and use in pediatric nephrology. *Pediatric Nephrology, 32*(1), 1–6.

Kasser, T., & Sheldon, K. M. (2000). Of wealth and death: Materialism, mortality salience, and consumption behavior. *Psychological Science, 11*(4), 348–351.

Konu, H. (2015). Developing forest-based well-being tourism products by using virtual product testing. *Anatolia: An International Journal of Tourism & Hospitality Research, 26*(1), 99–102.

Korgaonkar, P. K. (1984). Consumer shopping orientations, non-store retailers, and consumers' patronage intentions: A multivariate investigation. *Journal of the Academy of Marketing Science, 12*(1–2), 11–22.

Kotler, P. (1979). Axioms for societal marketing. In G. Fisk, J. Arndt, & K. Gronharg (Eds.), *Future directions for marketing* (pp. 33–41). Boston: Marketing Science Institute.

Kotler, P. (1987). Humanistic marketing: Beyond the marketing concept. In A. Firat, N. Dholakia, & R. Bagozzi (Eds.), *Philosophical and radical thought in marketing* (pp. 271–288). Lexington: Lexington Book.

Kozak, V. (2013). Analysis of reasons for beer consumption drop in the Czech Republic. *Ekonomie a Management, 16*(3), 130–138.

Kyureghian, G., & Nayga, R. M., Jr. (2013). Food store access, availability, and choice when purchasing fruits and vegetables. *American Journal of Agricultural Economics, 95*(5), 1280–1286.

Lee, C. K., & Benza, R. (2015). Teaching innovation skills: Application of design thinking in a graduate marketing course. *Business Education Innovation Journal, 7*(1), 43–50.

Lee, D. J., & Sirgy, M. J. (2004). Quality-of-life (QOL) marketing: Proposed antecedents and consequences. *Journal of Macromarketing, 24*(1), 44–58.

Loo, J., Shi, Y., Pu, X., & Loo, J. M. Y. (2016). Gambling, drinking and quality of life: Evidence from Macao and Australia. *Journal of Gambling Studies, 32*(2), 391–407.

Lowery, B. C., & Sloane, D. C. (2014). The prevalence of harmful content on outdoor advertising in Los Angeles: Land use, community characteristics, and the spatial inequality of a public health nuisance. *American Journal of Public Health, 104*(4), 658–673.

Lu, J. (2018). The value of a south-facing orientation: A hedonic pricing analysis of the Shanghai housing market. *Habitat International, 81*, 24–32.

Maynard, S., James, D., & Davidson, A. (2010). The development of an ecosystem services framework for South East Queensland. *Environmental Management, 45*(5), 881–895.

McKitterick, J. B. (1957). What is the marketing management concept? In F. M. Bass (Ed.), *The frontiers of marketing thought and science* (pp. 71–82). Chicago: American Marketing Association.

Mulki, J. P., Locander, W. B., Mairshall, G. W., Harris, E. G., & Hensel, J. (2008). Workplace isolation, salesperson commitment, and job performance. *Journal of Personal Selling & Sales Management, 28*(1), 67–78.

Nguyen, M. T., Rahtz, D. R., & Shultz, C. J. (2014). Tourism as catalyst for quality of life in transitioning subsistence marketplaces: Perspectives from Ha Long, Vietnam. *Journal of Macromarketing, 34*(1), 28–44.

O'Connor, G. E. (2018). The relationships of competition and demographics to the pricing of health insurance premiums in Affordable Care Act-era health insurance markets. *Journal of Public Policy & Marketing, 37*(1), 88–105.

Olbrich, R., Jansen, H. C., & Teller, B. (2016). Quantifying anti-consumption of private labels and national brands: Impacts of poor test ratings on consumer purchases. *Journal of Consumer Affairs, 50*(1), 145–165.

Olson, J. G., McFerran, B., Morales, A. C., & Dahl, D. W. (2016). Wealth and welfare: Divergent moral reactions to ethical consumer choices. *Journal of Consumer Research, 42*(6), 879–896.

Padua Filho, W., & Padua, G. (2016). How much should cost a medical consultation? A marketing analysis from the viewpoint of health sector in Brazil. *International Journal of Healthcare Management, 9*(2), 127–133.

Pantelic, D., Sakal, M., & Zehetner, A. (2016). Marketing and sustainability from the perspective of future decision makers. *South African Journal of Business Management, 47*(1), 37–52.

Parker, R. S., & Pettijohn, C. E. (2003). Ethical considerations in the use of direct-to-consumer advertising and pharmaceutical promotions: The impact on pharmaceutical sales and physicians. *Journal of Business Ethics, 48*(3), 279–290.

Pine, B. J., & Davis, S. (1993). Mass customization: The new frontier in business competition. *IBM Systems Journal, 32*, 40–64.

Porter, S. S., Comb, C. C., & Kraft, F. B. (2008). Salesperson wellness lifestyle: A measurement perspective. *Journal of Personal Selling & Sales Management, 28*(1), 53–66.

Powers, T. L. (2015). Forgotten classics: Marketing methods by Ralph Starr Butler (1918). *Journal of Historical Research in Marketing, 7*(4), 584–592.

Press, M., & Arnould, E. J. (2009). Constraints on sustainable energy consumption: Market system and public policy challenges and opportunities. *Journal of Public Policy & Marketing, 28*(1), 102–113.

Radford, S. K., Hunt, D. M., & Andrus, D. (2015). Experiential learning projects. *Journal of Macromarketing, 35*(4), 466–472.

Ridgway, N. M., Kukar-Kinney, M., & Monroe, K. B. (2008). An expanded conceptualization and a new measure of compulsive buying. *Journal of Consumer Research, 35*(4), 622–639.

Rook, D. W. (1987). The buying impulse. *Journal of Consumer Research, 14*(2), 189–199.

Rust, R. T., Moorman, C., & Dickson, P. R. (2002). Getting return on quality: Revenue expansion, cost reduction, or both? *Journal of Marketing, 66*(4), 7–24.

Salari, M., & Bhuiyan, N. (2018). A new model of sustainable product development process for making trade-offs. *International Journal of Advanced Manufacturing Technology, 94*(1–4), 1–11.

Sandeen, C. (2009). It's not easy being green: Green marketing and environmental consumerism in continuing higher education. *Continuing Higher Education Review, 73*, 93–113.

Sandhu, N. (2015). Persuasive advertising and boost in materialism: Impact on quality of life. *IUP Journal of Management Research, 14*(4), 44–60.

Sashi, C. M. (2012). Customer engagement, buyer-seller relationships, and social media. *Management Decision, 50*(2), 253–272.

Segar, M. L., Updegraff, J. A., Zikmund-Fisher, B. J., & Richardson, C. R. (2012). Physical activity advertisements that feature daily well-being improve autonomy and body image in overweight women but not men. *Journal of Obesity, 2012*, 1–19.

Shapiro, S. J. (2008a). An open source, controversies-based macromarketing: An initial step toward a free online macromarketing course? *Journal of Macromarketing, 28*(4), 426–428.

Shapiro, S. J. (2008b). Marketing, society, and controversy: An online course from a macromarketing perspective. *Journal of Macromarketing, 28*(2), 195–196.

Shapiro, S. J. (2012). Macromarketing teaching materials: A forty-year retrospective. *Journal of Macromarketing, 32*(4), 412–416.

Sharma, P., Sivakumaran, B., & Marshall, R. (2010). Impulse buying and variety seeking: A trait-correlates perspective. *Journal of Business Research, 63*(3), 276–283.

Shepherd, C. D., Tashchian, A., & Ridnour, R. E. (2011). An investigation of the job burnout syndrome in personal selling. *Journal of Personal Selling & Sales Management, 31*(4), 397–410.

Shultz, C. J. (2007). Marketing as constructive engagement. *Journal of Public Policy & Marketing, 26*(2), 293–301.

Siguaw, J. A., Simpson, P. M., & Baker, T. L. (1998). Effects of supplier market orientation on distributor market orientation and the channel relationship: The distributor perspective. *Journal of Marketing, 62*, 99–111.

Sirgy, M. J. (1996). Strategic marketing planning guided by the quality-of-life (QOL) concept. *Journal of Business Ethics, 15*(3), 241–259.

Sirgy, M. J. (2001). *Handbook of quality-of-life research: An ethical marketing perspective.* Dordrecht: Springer.

Sirgy, M. J., & Lee, D. J. (1996). Setting socially responsible marketing objectives: A quality-of-life approach. *European Journal of Marketing, 30*(5), 20–34.

Sirgy, M. J., & Lee, D.-J. (2008). Well-being marketing: An ethical business philosophy for consumer goods firms. *Journal of Business Ethics, 77*(4), 377–403.

Sirgy, M., Yu, G., Lee, D.-J., Wei, S., & Huang, M.-W. (2012). Does marketing activity contribute to a society's well-being? The role of economic efficiency. *Journal of Business Ethics, 107*(2), 91–102.

Sotamaa, Y. (2009). The Kyoto design declaration: Building a sustainable future. *Design Issues, 25*(4), 51–53.

Spector, R. (2005). *Category killers: The retail revolution and its impact on consumer culture.* Cambridge, MA: Harvard Business Press.

Spence, M. (1986). Cost reduction, competition and industry performance. In *New developments in the analysis of market structure* (pp. 475–518). London: Palgrave Macmillan.

Stewart, K. A., & Neumann, P. J. (2002). FDA actions against misleading or unsubstantiated economic and quality-of-life promotional claims: An analysis of warning letters and notices of violation. *Value in Health, 5*(5), 389–402.

Taylor, S. A., & Judson, K. (2014). The nature of stakeholder satisfaction with marketing education. *Higher Education Studies, 4*(4), 89–107.

Vargo, S. L., Maglio, P. P., & Akaka, M. A. (2008). On value and value co-creation: A service systems and service logic perspective. *European Management Journal, 26*(3), 145–152.

Vokey, M., Tefft, B., & Tysiaczny, C. (2013). An analysis of hyper-masculinity in magazine advertisements. *Sex Roles, 68*(9–10), 562–576.

Webb, K. L., & Hogan, J. E. (2002). Hybrid channel conflict: Causes and effects on channel performance. *The Journal of Business & Industrial Marketing, 17*(5), 338–356.

Weinstein, E. (2018). The social media see-saw: Positive and negative influences on adolescents' affective well-being. *New Media & Society, 20*(10), 3597–3623.

Witkowski, T. H., & Jones, D. G. B. (2016). Historical research in marketing: Literature, knowledge, and disciplinary status. *Information & Culture, 51*(3), 399–418.

Wong, F. K. Y., So, C., Ng, A. Y. M., Lam, P.-T., Ng, J. S. C., Ng, N. H. Y., et al. (2018). Cost-effectiveness of a transitional home-based palliative care program for patients with end-stage heart failure. *Palliative Medicine, 32*(2), 476–484.

Don R. Rahtz, Ph.D., is a marketing researcher and is the J.S. Mack Professor of Marketing at The College of William and Mary in the USA. He has traveled and worked extensively in the developing and transitional world. His expertise is in integrated marketing communication programs, international competitive intelligence, cultural intelligence, situational awareness, and market assessment. He has had a particular interest in Quality of Life (QOL), environmental issues, economic sustainable development, transitional economies, business/community interface evaluation, and health systems.

M. Joseph Sirgy, Ph.D., is a marketing professor and is the Virginia Tech Real Estate Professor of Marketing at Virginia Polytechnic Institute & State University in the USA. He has published extensively in the areas of consumer behavior, marketing and quality of life, and business ethics. He is also the executive director of the Management Institute for Quality-of-Life Studies (MIQOLS) and is currently helping organizations develop better policies and strategies to enhance consumer well-being, employee well-being, and community well-being.

Stephan Grzeskowiak, Ph.D., is an associate professor of marketing at the NEOMA Business School in France. His research interests include marketing and quality of life, consumer well-being, housing well-being, and marketing channels.

Dong-Jin Lee, Ph.D. is a professor of marketing at Yonsei University, Seoul, Korea. His research interests include consumer well-being and quality-of-life studies. His research has been published in the *Social Indicator Research, Journal of Business Ethics, Journal of Marketing, Journal of the Academy of Marketing Science, International Journal of Research in Marketing, Journal of Advertising*, and among others. He has served as the vice president for the International Society for Quality-of-Life Studies (ISQOLS).

Chapter 8
Training Statisticians in the Field of Quality of Life: A New Challenge for the University System. The Case of Qolexity in Italy

Filomena Maggino

"QoLexity" is a neologism, coined on the occasion of first international workshop of the Italian Association for Quality-of-Life Studies (AIQUAV) which was held in September 2011 in Florence (cfr. 2). It refers to a complex approach to Quality of Life (defined QoLexity), covering the issues of defining, measuring, monitoring and analysing the quality of life in quantitative terms, and involving different academic disciplines (philosophy, sociology, psychology, statistics, economics, politics sciences). Hence, the program was built adopting a logic leading from concept definition to statistical indicators, a guiding concept which is "complexity", and an approach that leads from research questions to data to analysis and communication of results.

The post-master program aimed at developing the well-known "knowledge triangle", putting into practice the linkage between innovation (new approaches and new skills in statistics), education(taking into account the need to provide methodologies to define, measure analyse and communicate new issue) and research (also through practical experiences and traineeships).

The Italian BES Project

Among all the initiatives that in this perspective are held around the world and in Italy, we would like to remind the national consultation started jointly by ISTAT and with the National Council for Economics and Labor (CNEL) to identify a shared set of indicators of the progress of Italian society.

A project, called Bessere Equo e Sostenibile – BES (Equitable and Sustainable Wellbeing), has been developed in Italy to identify a shared measurement of

F. Maggino (✉)
Sapienza University of Rome, Rome, Italy
e-mail: filomena.maggino@uniroma1.it

© Springer Nature Switzerland AG 2020   155
G. H. Tonon (ed.), *Teaching Quality of Life in Different Domains*, Social
Indicators Research Series 79, https://doi.org/10.1007/978-3-030-21551-4_8

well-being at the national level, to become a reference point for public debate and to be used to guide important democratic choices for the country's future. (Giovannini et al. 2012) In order to define the essential elements of well-being in Italy, the Italian National Council for Economics and Labour (Cnel) – whose members include representatives from associations, trade unions and the third sector, and the Italian National Institute of Statistics (Istat) set up a "Steering Committee for the measurement of progress in the Italian society" composed of representatives from social partners and the civil society aimed at defining the domains of societal wellbeing. Furthermore, Istat established a large and qualified Scientific Commission of experts with the aim of defining the indicators able to monitor wellbeing in the identified domains.

The institutional approach meets the wide shared idea that there are two crucial components allowing the wellbeing measurement: the first, strictly political, relates to the definition of the concept of well-being; the second, technical-scientific, concerns the definition of the element to be observed in order to measure the relevant concepts. As a result, CNEL, a constitutional body representing the civil society and Istat, an institution where experts operate in order to measure different domains (economic, social and environmental) of the country's life, combined their forces to define a process and construct a system of indicators.

The concepts adopted in order to define the country wellbeing try to conciliate

 (i) The individual level of wellbeing (*quality of life*, to be observed and monitored at individual/micro level)
(ii) The community level of wellbeing (*quality of society*, to be observed and monitored at societal/macro level).

The relationship between the individual (subjective and objective) wellbeing and the wellbeing of the society is explored by considering two issues. On one hand, even though the concept of "community wellbeing" could be covered by referring to aggregation of individual outcomes, the simple sum of all individuals' wellbeing composing that community cannot represent in itself the wellbeing of the whole community, which should include also other different characteristics. On the other hand, the discussion concerns if pursuing community's wellbeing requires a compromise between individuals' wellbeing. In other words, it should be verified whether any individual wellbeing is pursued at the expense of other individuals' wellbeing.

Two particular conceptual perspectives have been adopted able to monitor the quality of wellbeing, by considering the promotion and preservation of the fairness wellbeing distribution (*equity*) and the limits and opportunities of its promotion (*sustainability*).

Actually, equity and sustainability represent a particular lens allowing us to understand the limits and adequacy of wellbeing promotion and growth. In particular, the adoption of the two concepts allows the level of wellbeing to be monitored by checking if wellbeing is not distributed and has been promoted at the expenses of future generations' wellbeing.

The great innovation of BES is represented by the process of construction which involved both the civil society and several national experts.

In 2010, the Steering Committee defined the wellbeing domains. This process also benefited from the support of a survey on a representative sample of 45 thousand individuals (February 2011). Each interviewed expressed the importance – through a 0-to-10 score – of each domain included in a list of 15. Such a wide and representative consultation – involving all population strata – took place only in Italy. Following, the Steering Committee was able to approve the final list of 12 wellbeing domains by taking into account citizens' opinion and civil society' sensitiveness.

The domains are distinguished in two groups, those in which the wellbeing represents outcome of wellbeing (health, education, work, economic wellbeing, social relations, security, subjective wellbeing, environment, landscape and cultural heritage) and those which represent sectors functional to the promotion of country's wellbeing (politics and institutions, research and innovation, and quality of services). It deserves to be pointed out that BES has been the first national project identifying the landscape and cultural heritage as crucial domain for the wellbeing of a country.

The Scientific Committee selected and defined the indicators for each domain, by taking into account some general indications (such as, having both objective and subjective indicators in each domain, non ambiguity in measuring wellbeing, timeliness and continuity in production, national specificities, and so on).

The two committees discussed the list of indicators in order to reach the final selection (130) by assigning each indicator to only one domain, also in those cases allowing multiple assignments).

A permanent working group has been established at Istat aimed at monitoring the indicators also from the methodological point of view. A synthesis of the indicators belonging to each domain has been experimented by ensuring comparability across regional territories, over time and involving conceptually uncorrelated indicators. The synthesis methodology has been adopted by comparing different approaches and discussing the results not only in the ambit of the Scientific Committee but also in several scientific occasions.

A New Post–Master Program

The Need of New Training Project in the Field of Statistics

The lesson imparted by the BES project to all of us is that indicators are not enough. In order to let the idea of using new beyond-GDP indicators at any level of the society (including the political and policy level) can work and go on if also other actions are promoted and managed.

In this perspective, among others, two institutions are strategic, the National Institute of Statistics[1] from one hand and the education and university system on the other hand.

With reference to the latter, it is important to promote not only a wide culture about wellbeing measures and their statistical implications but also:

(i) A wide and continuous scientific debate involving scholars in a multidisciplinary environment.

(ii) New training projects allowing the complete the background of statisticians (and not only) which would need to manage systems of indicators monitoring the wellbeing of population in the ambit of official statistics and not only.

Following this idea, in 2010 the Italian Association for Quality-of-Life Studies (AIQUAV) has been founded (www.aiquav.it) and since then it organizes regular annual conferences as well as other activities also in partnership with other organizations.

In September 2011, AIQUAV organized its first international workshop in Florence a workshop (http://www.aiquav.it/index.php/aiquav-lab/workshop) for which a neologism was coined, "QoLexity".

It refers to the complex approach to Quality of Life definition, analysis and communication and has been discussed at that workshop by many scholars and experts. The discussion produced a new interdisciplinary approach (defined QoLexity), identified in order to define, measure, monitor and analyse the quality of life in quantitative terms, and involving different academic disciplines (philosophy, sociology, psychology, statistics, economics, politics sciences).

The Knowledge Triangle: Innovation, Education and Research

Following that discussion, the University of Florence and the Italian National Institute of Statistics agreed upon the necessity to build a new educational program, which takes into account that complexity. They identified in the second level post-master program[2] the right formula addressing that need.[3]

---

[1] The Institute is different from the Office since it institutionally has a relative more independency from the government. In fact, it has a President while the Office has a Director General.

[2] According to the Italian University system, the access to the second level master is possible to anyone in possession of a qualification corresponding to bachelor's degree (3-year degree) + master degree (2-year degree).

[3] An interesting experience provided some inspiration for this proposal. During the IX conference of the International Society of Quality of Life Studies (ISQOLS), held in Florence in 2009, July 19–23 (among the special collateral events, a training course was organized on 'Statistics, Knowledge and Policy', fruit of a cooperation between the OECD – Global Project on Measuring the Progress of Societies, Joint Research Centre (JRC) of the European Commission and the International Society for Quality of Life Studies (ISQOLS). The training course was held from 14th to 17th of July and attended by people from 12 different countries and with many different professional backgrounds (economic, social and statistical).

The program tried to develop the well-known "knowledge triangle", describing the linkage between innovation, education and research.

Innovation: The Goal of the University Program

The debate on defining new measures of societal progress and well-being (*beyond GDP* movement) highlighted a new role for the National Statistical Offices (NSOs).

To this end, we can remind the Istanbul Declaration, signed during the II OECD World Forum on "Statistics, Knowledge and Policy" (2007) by the representatives of the European Commission, the Organisation for Economic Cooperation and Development, the Organisation of the Islamic Conference, the United Nations, the United Nations Development Programme and the World Bank, who agreed on the need for "statistical offices, public and private organisations, and academic experts to work alongside representatives of their communities to produce high-quality, facts-based information that can be used by all of society to form a shared view of societal well-being and its evolution over time. Official statistics are a key "public good" able to foster the progress of societies. The development of indicators of societal progress offers an opportunity to reinforce the role of national statistical authorities as key providers of relevant, reliable, valid, timely and comparable data and the indicators required for national and international reporting."

New challenges for NSOs arose also in terms of new and additional skills to be acquired. In other words, future statisticians working in NSOs should be able to develop new accurate and representative sets of progress measures for a society, particularly in the field of quality of life.

These new perspectives urged the need of new training programs (especially at academic level), providing new competences, requiring an interdisciplinary approach and new skills in managing statistics (at analytical, management and communication levels).

- Education: the organization of the university program

The conceptual leading idea used in order to frame the activities of the university program is related to "complexity": the measurement and analysis of quality of life and societal wellbeing need a compound narrative of the reality which needs to be (i) defined, (ii) measured, (iii) analysed, and (iv) communicated.

- Research: the university program as a cooperative experience

The post-master program provided students with specific research competences, also through practical experiences and traineeships, held in cooperation with prestigious institutions and organizations (such as, ISTAT, Eurostat, OECD). This experience allowed not only students to experience a direct work on official data but also the institutions and organizations to develop particular activities (e.g., deeper analyses of existing data). This was accomplished in cooperation between experts from NSOs and academic researchers by taking into account the emerging new needs.

QoLexity: Contents and Didactic Organization

The university post-master program developed four main topics, addressing different questions as represented in Table 8.1.

Access to the post-master program was reserved to students in possession of any second level degree (master degree) who had in their curriculum studiorum at least one exam in Statistics.

The post-master program provided 60 Credits[4] composed by

- 42 credits provided by didactics (252 h)[5]
- 13 credits provided by traineeship (13 credits × 25 h = 325 h)
- 5 credits provided by the thesis.

A mixed didactic formula was developed, (i) traditional lesson (first part: teacher's lesson; second part: open discussion), (ii) work exercise (first part: teacher's illustration of the work to be accomplished; second part: group work).

The 42 credits provided by **didactic** were developed in **four areas**.

A. Concepts and tools Total: 7 credits – 42 h

- Towards a common language: general concepts and their meanings
- Quality of life and related concepts

Table 8.1 QoLexity: topics addressed by the post-master program

Quality of life	Conceptual definitions	How can complexity be conceptually revealed and constructed?
		How can QoL be defined?
		How can QoL be defined through indicators?
	Data sources and collection	How can data be found?
		How can data be collected?
		What are the main technical issues?
	Analytical tools and strategies	How can the observed pictures be reconstructed?
	Allowing the whole picture to be reconstructed	How can the whole picture be simplified and shown?
	Findings' comunication and dissemination	How can the whole picture be represented?
		How can the whole picture be communicated?
		How can knowledge be transferred into policy?

---

[4] In the Italian University System, each credit corresponds to 6–12 h of work (lessons, individual study, laboratory, and so on).

[5] According to the University-of-Florence rules, the 42 credits should be delivered by professors belonging to the University of Florence (at least for the 60%, 25, of the credits) and external teachers (max. 40%, 17, of the credits). Moreover, a minimum of 6 credits are assigned to each subject.

B. Data Total: 12 credits – 72 h

- Quality-of-Life data
- Data collection:

C. Analytical approachesTotal 15 credits – 90 h

- Indicators: from reality to reading the reality
- Indicators: analytical tools and strategies
- Quality-of-life data analysis: pathways to modelling
- Quality-of-life data analysis: looking for explanations
- Making all concrete

D. Representing and communicating Total 8 credits – 48 h

- Representing quality-of-life data and results
- Communicating quality-of-life results
- Putting all together

The 13 credits provided by **traineeship** were obtained through not-paid stages. Different organizations offered their availability in this perspective, of course the Italian National Institute of Statistics (ISTAT), but also EUROSTAT (2 positions per Academic Year), OECD, EUROFOUND, Region of Tuscany (different agencies: IRPET ARS, ARPAT). Students were free to contact also other institutions and organizations if available.

Students started their traineeship against the submission of a project illustrating the activity to be realized at the identified external organization. Generally, the student's project was shared by the coordinator of the post-master program and the officials belonging to the external organization. The traineeship could started after the approval of the submitted project.

The involved professors were mainly from the University of Florence and the Italian National Institute of Statistics but also from other academic (and not only) institutions (European Commission, LUISS – Rome, OECD, University "Bocconi", University of Milan – Bicocca, University of Pisa, University of Rome "La Sapienza", University of Rome "Tor-Vergata", University of Siena, and others).

Lessons

The lessons were organized on weekends (one per month) starting from January to October. Part of them were held in Florence and the other part in Rome.

Individualized Paths

In order to get the final certification, students had to attend the whole program. In specific cases, the students decided (according to the University's rules) to attend only one or two modules, according to their individual needs and interests. In this case, the certification could not be granted.

QoLexity: Lessons from This Experience

The university post-master program QoLexity lasted for three academic year. Many changes in their role of the key players of the initiative[6] … demonstrating how much is important the individual involvement much more than institutional involvement.

Cooperating Perspectives

- Students had the opportunity to start a cooperation with AIQUAV, in which academic competences and professional experiences found a confluence with an open discussion and continuous improvement; in other words, synergies with AIQUAV created opportunities for jointly organizing workshops, lecturers, conferences, seminars;
- The convergence of numerous research skills and competences and different training experiences created occasions of interaction between the academic world and NSIs;
- The experiences could found a natural way out in different PhD programmes, where students, solidly trained in fundamental statistics and/or social research methodology, have the opportunity to get into more depth by focusing on issues strictly related to social statistics;
- Creating an interaction with the ISTAT and other international programmes, such as the European Master in Official Statistics, in the perspective of common training initiatives on specific aspects of this topic.

---

[6] During the third year of this experience the Rector of the University of Florence changed, the President of Istat changed and the coordinator left the University of Florence.

Working Perspectives

The post-master program provided the participants with professional expertise with reference to quality-of-life studies from the theoretical, methodological and practical point of view.

In particular, the **professional profile** addressed by the post-master program concerned an expert able to (i) manage quality of life concepts, (ii) handle existing data sources and plan new data collection, (iii) apply proper statistical methods and models, (iv) communicate relevant results in different contexts and to different audiences.

The reference **labour market** for this professional profile includes private companies and agencies as well as public institutions and organizations dealing with quality-of-life-related issues both at national and international levels.

The post-master program provided the participants with professional expertise with reference to quality-of-life studies from theoretical, methodological and practical point of view. This expertise can improve the professional profile of statisticians and communicators and can represent a good starting point also for future researchers in the field of quality-of-life studies.

Reference

Giovannini, E., Morrone, A., Rondinella, T., & Sabbadini, L. L. (2012). "L'iniziativa CNEL-ISTAT per la misurazione del Benessere Equo e Sostenibile in Italia" in *Autonomie locali e servizi sociali*, n. 1, Il Mulino, Bologna.

Filomena Maggino is Professor of Social Statistics at the Sapienza University of Rome, Italy. Counsellor of the Prime Minister Office (Italian Government – Conte's cabinet). Editor-in-Chief of *Social Indicators Research* and *Encyclopedia of Quality-of-Life and Well-being Research* (Springer). President and co-founder of the *Italian Association for Quality-of-Life Studies* (AIQUAV). Past-president of the *International Society for Quality-of-Life Studies* (ISQOLS). In the field of quality of life research and wellbeing measurement, she is expert in definition and construction of indicators and systems of indicators, statistics and complexity, synthesis of indicators as well as social indicators, Big Data and Official statistics, and representing and communicating complex data.

Chapter 9
Learning from Experience: Non-technical Teaching to Promote Quality of Life Statistics

Jon Hall

Measurements are important in determining national directions. As the economist Joseph Stiglitz remarked in 2009, "What we measure affects what we do. If we have the wrong metrics, we will strive for the wrong things. In the quest to increase GDP, we may end up with a society in which most citizens have become worse off" (Stiglitz 2009).

For a good deal of the twentieth Century many countries – and decisions-makers – worked with the tacit belief that national progress was synonymous with a growing economy. That is, if the GDP was up then quality of life should surely follow[1] (see for example Costanza et al. 2009). But recognition of the dangers of an overreliance on GDP have grown steadily more vocal in recent years with a good deal of work around the world underway to challenge GDP's hegemony, such as that from Stiglitz et al. (2009). Statisticians, economists and policy makers around the world are working to design and use alternative measures of human progress: measures which focus on outcomes of life quality, rather than simply inputs like economic activity. This chapter discusses some of the ways in which education and training can foster and support this work.

Any views expressed in this Chapter are of the author and are not representing views of the United Nations Development Programme, the Human Development Report Office nor of any other organization, agency or programme of the United Nations.

---

[1] To read more about these issues you can turn to Costanza et al. (2009) for example.

J. Hall (✉)
United Nations Development Program, New York Office, New York, NY, USA
e-mail: jonathan.hall@undp.org

© Springer Nature Switzerland AG 2020
G. H. Tonon (ed.), *Teaching Quality of Life in Different Domains*, Social Indicators Research Series 79, https://doi.org/10.1007/978-3-030-21551-4_9

Introduction

I start from a position that the world would be a better place if many decisions – by government, individuals and organizations – were shaped through greater attention to quality of life than they are at the moment. I also take it as self-evident that good decisions must be based – at least in part – on solid evidence. That in turns requires:

1. The production of quality of life statistics (QOLS); and
2. That the data are subsequently used appropriately to shape decision making.

What role can learning play in increasing both the supply and use of QOLS?

There are doubtless many ways in which education and training can and does play a role. There is plenty of quite focused – more traditional – technical training provided on subjects like "how to design a health survey" (Unite For Sight, 2018) that seek to improve the supply of data. Education is also important for promoting the informed analysis of available data, with professorships in disciplines such as quantitative social research methods (London School of Economics 2018), and universities offering courses in subjects like "Applied Urban Science and Informatics", "Data Analytics for Public Policy" and "Social Data Analytics" (Masters in Data Science 2018).

My focus here is on other forms of learning, primarily 'experiential learning' (learning through doing): after 20 years spent working in two governments and two international organisations I believe that the largest barriers to a greater use of QOLS in decision making are not created by a lack of technical capacity to produce or use the data. Nor do the barriers stem simply from a lack of demand, or a lack of supply. Rather, the roadblocks arise from a complex interplay of supply <u>and</u> demand and from the people and organisations that determine how statistics are produced and used. Education and training can, I believe, help overcome these challenges. This chapter describes some possible approaches.

I talk throughout this chapter about quality of life statistics, using that phrase as an umbrella term for a basket of data that encompasses broad themes such as 'societal progress' (OECD 2018), 'human development' (UNDP 2018) or 'well-being' (OECD 2017) all of which are variations on a similar theme, a theme that could be described as 'quality of life'. Each theme is a different prism through which to consider human progress in ways that go beyond a simple focus on metrics based on dollars and cents.

Supply and Demand and Demand and Supply

National Statistical Offices (NSOs) remain the prime source of data for government policy making. Their statistical collection and dissemination is organized and governed in different ways. Some, such as the Australian Bureau of Statistics operate as independent statutory authorities, with a good deal of independence from government (Australian Bureau of Statistics 2018). Others work in a closer relationship with government which can help to ensure the statistical work program is quicker to react to policy-makers changing demands but can also open the way to charges of politicization of official numbers, such as those levelled against Greece in 2009 (Willis 2010). But in almost all cases a national statistical office's work program – including the production of QOLS - is influenced, albeit to varying degrees, by the priorities of government and other data users. Indeed, if the work program is not influenced by user requirements it really ought to be (United Nations 2003). In other words, the supply of QOLS is influenced, at least in part, by the demand for them.

At the same time, it can be difficult for policy makers to see a value in something that they have no experience of using because it does not yet exist. And so the demand for quality of life statistics also depends on their supply.

How can we use training and education to square that circle and simultaneously encourage a demand for – and supply of – QOLS?

Education and Training for Whom?

Consider any topic, or situation, for which there is scope to make better use of QOLS. This might range from determining national economic policy through to the sort of information prospective homeowners ought to be aware of when considering a move to a new suburb. A useful first step is to consider why quality of life is not being sufficiently considered in decision making. Two questions are fundamental.

Question 1: If the data exists then why isn't it being used?

  (a) Is there a failure of analytical capacity? Potential users do not have the skills to analyze or interpret the existing data.
  (b) Is there a failure of communication? Potential users do not know the data is out there.
  (c) Is there a failure of demand? Potential users are not interested in considering the data. This might be from a resistance to change ("we've never looked at this in our briefing papers before"), a reluctance to upset the status quo ("the department of finance won't like this"), or from political considerations ("this government is interested in economic growth not wellbeing").

Question 2. If the data does not exist, then why isn't it being collected?

  (a) Is there a failure of statistical prioritization? Does the NSO feel the data is insufficiently important to be collected?
  (b) Is there a failure of political authorization? Is the NSO persuaded of the importance to collect the data, but feel the government would oppose the move?

Many other factors can also come into play. And it is very likely that the statistical landscape in any country has been carved out from these factors and many more including historical and cultural or from key personalities. But during conversations I have had over the past 20 years with data users and producers, from many sectors and many countries, these "failures" to produce or use QOLS seem common place. Sometimes the issues are real. Sometimes they are perceptions. Education and training can help tackle them. Here are some examples.

Putting a Spotlight on National Statistical Office Success

In 2002 the Australian Bureau of Statistics (ABS) released Measuring Australia's Progress (ABS 2002) "a publication built around a set of headline indicators that spanned economic, social and environmental concerns." (Hall 2005). The foreword to the publication notes that "Measuring Australia's Progress (MAP) is about Australia's progress. It is intended to help Australians address the question, 'Has life in our country got better, especially during the past decade?'", (ABS 2002), and goes onto claim that "Measuring a nation's progress – providing information about whether life is getting better – is one of the most important tasks that a national statistical agency can take on. For almost 100 years, the ABS has been measuring Australia's progress through the multitude of statistics we publish relating to Australia's economy, society and environment. However, for the most part, our statistical publications have tended to focus on each of these three broad areas in isolation."

This was a groundbreaking project for a government statistical agency: the first time that an NSO had sought to define and measure national progress by producing a "diverse collection of national progress indicators" (Pink et al. 2014). Not long after MAP was released I wrote, while working for the ABS, that the publication would likely not have been written had the ABS not had such a strong tradition of independence. I argued that as MAP was "quite politically sensitive" and required "some subjectivity" in its construction, "it would almost certainly have been very difficult to prepare a publication such as MAP without compromising our statistical integrity." (Hall 2005).

In other words, a less politically independent NSO might have been reluctant to undertake similar work for fear of a backlash from government, the media or others.

The publication was influential overseas. The ABS talked about the MAP experience in major international fora including the OECD's World Forum on Key Indicators in Palermo (Sicily) in 2004 (OECD 2005). And several organizations – including NSOs – went on to cite MAP as a key influence for related initiatives. For example, Measuring Ireland's Progress (Central Statistical Office 2003), the OECD's Global Project on Measuring the Progress of Society's (OECD 2018) and the Canadian Index of Wellbeing (Canadian Index of Wellbeing 2016) were all inspired at least in part by MAP. And this work in turn inspired others.

Inspiration for NSOs came – I believe – on at least two fronts. First, MAP helped convince NSOs that it was important for society to have a broader public debate about national progress and quality of life beyond measures of economic performance. Second, MAP demonstrated that NSOs had a legitimate role in promoting and informing such a debate. Statistical offices could turn to the Australian example to justify embarking on this work. See, for example, the foreword to Measuring Ireland's Progress which notes "There has been a considerable focus in the past couple of years at national, EU and international level in trying to devise a set of indicators which, taken together, broadly summarize the progress being made in achieving desirable outcomes for society". (Central Statistical Office, 2003)

> **Recommendation**
> The international official statistical community is a well-connected network. It is also the major source of QOLS. Showcasing the work of well-respected NSOs who have produced QOLS and demonstrating why that work is an important and a legitimate part of a statistical office's mission, is one important element of a strategy to educate about QOLS.

Bridging the Divide Between Users and Producers

Improving the dialogue between the users and producers of statistics is an important issue in many areas of statistics (see for example Medstat III 2013), including QOLS.

As the Medstat guidelines note "The value – for society – of an effective statistical system stems from the improvement it generates in informing debate and decision-making: statistics are only useful if they are used. That is not to say that statistics that are not used are necessarily useless: rather they may represent a wasted opportunity to shed light on important issues. It follows, therefore, that statisticians have a duty to ensure their numbers are used. That, in turn, requires engaging with users of statistics, to ensure that the following holds true: the outputs of a NSS are relevant and of appropriate quality for users' needs, and users are aware of those outputs and are able to use them appropriately." (Medstat III 2013).

This holds true for QOLS. But why is there not more engagement already?

My impressions – largely anecdotal but widespread – are that official statisticians in many countries often view policy public servants as

(a) Overly political (by which I mean acting in the best interest of their minister rather than the country);
(b) Holding unrealistic expectations about the speed with which data can be produced, or its accuracy.

Meanwhile many policy makers I have interacted with around the world view the government's statisticians as

(a) Cut off from the "real world" of having to answer to a minister;
(b) Slow, ponderous and overly cautious.

And, though my impressions are anecdotal, others have recognized a similar pattern of misunderstanding. In a 2007 report on using official statistics the United Kingdom's Statistics Commission wrote that "a few believe that, currently, ONS is insular in its way of working and would benefit most from improved consultation practices. '…ONS is a closed shop, that's the opinion from the contact I've had. What's done in ONS is done in ONS and the figures are produced and that's it – you live with them and they're the official statistics and that's the end of the discussion…'. The same report recommended that "improved communication between [statistical] producers and users would enhance mutual understanding of the pressures and constraints faced by each group." (Statistics Commission, 2007).

This is an important issue for efficient and effective government generally, but – for this paper – it is important for anyone seeking to encourage greater use of quality of life statistics.

Public servants, like statisticians, are usually working to achieve the same goal: working to make their country a better place. Yet when both groups have little interaction with each other this common purpose can be forgotten, and misunderstanding – even mistrust – can arise. When statisticians and policy makers collaborate on a report to assess quality of life it can increase the trust between the two groups. Teaching can also play a role.

> **Recommendation**
> I have run workshops specifically aimed at bridging the gap between the users and producers of statistics in Europe, North Africa and Sub-Saharan Africa. I have run many other workshops that have involved both users and producers of statistics. And the challenges I saw in Australia seem to play out just about everywhere: policy makers see statisticians as overly cautious and dogmatic; statisticians see policy makers as reckless and seeking political approval.

To tackle these stereotypes, I have run exercises that bring together statisticians and policy makers in a simulated meeting in which the government urgently needs data to respond to a political crisis. Data that the statistical office cannot produce quickly. The twist of the exercise is that the (real) policy makers play the statisticians in the meeting and vice versa. Participant feedback consistently suggests this is a popular exercise in many different places. It can have at least three outcomes.

First, people enjoy the role play: the exercise encourages participants to act out the meeting with wit, humor and exaggeration. This creates a lot of laughter.

Second, beyond the laughter, participants seem to finish with greater empathy for the other side: it is frustrating for bureaucrats (played by statisticians) to hear the numbers they require urgently will not be ready for at least a year; it is frustrating for statisticians (played by the bureaucrats) when those demanding the numbers don't understand how long it takes time to gather accurate statistical information.

Third, and perhaps most importantly, the enjoyment people take from working together on exercises like this can lead to new friendships and networks across the user-producer divide. This is good for increasing trust. It is good for dialogue. And ultimately good for the chances of using and producing more QOLS.

Valuing the QOLS Process (Not Just the Product)

Teaching QOLS often focuses on the product (the data and its analysis) and/or its uses. However the process of selecting the data – and analyzing it – can also be valuable, especially when it is undertaken in collaboration with a diverse group of stakeholders, including the wider community, whose quality of life you seek to measure. The benefits of this process can be attractive for policy makers and others, even if those same people might not be convinced by the value of QOLS alone. This can create a stronger demand for QOLS and so should be stressed when promoting QOLS.

A broad consultation process around a set of QOLS is desirable in both improving the quality of the product though "tapping into some of a nation's leading thinkers"; guarding against relying on the "potentially narrow viewpoint" of statisticians or bureaucrats"; and promoting the end use of the QOLS by fostering "a wider level of ownership and support for a project, which can help to ensure it achieves outcomes." (Hall et al. 2005)

A paper I co-wrote, published by the Bertelsmann Foundation in 2013, discusses such processes in detail, going beyond the direct benefits of a consultation process to consider a set of further – indirect and 'serendipitous' – benefits. It begins with the "belief that some of the most significant benefits of indicator initiatives are those that reach beyond the measures themselves. These benefits include those that arise from the exchanges that take place within a group that comes together to discuss the meaning of progress and how it should be measured. These exchanges can generate new relationships that yield unforeseeable gains for all." (Hall and Rickard 2013).

Our paper identified seven key "serendipitous" benefits that we grouped in into three clusters.

1. Strengthening the machinery of democracy: discussions on quality of life can facilitate deliberative democracy and the development of new paradigms of thinking. "They do so by providing citizens and policymakers alike new opportunity to discuss relevant concerns within a community, as well as the goals, values and future direction of society more generally."

2. Making the business of government easier: processes around selecting quality of life statistics often "require stakeholders to find common ground on sensitive and divisive issues. By rendering transparent the societal tradeoffs inherent to the political economy of reform, these processes help raise awareness regarding the often difficult choices that need to be made. These processes also involve infor-

mal networks and cross-cutting relationships that ultimately encourage joined-up thinking in government."
3. Building a society's capacity to advance well-being (or quality of life). Projects measuring progress or quality of life "build a society's capacity to effectively develop capabilities (i.e., the opportunity to do and be what is deemed valuable in a community) and advance accountability among individuals and institutions alike. They do so in part by providing the framework and resources by which members of a community develop skills in debate, mediation and consensus-building. Regular reviews and benchmarking help ensure that the community as well as government agencies remain accountable for their decisions and actions. Because the processes driving these indicator initiatives frequently involve friction and exchange among different or competing interests, they often spark innovations in social organization or technology and result in changed behavior."

These benefits might be attractive to policy makers in different ministries, including many who might not have any particular interest in otherwise measuring quality of life. Moreover, the very act of teaching quality of life – do a broad group of stakeholders – might also create some of these benefits.

> **Recommendation**
> Stressing the many potential benefits of the process of compiling a set of QOLS can help sell the idea inside and outside government. Moreover, the very act of educating a broad group of stakeholders about QOLS can begin to create some of these benefits.

Creating an International Community

Running workshops in dozens of countries around the world has persuaded me that many of the issues faced by those seeking to use or produce QOLS are common across countries. Talking to an international group of practitioners can be a powerful way to teach QOLS, but in these situations I believe the most important learning comes from peer to peer conversations among the participants rather than from facilitator to participant. Hearing a lecturer say "In such and such a situation, one should do this" may or may not be helpful. Hearing a participant say "The same thing happened in our country. We ended up doing X and Y and the problem was resolved." seems to resonate far more with workshop participants. And so building an international community can provide a source of ongoing advice which participants can benefit from during the workshop and beyond if they stay in contact. Maintaining the network after the workshop finishes is not always easy: it requires ongoing effort and follow up conversations and more opportunities to meet face to face.

Networks can range from informal Facebook groups and email lists, through to a stream of work and events such as the OECD's Global Project on Measuring the Progress of Societies (OECD 2007a).

> **Recommendation**
> Regional or global workshops can create communities that become an important source of advice and experience upon which others can draw. Maintaining and growing such communities can take some effort and resources, but a face to face meeting is an important element to getting them off the ground.

From Data to Action: The Importance of Communication

Promoting the use of QOLS goes beyond simply encouraging supply and demand. Ensuring the necessary statistics are available, and that there is a demand for them from policy and decision makers is a necessary step. But it is not sufficient to ensure the statistics will be used. Many other factors will determine whether this will happen. Societies need, for instance, policy makers who value data and can readily obtain the statistics they require and easily understand the numbers and their limitations. This is sometimes not the case.

I argued earlier that data producers have an important and legitimate role in seeking to ensure the data they produce are used because statistics are only useful if they are used. (Medstat III 2013). The United Nation's Fundamental Principles of Official Statistics are a touchstone for NSO's around the world. The principles deal primarily with the production of statistics rather than their use. And when they do discuss use, the emphasis is on minimizing the risk of user-error, rather than maximizing the use of the data. For example, Principle 3 states "To facilitate a correct interpretation of the data, the statistical agencies are to present information according to scientific standards on the sources, methods and procedures of the statistics". And Principle 4 states "The statistical agencies are entitled to comment on erroneous interpretation and misuse of statistics." (United Nations Statistics Commission 2018).

These principles do not in any way prevent statistical offices from encouraging the use of statistics. But I believe they do point to a mindset among some NSOs that their performance should be assessed by their statistical outputs – such as the quantity of data released – rather than the outcomes – such as increased evidence-influenced decision-making – that NSOs are ultimately working to generate. Perhaps in part this mindset comes from a recognition that such outcomes are much more difficult to quantify. But, whatever the reason, some NSOs appear to see that their role in the statistics-policy cycle ending when a data set is made public.

Statistical communication is an important element in ensuring that statistical outputs are translated into outcomes. And yet it is something that is seldom taught during statistics courses and which few would rate as a strength of most NSOs. In 2008 I heard the late Professor Hans Rosling, a successful statistical communicator and founder of the GapMinder software (GapMinder 2018), speak about the lengthy journey statistical data takes from collection in the field, through processing in the NSO to eventual publication and dissemination. And yet, he observed, it was the final 2 cm of the journey – the stage during which the numbers reach our eyes and thence travel to our brain – that was the most difficult hurdle. Poor communication was, he argued, to blame (Rosling 2008).

There are many ways to improve statistical communication, and many new software packages are available to present data to better reach, influence and serve users. What I think is important for this chapter is to recognize that good statistical communication is an important element of any toolkit aiming to promote QOLS. It is also important to recognize that different communication styles suit different audiences. Policy makers and the media for instance might require information in very different ways. Taking the time to talk to users will provide the most useful insights into how best to do this.

As more and more statistical information becomes available, from both traditional and official – as well as new and unofficial – data sources, those who release QOLS must – more than ever – move beyond what I like to call a 'Field of Dreams mentality'- "If you build it, he will come"[2]. Simply releasing statistical information is not enough to ensure it reaches an audience, let alone to ensure it is used by them. Statisticians have a role in ensuring – partly through strong communication – that their data are used.

Recommendation
Promote the importance of statistical communication among those who publish QOLS, and ensure they consult with key audiences to ensure the communication they eventually use is appropriate. Including sessions in a user-producer workshop to facilitate this dialogue can be helpful.

Working with the Media

There are different audiences for QOLS. But many quality of life projects seek – at least in part – to engage the public and promote a more informed facts-based public debate about quality of life. As the Istanbul Declaration, signed by the OECD, the United Nations and many other organizations during the OECD's Second World Forum on Statistics, Knowledge, Policy declared "The availability of statistical indicators of economic, social, and environmental outcomes and their dissemination to citizens can contribute to promoting good governance and the improvement of democratic processes. It can strengthen citizens' capacity to influence the goals of the societies they live in through debate and consensus building, and increase the accountability of public policies" (OECD 2007b).

---

[2] Hollywood Movie

The "public", however, do not usually get their information direct from statistical offices but via the media. And so journalists are an important ally in promoting QOLS. However, in my experience very few statisticians receive training in how to work with the media. Moreover, many statisticians are nervous about interacting with the media, largely for fear of making a mistake and 'getting into trouble". This seems to be driven by a fear that journalists want "to trap" those they interview.

In reality this seldom seems to be the case, at least not when journalists interview statisticians about QOLS. The media may occasionally push those they interview to try to make political pronouncements from the data, but in general reporters are usually looking primarily for guidance in how best to (accurately) tell a story from the statistics. Promoting the idea that the media should be seen as a statistician's friend and not their enemy is an important message to get over during QOLS workshops.

It is also important for statisticians to better understand the sort of information and support the media require to prepare an accurate report, and that this will likely vary according to how sophisticated a data-user the journalist is. In some workshops for statisticians I have collaborated with a local journalist or press officer to run a session to discuss these ideas in detail. These sessions are usually well-received, especially when they have included a role play "press conference exercise". In this exercise participants play the roles of both statisticians and journalists to simulate a press conference about a new (poorly communicated) QOLS publication. Participants finish the exercise with a better understanding of working with the media and a clear understanding of how frustrating it can be – for journalists – to try to extract a story from complex statistical data.

Recommendation
Media coverage is important to ensuring QOLS have an impact. It can be productive to develop statisticians' skills in working with the media. Key components of the training are.

1. Helping data producers to better understand what journalists need to write an article; and
2. Encouraging data producers to view the media as a friend not a foe.

Working with University Professors

Last, but not least, I should mention the importance of working with academics to teach students about QOLS, an area that is often overlooked. Today's students will be the leaders of tomorrow, and it is a privilege to have an opportunity to instill ideas around quality of life, and moving beyond GDP, in their minds and to discuss this with them.

Students are often receptive to these ideas and excited by them. I have worked with academics to run workshops for (usually) master's degree program students in different countries, as well as for international groups of students from multiple institutions and multiple disciplines.

The following ideas usually resonate well with such groups and can generate an interesting discussion.

1. The question "How do we know if we are developing as a society?" is not straightforward and has no single answer.
2. The statistics we produce and chose to pay attention to have an influence over the directions a society heads.
3. The importance of strong communication in ensuring that statistics are used. This leads to a discussion on the need to challenge the boundaries of what is seen as "appropriate communication" in organizations that release statistics.
4. The importance of challenging the status quo: we need new statistics, presented in new ways, to new audiences if we are to take new directions.

In addition to presenting these ideas in person it can also be useful to prepare material that can be shared with academics anywhere. Many professors are interested in these ideas but may not have time in their busy teaching schedules to prepare lectures. Offering them material – in the form of say a fully-scripted power point – can make all the difference.

> **Recommendation**
> Talking to students is both an investment in the future, and a chance to think in fresh ways about old concerns. Providing material to academics to include in economics, statistics and public policy courses can also be beneficial.

Conclusions

This chapter has described some of the barriers – largely behavioral and cultural – that present an obstacle to nations paying greater attention to QOLS in their decision making.

Having QOLS and people who can use that data to inform policy is fundamental. But, while resource and capacity constraints to achieving this exist in many countries, there are a variety of other stumbling blocks that get in the way, including a national statistical office's belief about their role in government. Even when the data already exist, the relationship between those who produce it and those who should use it can prevent it from being used properly. How data are communicated can also determine whether data ultimately have an impact. Formal teaching can play a role in tackling these challenges. But I believe experiential learning – through workshops and networks – can be much more effective.

References

Australian Bureau of Statistics. (2002). *Measuring Australia's Progress*. Canberra: ABS.
Australian Bureau of Statistics. (2018). *ABS Legislative Framework*. Retrieved from http://www.abs.gov.au/websitedbs/D3310114.nsf/Home/ABS+Legislative+Framework
Canadian Index of Wellbeing. (2016). *How are Canadians really doing? The 2016 CIW National Report*. Waterloo: Canadian Index of Wellbeing and University of Waterloo.
Constanza, R., Hart, M., Posner, S., & Talberth, J. (2009). *Beyond GDP: The need for new measures of progress* (Pardee Paper No. 4). Boston: Pardee Center for the Study of the Longer-Range Future.
GapMinder. (2018). *GapMinder.Org homepage*. Retrieved from https://www.gapminder.org/
Hall, J. (2005). Measuring progress: An Australian travelogue. *Journal of Official Statistics, 21*(4), 727–746.
Hall, J., & Rickard, L. (2013). *People, progress and participation. How initiatives measuring social progress yield benefits beyond better metrics*. Global Choices 1 | 2013. Bertelsman Foundation.
Hall, J., Carswell, C., Jones, R. and Yencken, D. (2005). Collaborating with civil society: reflections from Australia. In *Statistics, knowledge and policy: Key indicators to inform decision making*. Paris: OECD Publishing. https://doi.org/10.1787/9789264009011-en.
Ireland's Central Statistical Office. (2003). *Measuring Ireland's progress, Volume 1–2003*. Government of Ireland.
London School of Economics. (2018). *Professor Kenneth Benoit*. Retrieved from http://www.lse.ac.uk/Methodology/People/Academic-Staff/Kenneth-Benoit/Kenneth-Benoit
Masters in Data Science. (2018). *Data analytics degrees for public policy*. Retrieved from https://www.mastersindatascience.org/specialties/best-data-analytics-degrees-for-public-policy/
Medstat III. (2013). *Supporting the dialogue between the users and producers of statistics with a special focus on social statistics in the Southern & Eastern Mediterranean Countries*. European Commission. Available at https://circabc.europa.eu/sd/a/9dab4cbb-4539-4b35-87a2-68dc5efd6b11/EN_Regional%20Guidelines%20for%20Users-Producers%20Dialogue_HD.pdf
OECD. (2005). *Statistics, knowledge and policy: Key indicators to inform decision making*. Paris: OECD Publishing. https://doi.org/10.1787/9789264009011-en.
OECD. (2007a). *Measuring the progress of societies*. Paris: OECD. Retrieved from http://www.oecd.org/site/worldforum06/37014829.pdf.
OECD. (2007b). *The Istanbul declaration*. Paris: OECD. Retrieved from http://www.oecd.org/site/worldforum/49130123.pdf.
OECD. (2017). *How's life? 2017: Measuring Well-being*. Paris: OECD Publishing. https://doi.org/10.1787/how_life-2017-en.
OECD. (2018). *Measuring the progress of societies*. Retrieved from https://www.oecd.org/site/progresskorea/measuringtheprogressofsocieties.htm
Pink, B., Taylor, S., Wetzler, H. (2014). Measuring progress: The international context. In Podger A. & Trewin D. (Eds.), *Measuring and promoting wellbeing: How important is economic growth?* (pp. 163–190). ANU Press. Retrieved from http://www.jstor.org/stable/j.ctt6wp80q.10
Rosling, H (2008). *From dissemination to access – Promote innovation!* Presentation to the Seminar on Innovative Approaches to Turning Statistics into Knowledge 26–27 May 2008, Stockholm Sweden. Available at http://www.oecd.org/site/worldforum06/40009289.pdf
Statistics Commission, 2007. *Report no. 33 the use made of official statistics*. Statistics Commission. UK.
Stiglitz, J. (2009, September 13). Towards a better measure of wellbeing. *The Financial Times*.
Stiglitz, J., Sen, A., & Fitoussi, J.-P. (2009). *Report by the commission on the measurement of economic performance and social progress* (French Commission on the Measurement of economic Performance and social Progress).
UNDP. (2018). *Human development reports*. Retrieved from http://hdr.undp.org/en

Unite For Sight. (2018). *Designing quality healthy survey questions*. Retrieved from http://www.
   uniteforsight.org/global-health-university/quality-survey
United Nations. (2003). *Handbook of statistical organization, third edition: The operation
   and organization of a statistical agency*. https://unstats.un.org/unsd/publication/SeriesF/
   SeriesF_88E.pdf
United Nations Statistics Commission. (2018). *Fundamental principles of official statistics*.
   Retrieved from https://unstats.un.org/unsd/dnss/gp/fp-english.pdf
Willis, A. (2010). EU report slams Greece over false statistics. *EUobserver*. https://euobserver.
   com/economic/29258

Jon Hall is a Policy Specialist for the United Nations Development Program, New York, USA. Jon has been thinking about how to quantify – and influence – quality of life since 2000. His 2002 work for the Australian Bureau of Statistics on Measuring Australia's Progress won a national award as the "smartest" social project of the year. From 2005 – 2009 he led a project at the O.E.C.D promoting these ideas around the world and since 2012 has been working on strengthening national human development reporting. Jon has a master degree in applied statistics and econometrics, and another in public service administration. He has lectured in over 50 countries and has a particular interest in measuring happiness. In 2013 he was one of ten "global opinion leaders" to meet with German Chancellor Angela Merkel to discuss his work.

Chapter 10
Teaching Nonviolent Economics as a Path for Achieving Quality of Life

Jorge Guardiola

Introduction

When teaching economics, substantial attention should be given to quality of life. In the course presented in this chapter, quality of life is understood as happiness and sustainability. The definition of sustainable development comes from the Brundtland report (World Commission on Environment and Development 1987). This report coined and popularized the term sustainable development, defined, in a nutshell, as the type of development that meets the needs of people today without compromising the needs of future generations. Sustainable development is essential for achieving happiness for people in the future; therefore, sustainability should be understood as one of the principal dimensions of the many incorporated in the definition of quality of life (see for instance Tonon 2010). The definition of quality of life in this course takes a pacifist view, using a nonviolent approach that is to an extent inspired by the work of Gandhi and other famous pacifists. This enables a pacifist orientation to quality of life, viewing quality of life and nonviolence as very similar concepts, as we argue below.

In fact, the experience on the course builds from my definition of Nonviolent Economics, which is as follows: a vision of the economy in which people, companies and the State produce and distribute sufficient goods and services from a scarcity of natural resources to meet the needs of all people without compromising the needs of future generations and while respecting all other living beings and the environment. Therefore, quality of life and Nonviolent Economics go hand-in-hand, as a common feature is the satisfaction of human needs (which is central to achieving happiness and sustainable development). Nonviolence is not interpreted as a

J. Guardiola (✉)
Instituto de la Paz y los Conflictos, Departamento de Economía Aplicada,
Universidad de Granada, Granada, Spain
e-mail: jguardiola@ugr.es

© Springer Nature Switzerland AG 2020
G. H. Tonon (ed.), *Teaching Quality of Life in Different Domains*, Social
Indicators Research Series 79, https://doi.org/10.1007/978-3-030-21551-4_10

means of achieving quality of life, or vice versa; rather, they are complementary elements on the same path. Given that quality of life is about perceptions (Tonon 2010), nonviolence, which is articulated around sustainability and the achievement of happiness, is a crucial component that permits people to perceive their lives as good lives worth living. Living in poverty or surrounded by violence is not a conducive environment for quality of life, as relations with the environment and with others are a crucial element in this regard (Patrick et al. 2002). Happiness is related to needs satisfaction (e.g. Fuentes and Rojas, 2001), and future generations should also be given the opportunity to satisfy their human needs (Guillén-Royo et al. 2017).

This chapter presents an experience of addressing quality of life, through a non-violence framework, in an Economic Policy course delivered to students of Social Work, Politics, and Sociology. The rest of the chapter is structured as follows: Section "Challenges in designing an alternative course in economics" presents the challenges experienced when adopting this approach to economics. Section "Presenting quality of life: A nonviolent approach" is devoted to exploring what violence really is and, most importantly, what nonviolence is. Several examples used to illustrate to the students the violence inherent in the economy and how quality of life can be achieved without harming; others are presented in section "Teaching nonviolent economics for quality of life". Section "Course syllabus" outlines the course syllabus. Finally, section "Conclusions and final recommendation" concludes and includes a brief discussion.

Challenges in Designing an Alternative Course in Economics

The main challenges experienced with this particular view in economics are mostly structural, relating to the cultural conception of what economics should be. This is because a nonviolent or quality-of-life conception in economics sometimes defies the theories found in textbooks and faculty members' conceptions of economics.

Textbooks

Textbooks normally have a neoclassical orientation, which is related to neoliberal ideology. They also incorporate a Keynesian approach, fused or synthetized with the neoclassical approach. Economics textbooks normally provide a point of reference for the design of the curriculum and the approach used during the course.

It should be borne in mind that many economic axioms are in fact political ideology based on ideas that are open to argument and far from settled. For instance, considering people as selfish, competitive and insatiable individuals (homo oeconomicus) is closely tied to the Hobbesian perception of man, and contrary to the empirical idea of what a person is. As well as being untrue, this approach disregards the importance of friendships and good relationships to human beings, while it is in fact one of the most important drivers of happiness (Becchetti et al. 2008, 2011; Guardiola et al. 2013).

In economics textbooks, companies are also considered as profit maximizes that disregard any ethical issue regarding society or the environment. This may be in accordance with the behaviour of some companies that only care about money regardless of any social or environmental impact. However, in a perspective that promotes the pursuit of happiness in society, this kind of action should be considered more as a threat to the achievement of present and future generations' happiness than a theory to teach in class. Also, the increasing implementation of other business models beneficial to the common good should be taken into account (Felber 2015).

There is some empirical evidence that economics students cooperate less, are more likely to cheat to gain an advantage and are more self-interested than students in other disciplines (Frank and Schulze 2000; Frank et al. 1993, 1996). This suggests that in fact the kind of culture we are presenting in the classrooms may influence students, or it may be the case that economics courses attract people who are more antisocial than average. Anyhow, action should be taken to present healthier values in economics courses.

Relationships: Teaching Staff and Students

Economic paradigms are typically communicated and upheld by economics lecturers. In this vein, some faculty members may not be content if a younger colleague takes a different approach to teaching the course contents. The challenge here is to try to learn, through discussion, from this faculty member's point of view, as well as showing him/her the reasons for following a different path.

For the younger faculty members, having a different approach may also prove an obstacle to achieving working stability, as some older colleagues may dislike the incorporation into the department of someone who thinks so differently. This also goes for the students: my personal experience with the students of Politics, Social Work and Sociology has always been positive regarding the vision I share in the classroom but I think that if I followed the same approach with economics students (a subject I do not teach at the present moment), I could have some problems.

Motivation

Economics should be considered and taught as a tool for life, and should impart healthy values that are good for individuals and for society as a whole. Changing economic ideas is a utopian objective difficult to achieve; nevertheless, this objective spurs me to keep going on this path. The philosopher of science, Thomas Kuhn (2012), clearly warned about the difficulty of changing paradigms in sciences. Indeed, in order to convince others to accept a new paradigm, new evidence is needed (which we already have) and a state of crisis in the scientific discipline (we are still a long way off that point in economic thought). But changes start with each individual, so everyone should internally transform his/her ideas and behaviour, aiming to inspire others.

In the classroom, teachers tend to reproduce what we have been taught: if we have been taught economics in a certain way as learners, we tend to reproduce it through our actions. In economics, this creates a pernicious multiplicative effect if we as teachers reproduce neoclassical messages in the classroom. In short, if we received anti-social and anti-environmental information from our teachers, this would shape our approach when it comes to relating with other people and the environment.

Presenting Quality of Life: A Nonviolent Approach

What Is Violence and How Is it Present in Economics?

According to Johan Galtung (2004), there are three types of violence (see Fig. 10.1): cultural, structural and direct violence. The first two types are subtle and even invisible, in contrast with direct violence, which is more evident.

Cultural violence refers to a particular way in which we think and see the world that involves violence such as racism, machismo or extreme selfishness. It can encourage the other two forms of violence through complex channels. Cultural violence is normally present in mainstream economics culture. For instance, the utopian idea of perfect competition in markets is not desirable as it involves cultural violence. Firstly it does not really exist and thus presents a distorted reality. Secondly, and most importantly, because it renders certain corporate actions invisible, such as environmental damage, bad working conditions and other abuses that

Fig. 10.1 Three types of violence

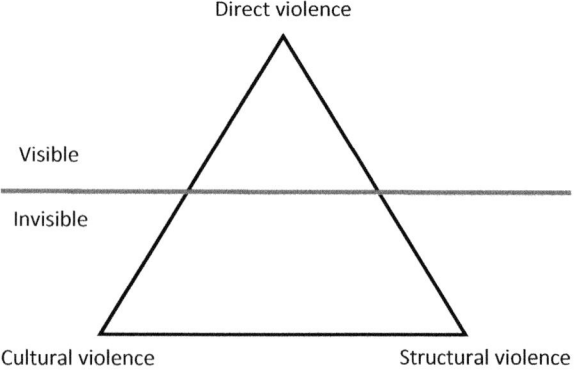

some companies commit when they are excessively powerful. As presented in the previous Section, the idea of homo oeconomus is also a very violent one, as it disregards what is really important in life.

Structural violence refers to the institutions in society that generate violence and permit inequality, poverty, marginalization, or environment degradation. Though we do talk about poverty and inequality in economics, it does not receive enough attention. Environmental degradation is the most significant omission in most curricula, which is surprising given the importance that natural resources have in life and for future generations.

An important example of structural violence is the norms involved in international trade. In most economics classrooms, discussions of international trade include almost no consideration of how it harms people and nature. There is little discussion about how some powerful multinational companies undermine many people's quality of life, and few references to how international trade rules have tolerated high levels of poverty and hunger in the world, in spite of the fact that some decades ago it was presented as a powerful tool to prevent or remedy these social problems.

Another crucial aspect of structural violence that is absent from economic textbooks is military expenditure. Spending on weapons and defence has a doubly harmful effect on quality of life: (1) it enables direct violence through the use of weapons; and (2) it entails an opportunity cost (see the next section for a definition of opportunity cost) as the money devoted to weapons spending could be redirected to more important budget items such as health and education.

Finally, direct violence refers to insulting, physically harming or killing others, and it takes its most dramatic shape in war. Direct violence may infringe not only on people but also on other forms of life; for example, through the destruction of biodiversity. Resource-extraction activities, such as intensive agriculture, fishing or mining, which are mostly located in countries in the Global South, are examples of the destruction of nature, which in turn creates structural violence affecting the inhabitants of those areas. Natural disasters stemming from climatic change are also instances of direct violence.

Wars have multiple causes, and some wars are driven by economic motives, such as control of natural resources or gaining economic and political advantage over others. Examples of wars that had an important economic cause are the Opium War, when the United Kingdom forced China to accept opium trade, or the Iraq wars aimed at controlling its oil reserves.

The triangle of violence adopts an important role in my courses. The description above is only an overview of what violence is and gives some hints as to how it is present in reality, viewed from an economics perspective. If we turn our focus to pinpointing violence, we discover that it is very present. In order to achieve quality of life, it is necessary to recognize what prevents people from obtaining it. The violence perspective allows us to identify the obstacles, and a nonviolence approach may help to overcome them.

A Nonviolent Approach for Quality of Life

We understand nonviolence as a commitment to the search for justice and wellbeing without having to use violence. Following the pacifist and historian Mario López Martínez (2017), nonviolence consists not only in the rejection of violence, but primarily in the search for alternatives to resolve conflicts. Through nonviolence, these alternatives should ensure greater freedom and well-being for the people involved in the conflict, which does not foster quality of life, nor is nonviolence passive resistance. Gandhi went to great lengths to show that nonviolence is a very active approach, because it allowed conflicts to be energized in order to find solutions that dignify not only the oppressed, but also the oppressors. In fact, the lives of activists like Gandhi were not passive at all, but very active.

Nonviolence is a means and an end in itself, and involves a series of moral practices that translate into actions that seek to free people (not only the oppressed, but also the oppressors) from cultural, structural, and direct violence. The path of nonviolence sometimes involves resistance and civil disobedience, in order not to cooperate with what is considered an evil.

To the best of my knowledge, there is no empirical evidence linking nonviolence with quality of life, but it seems reasonable to assume that violent societies are unhappy ones, and that joy and satisfaction with life can be achieved more easily in peaceful ones.

López Martínez (2017) identifies four characteristic principles of nonviolence: (1) a prohibition on killing: life should be preserved, defended and respected—not only human life but also animal and plant life; (2) a search for truth, which allows us to shed light on conflicts and their resolution; (3) dialogue and active listening, to maintain contact with the other party and avoid dehumanizing the relationship; and (4) alternative and creative thinking, becoming aware that other models and other paradigms of reality, which bring people well-being and freedom, are possible and necessary.

Following those principles, quality of life viewed through a nonviolent perspective means a search for truth, dialogue, and the possibility of thinking in an alternative way, in order to create new healthier paradigms. Through this nonviolent path, it is necessary to have a scientific perspective of economics encompassing a truth that allows conflict resolution, is active in listening, and is enriched with alternative ideas. This is of crucial importance, since economics shapes the way in which we relate to other people, to other living beings and to the planet; and this is also crucial for quality of life. In order to improve quality of life, a transformation is needed that is reflected in the way we act and how public policies are designed (Michalos and Zumbo 1999).

This perspective implies a change of paradigm and a change of priorities, which must be based on an ethic that enhances people's quality of life and allows the preservation of the environment and other living beings. Most importantly, it is necessary to proclaim the economy as a means rather than an end, as human societies were not created to conform to the economy, but vice versa. Therefore, economics should be seen as a means that is at the service of people and the environment (the satisfaction of human needs and respect for life, both present and future). This conception is transformative, since it clashes with the conventional model of the economy.

Teaching Nonviolent Economics for Quality of Life

In this Section, I present some examples of my personal experience of following the path described above in an economics course. Given the limitations of space, this is not intended to be an exhaustive list.

The Proposed Change of Paradigm: Do Not Confuse Means with Ends

The greatest challenge in economics is to recognize that money is a means to guarantee a certain end: the well-being of humans and other sentient beings, so that people can satisfy their needs and live in harmony. The capitalist paradigm, the one to overcome, interprets it the other way around, so a change is necessary. Figure 10.2 graphically depicts the cultural change that needs to be implemented.

The description of what needs to be changed is simple, but making the change is complicated. Recognizing that people are much more than human resources, and nature more than natural resources, implies a change in the language and a decolonization of ideas. It is necessary, therefore, to create new thoughts, new action and subtly begin to generate new emotions in line with the new paradigm, which is much healthier, not only for society as a whole but also for individuals.

Which Interpretation of Economics?

Nonviolent Economics is presented in the classroom as an ideological perspective for seeing life through the lens of economics. In accordance with the paradigm explained above, the interpretation of Nonviolent Economics applied in the

	Means	Ends
Paradigm to overcome	Human resources	Companies: Maximize profits
	Natural resources	People: Pursue money or status
New paradigm	Economic sustainability	Human needs
		Respect for nature

Fig. 10.2   The cultural change to avoid violence and achieve happiness

classroom is a vision of the economy in which people, companies and the State produce and distribute sufficient goods and services from a scarcity of natural resources to meet the needs of all people without compromising the needs of future generations and while respecting all other living beings and the environment. This definition is inspired by the one from the World Commission on Environment and Development (1987).

This definition of Nonviolent Economics shares some points with the standard definition of economics: the science of how scarce resources are managed to meet people's needs. However, this definition of Nonviolent Economics incorporates some different conditions: firstly, that all people should be able to satisfy their needs, without facing situations of abuse of power, oppression and exploitation; and secondly, that people who have not yet been born have the right to enjoy the environment, meaning that we cannot leave them a devastated planet as a legacy. Therefore, in order to ensure these conditions are met, empathy, love and respect for other people are essential, as well as sustainability and respect for other animals and plants.

In the classroom, different schools of economics are also introduced, and the Nonviolent Economics perspective is used transversally to identify how each school relates to this definition. The schools of thought presented are Neoclassical, Post-Keynesian, Neo-Marxist, Ecological, Feminist, New Institutional Economics and Behavioural Economics. Of course, it is impossible to deal with all schools of thought, so the most important ones have been selected. The first three schools of economics are the most widely known, and their originators are perhaps the best known economists (unfortunately there are few women in this list of "famous economists"). These economists are Adam Smith ((Neo)Classical), John Maynard Keynes ((Post)Keynesian) and Karl Marx ((Neo)Marxism).

Most schools incorporate cultural violence, generally because they render important issues invisible which harms quality of life. Others do so due to other particular issues, for instance Marx advocated direct violence to achieve social revolution that would lead to communism, and direct violence is necessarily detrimental to quality of life. The exceptions are Feminist and Ecological Economics, which put life and the care at the centre of the discussion, which is closely compatible with our notion of Nonviolent Economics.

In reality, there is something to be learned from all these schools, and some aspects of each school's thinking can contribute to a society that is more cohesive and respectful of the environment and people, even if other aspects may run counter to such a goal. To the extent that they can contribute to a more peaceful society, each of these ideologies is interpreted as rivers that flow into the sea. This sea is quality of life and nonviolence, concepts that I believe have much in common. Each river reaches this sea, so each ideology has something to say and contribute. The rivers of some ideologies are wider and faster flowing, while others are more of a trickle. That is why we try to identify that flow in the classroom. We hope that, even when it comes to making the narrow channels visible, discussion and reflection enables us to increase the flow of these ideologies.

The Opportunity Cost in Terms of Happiness

During their lifespan, different agents (individuals, households, companies or the State) have to make decisions, which are sometimes multiple and difficult, involving a sacrifice. The opportunity cost is defined as the cost that an agent must bear in order to undertake a specific action when renouncing their second-best option. Therefore, it is evaluated as the benefit (or joy or utility) that an agent would have obtained by opting for the second-best action. Take the example of deciding between studying for an exam or going out with friends. If in the end the person decides to go out with friends, their opportunity cost is the good grade they could have obtained if they had stayed at home studying. On the other hand, if he/she decides to study, the opportunity cost would be how much fun he/she would have had with the friends if the other option had been chosen. From a business perspective, a company can decide whether to invest in a new technology or not. Each of the options will have costs and benefits. The benefits of the option not chosen determine the opportunity cost.

The opportunity cost, therefore, conditions decision-making, and it is a very powerful tool to identify violence and understand how reallocation of resources would impact people's quality of life. In this vein, the following example is presented in the classroom:

> You are visiting a museum, which suddenly explodes into flames. You have to run for your life. In one room there is a painting by Cézanne of great economic value, and a little child. You have to choose between carrying the child to safety or the painting. You can only carry either the child or the painting!

Most students raise their hand when they are asked if they would have picked up the child, and almost none raise their hand to show that they would have chosen the painting. The Cézanne painting, shown in class, was bought by a millionaire for 191 million euros. On the other hand, a mesh coated with repellent, which can save the life of a child living in a malaria-endemic country, can cost about 200 dollars (around 180 euros), taking into account production and distribution costs. If we divide the cost of the painting by the cost of the mesh (191,000,000/180) we get a total of 1,061,111 children who can be saved from malaria with that amount of money.

Another example is used, this time at the State level: the Spanish economist Arcadi Oliveres criticizes the fact that many banks around the world have received 4.6 trillion dollars in loans (some of them difficult to return) as a direct aid from governments, in the period between the beginning of the crisis in 2008 and 2012 (the figure has risen even higher since then). In Spain, the banks that received public aid during the crisis did not stop their eviction policy, seizing houses from people suddenly afflicted by poverty, thereby exacerbating their situation. Olivares estimates that if this amount of money had been invested in the fight against hunger, it would have been enough to end hunger 92 times. The opportunity cost of rescuing banks instead of saving lives is incalculable, and it should be considered a crime against humanity.

A third example used to illustrate this is the following: In economic terms, the cost of containing violence is the cost of any activity that is related to preventing or dealing with the consequences of direct violence. It includes direct costs such as the cost of healing a victim (medical care and medication), as well as indirect costs such as brain drain because of direct violence. The cost of containing direct violence in the world amounts to $9.46 trillion (Institute of Peace and Economics 2015), which is about nine times everything Spain produces in a year, 75 times what the world spends on development cooperation, and almost double the world's agricultural production. It is not only moral arguments but also economic ones that point to the need for a nonviolent economy.

Those examples put into perspective the terrible cost borne in terms of quality of life in society, due to poor allocation of resources and failures in the distribution of property rights.[1] At this point, we raise the question of whether we are really being rational and coherent in the decisions we make as individuals or as society. Considering the way the economic system is organized and the way we act, the answer is undoubtedly no. The more resources that are allocated to satisfying human needs, the lower the social costs and the violence caused.

Many day-to-day decisions have a high opportunity cost in terms of quality of life, and generate a great deal of violence, but they are accepted because they are commonplace; or it may be the case that they are not accepted at first, but people simply resign themselves to the situation and adapt accordingly. Examples are prisons, prostitution, poverty, police repression and sexual and labour exploitation. We get used to living with violence. Unfortunately, one of the triumphs of the violent system is that people perceive violence as normal.

Different Kinds of Motivations

In the classroom, basic needs and markets are analysed, and as part of these subjects, there is a focus on motivation. There are two ways that our motivation in life can guide us, according to our values. Our behaviour can be motivated by extrinsic or intrinsic values: people with extrinsic values seek status, money, power, fame and beauty, while those driven by intrinsic motivation do things for the pleasure of doing them. Intrinsic motivation is linked with healthy relationships and community living, whereas extrinsic motivation is related to materialism.

In addition, we deal with behaviours both inside and outside the market, which lead to a healthy society. In this vein, there are numerous empirical investigations that confirm that pro-social behaviour (such as donating money) and pro-environmental behaviour (such as recycling and buying organic products) increase the happiness of those who engage in them, in addition to generating a beneficial

---

[1] More examples and information on those quality of life costs can be found in Singer (2010).

impact on society and the environment.[2] Studies on mindfulness and meditation, which aim to increase people's empathy, show that welfare levels also increase (Ericson et al. 2014). In terms of a paradigm shift, empathy and generosity towards others imply treating others as an end rather than a means. It is much more beneficial to change the paradigm than to stick with economists' misinterpretation about social ends and their means.

Studies by psychologist Tim Kasser and co-authors have determined that materialism is associated with lower levels of well-being, poorer mental health and lower self-esteem, as well as lower levels of pro-social and pro-environmental behaviour (Kasser 2002). The more materialistic people there are, the greater the consumption, and therefore the greater the profit levels of companies, the greater the economic growth and the greater the tax revenues. On the other hand, intrinsic motivation is related to greater self-satisfaction, which results in higher levels of happiness and generosity. So there seems to be a paradox here. In the same vein, psychologist Joseph Sirgy presents materialistic people as more dissatisfied (Sirgy 1998). How can the economic system, designed by human beings, encourage extrinsic motivation, while it has been scientifically demonstrated that extrinsic motivation brings about anti-social and anti-environmental behaviour? It is not better to design an economic system that results in pro-social and pro-environmental behaviour?

The paradigm to overcome, which regards people and nature as means, is associated with extrinsic motivation, while the new paradigm that upholds life as an end is conceptually linked to intrinsic motivation.

What to Produce? Producing Guns Is Not the Same as Producing Butter

When explaining the production options of a company or nation, the Nobel laureate in economics, Paul Samuelson, uses the illustrative example of agents being able to decide between two options for production: guns or butter. If all resources are devoted to producing butter, no guns can be produced. But if only part of the resources is used to produce butter, then some guns can be produced. When all resources are devoted to production, different combinations of production are possible. This is referred to as the production-possibility frontier.

The problem is that the production and consumption of butter has a quite different impact on society and the environment than the consumption of guns. Butter is a source of nourishment, although it can be harmful in excess, whereas guns kill. It is not the same to produce goods and services that can kill or harm, such as weapons or speculative financial tools (for instance, derivatives that speculate with food

---

[2] Several research papers examine pro-social and pro-environmental behaviors and link them with greater happiness. For examples of the former, see Aknin et al. (2013) or Aknin and Dunn (2013). Examples of studies on pro-environmental behavior are Binder and Blankenberg (2016), and Suárez-Varela et al. (2016).

prices), as it is to produce goods and services that create well-being, such as medicines, education or art. Violent production is associated with the old paradigm, which makes no distinction between certain types of production in terms of their effect on life on earth.

On the other hand, if we see people and the environment as the ultimate goal, the production of weapons is meaningless. We must consider the fact that production implies a previous destruction. To make butter or guns, it is necessary to destroy nature. Through the production process and by means of manpower, nature is transformed into something that, in theory, should be more valuable than what has been destroyed.[3] But how can producing something as destructive as weapons can be more valuable than what was previously destroyed for their production? Putting people and the environment at the centre gives us a theory of value that could orient production towards social welfare.

In this theory of production and value creation, the value of what is produced has to be greater than the value of what is destroyed. But the value of production is determined by the use, therefore the products must reach the right hands. The people who can give more value to production are the most disadvantaged, those who are not satisfying their needs. That is why appropriate distribution mechanisms, which go far beyond markets, are required to successfully satisfy needs. It should not be forgotten that markets can only be accessed by people who have money, regardless of their level of need satisfaction. This vision of production seems to be in accordance with a new healthier paradigm that improves people's quality of life.

How to Measure Societies' Progress and Orientate Public Policy Towards Achieving It?

The indicator most commonly used to measure societies' progress is the macroeconomic variable Gross Domestic Product (GDP). This is a monetary valuation of the goods and services that a country produces (in principle, legally) in a given period. That is, GDP is obtained by multiplying the amount of goods and services produced in a country in a given period by the price of each one.

In mainstream economics it is viewed as the key indicator to proxy quality of life and social prosperity. In ancient times, our ancestors looked up at the sky and thus predicted whether there would be a good or a bad harvest. In this way, they judged whether the community was likely to be well, remain united, and avoid hardship. These days, we look at GDP growth forecasts to see how well or badly we are going to do in the near future. If positive GDP growth is forecast, we will be happy. But if the growth is less than expected or negative, then we have lower expectations of a happy future.

---

[3] For further discussion on this see Ruskin (1985).

In the classroom, we question the extent to which GDP reflects a country's prosperity and quality of life, and whether we are omitting important aspects along the way. After explaining the origins and measurement of GDP, we examine the advantages and disadvantages of this indicator as a measure of social progress. Among the advantages of GDP, we identified the following:

- An increase in production means an increase in employment, that is, the more production there is, the greater the need to recruit people.
- It favours the Welfare State, as the greater the production and consumption, the greater the tax revenues, which—given the correct economic policy—can be devoted to social spending.
- However, GDP also presents many disadvantages[4] in proxying an idea of progress based on quality of life that avoids violence:
- It does not include care work and, in general, unpaid work, which remains invisible.
- It encourages the destruction of nature, as the greater the production the greater the need for natural resources.
- It fails to account for the well-being of subsequent generations, as the destruction of nature jeopardizes their quality of life.

It renders inequality and poverty invisible, as GDP growth is compatible with high poverty and inequality rates, unless certain economic policies are implemented.

- It gives equal weight to all products or investments (what to produce?) regardless of their social and environmental impact; it does not distinguish between the production of butter and the production of guns.
- It gives equal weight to all ways of producing goods (how to produce?), therefore GDP can increase even while people are working in unfavourable conditions (salaries below the living wage, long working hours, health risks, etc.) and while nature is being destroyed or contaminated.
- Consumerism and materialism contribute positively to GDP, which, as explained above, contributes to anti-social and anti-environmental behaviour and low quality of life.
- GDP can grow despite increased stress and decreased happiness. In fact, there is evidence of the Easterlin paradox in several countries (Easterlin et al. 2010).
- It does not include the things in life that make life worth living. GDP encourages the satisfaction of human needs through the market. For instance, if a relative is sick, hire a caregiver; if you have a conflict with someone, hire a lawyer; if you are afraid, hire security; if you are generally unhappy, go shopping.

Due to GDP's numerous flaws as a measure of quality of life, it is necessary to explore alternative indicators that are consistent with a nonviolent economy and better approximate prosperity and the common good (Land and Michalos 2018). The next step is to explore those alternative indicators, four of which are presented in class: the Real Progress Index, subjective well-being, the ecological footprint and

---

[4] More on this can be found in Bartolini (2014) and Jackson (2009).

the Happy Planet Index. Those indicators are explained, with the caveat that a single indicator cannot capture the complexities of progress (Michalos 1997).

We then talk about economic policies that aim to improve quality of life and avoid violence. We argue that fiscal, monetary, and trade policies should better address the kind of influence they are creating in society and on the environment, rather than focusing only on the economic impact. We also discuss how the 2008 economic crisis was a lost opportunity to learn how to achieve happier societies.[5]

Course Syllabus

Unit 1. Basic principles of economics

1. Definition and scope of Economics

    1.1. Agents and economic goods. The circular flow of income
    1.2. Resources, scarcity and choice: the opportunity cost

2. Methodology of economics

    2.1. Economic theory and the different branches of economics.
    2.2. Microeconomics and Macroeconomics
    2.3. Positive analysis and normative analysis

Unit 2. Supply and demand: the market mechanism

1. Formulation of the supply and demand model
2. Demand

    2.1. Individual and market demand
    2.2. Movements along the demand function
    2.3. Shifts in the demand function

3. Supply

    3.1. Individual and market supply
    3.2. Movements along the supply function
    3.3. Shifts in the supply function

4. Quantity and equilibrium price
5. Elasticities of demand and supply

Unit 3. Production

1. Production and costs
2. Degrees of competition and market rates
3. Perfect competition
4. Imperfect competition: monopoly, oligopoly and monopolistic competition

---

[5] See more in Guardiola, Picazo-Tadeo, & Rojas (2015).

Unit 4. The public sector and markets

1. Limitations of the market economy

    1.1. Allocation inefficiency
    1.2. Economic instability
    1.3. Inequity

2. Public sector intervention in the economy and quality of life

Unit 5. Macroeconomics, a global vision

1. Concept and origin of macroeconomics

    1.1. The scope of macroeconomics
    1.2. Target macroeconomic variables and quality of life: economic growth, unemployment and inflation

2. Measuring economic activity

    2.1. Measuring GDP
    2.2. Nominal and real GDP

3. Measuring prices and unemployment
4. Macroeconomic identities

Unit 6. Aggregate demand and fiscal policy

1. The Keynesian model of aggregate demand
2. Aggregate consumption
3. The demand for investment
4. Public expenditure and revenue
5. The public budget and fiscal policy
6. The equilibrium in the market for goods in an economy with a public sector and an external sector

Unit 7. Money and monetary policy

1. Money in the economy
2. The demand for money and the money supply
3. Bank money and the creation of bank money
4. The Central Bank and monetary policy

Unit 8. The external sector and the foreign exchange market

1. International economic relations: the comparative advantage
2. The balance of payments
3. The foreign exchange market

Conclusions and Final Recommendation

The so-called father of economics, Adam Smith, is widely known for his defence of selfishness, due to an unfortunate paragraph in the book The Wealth of Nations (1776), where he identified selfishness as the motivation of market sellers. However, he dedicated an entire book to dealing with values such as empathy and unselfish self-esteem, called the Theory of Moral Sentiments (1759), which went unnoticed among the economists. This is an illustration of how a misinterpretation can shape a culture of economics, which can then be improved.

It is important to change our understanding of economics to build better societies, avoiding violence and suffering. It is necessary to recognize new ways of interpreting the economy that are more human, feminist and ecological, because these interpretations better enable us to guarantee the individual and collective well-being, by relying on new healthier paradigms. We need a new conception that prevents harm to third parties occurring through our actions. We need a nonviolent perspective that allows us to achieve quality of life, with special consideration for the most disadvantaged people. The way we teach economics in the classroom is critical to this endeavour, and we need more information that helps point our societies in a healthier direction.

In order to achieve this, a cultural shift is required from economic agents, so that people and nature can be an end in themselves instead of a means to the end of maximizing profits or welfare. People should seek to find intrinsic rather than extrinsic motivation, in order to be happy and make others happy. Companies should have better moral codes to avoid harm and create well-being, and the State should aim to guarantee all people's needs, which means paying special attention to economically-disadvantaged people.

The initiative must go beyond mere words in a text: global transformation begins with an internal transformation of our thoughts, emotions and actions, and must be translated into collective actions and policies to create a strong impact on society. We have to keep in mind that nonviolence is not a means to achieving quality of life, or vice versa; rather the two are complementary elements on the same path. Nonviolence is the best path to achieving sustainability and happiness, which are important components of quality of life (Michalos 1997). But to achieve sustainability and happiness, many cultural and institutional changes are required, which in turn entail the avoidance of cultural, structural, and direct violence. As Gandhi said, we must be the change we want to see in the world; and that change must begin with each person according to their possibilities. How to effect change is a major challenge. The answer seems to be a combination of thought (imagination and knowledge) and willingness, in order to generate love for oneself and all other life forms.

Funding

This research has been partially supported by the Ministry of Economy, Industry and Competitiveness, the State Research Agency (SRA) and European Regional Development Fund (ERDF) (project reference ECO2017–86822-R).

References

Aknin, L. B., Barrington-Leigh, C. P., Dunn, E. W., Helliwell, J. F., Burns, J., Biswas-Diener, R., et al. (2013). Prosocial spending and well-being: Cross-cultural evidence for a psychological universal. *Journal of Personality and Social Psychology, 104*(4), 635–652. https://doi.org/10.1037/a0031578.

Aknin, L. B., Dunn, E. W. (2013). Wealth and subjective well-being: Spending money on others leads to higher happiness than spending on yourself. *Activities for Teaching Positive Psychology: A Guide for Instructors*, 93–97. https://doi.org/10.1037/14042-015

Bartolini, S. (2014). Building sustainability through greater happiness. *Economic and Labour Relations Review, 25*(4), 587–602. https://doi.org/10.1177/1035304614559436.

Becchetti, L., Pelloni, A., & Rossetti, F. (2008). Relational goods, sociability, and happiness. *Kyklos, 61*(3), 343–363. https://doi.org/10.1111/j.1467-6435.2008.00405.x.

Becchetti, L., Trovato, G., & Bedoya, D. A. L. (2011). Income, relational goods and happiness. *Applied Economics, 43*(3), 273–290. https://doi.org/10.1080/00036840802570439.

Binder, M., & Blankenberg, A. K. (2016). Environmental concerns, volunteering and subjective well-being: Antecedents and outcomes of environmental activism in Germany. *Ecological Economics, 124*, 1–16. https://doi.org/10.1016/j.ecolecon.2016.01.009.

Easterlin, R. A., McVey, L. A., Switek, M., Sawangfa, O., & Zweig, J. S. (2010). The happiness-income paradox revisited. *Proceedings of the National Academy of Sciences of the United States of America, 107*(52), 22463–22468. https://doi.org/10.1073/pnas.1015962107.

Ericson, T., Kjønstad, B. G., & Barstad, A. (2014). Mindfulness and sustainability. *Ecological Economics, 104*, 73–79. https://doi.org/10.1016/j.ecolecon.2014.04.007.

Frank, B., & Schulze, G. G. (2000). Does economics make citizens corrupt? *Journal of Economic Behavior & Organization, 43*(1), 101–113. https://doi.org/10.1016/S0167-2681(00)00111-6.

Frank, R. H., Gilovich, T. D., & Regan, D. T. (1996). Do economists make bad citizens? *Journal of Economic Perspectives, 10*(1), 187–192. https://doi.org/10.1257/jep.10.1.187.

Frank, R. H., Gilovich, T., & Regan, D. T. (1993). Does studying economics inhibit cooperation? *Journal of Economic Perspectives, 7*(2), 159–171. https://doi.org/10.1257/jep.7.2.159.

Felber, C. (2015). *Change everything: Creating an economy for the common good*. Zed Books Ltd.

Galtung, J. (2004). Violence, war, and their impact: On visible and invisible effects of violence. In *Polylog: Forum for intercultural philosophy*, 5.

Fuentes, N., & Rojas, M. (2001). Economic theory and subjective well-being: Mexico. *Social Indicators Research, 53*(3), 289–314.

Guardiola, J., González-Gómez, F., García-Rubio, M. A., & Lendechy-Grajales, A. (2013). Does higher income equal higher levels of happiness in every society? The case of the Mayan people. *International Journal of Social Welfare, 22*(1), 35. https://doi.org/10.1111/j.1468-2397.2011.00857.x.

Guardiola, J., Picazo-Tadeo, A. J., & Rojas, M. (2015). Economic crisis and well-being in Europe: Introduction. *Social Indicators Research, 120*(2), 319. https://doi.org/10.1007/s11205-014-0594-x.

Guillen-Royo, M., Guardiola, J., & Garcia-Quero, F. (2017). Sustainable development in times of economic crisis: A needs-based illustration from Granada (Spain). *Journal of Cleaner Production, 150*, 267–276.

Institute of Peace and Economics. (2015). *The economic cost of violence containment.* (Institute of Peace and Economics). Available at: http://economicsandpeace.org/wp-content/uploads/2015/06/The-Economic-Cost-of-Violence-Containment.pdf

Jackson, T. (2009). *Prosperity without growth.* London: Earthscan.

Kasser, T. (2002). *The high price of materialism.* Cambridge, MA: The MIT Press.

Kuhn, T. S. (2012). *The structure of scientific revolutions.* Chicago: University of Chicago press.

Land, K. C., & Michalos, A. C. (2018). Fifty years after the social indicators movement: Has the promise been fulfilled? *Social Indicators Research, 135*(3), 835–868.

López Martínez, M. (2017). *Noviolencia o barbarie.* Dyckinson.

Michalos, A. C. (1997). Combining social, economic and environmental indicators to measure sustainable human well-being. *Social Indicators Research, 40*(1–2), 221–258.

Michalos, A. C., & Zumbo, B. D. (1999). Public services and the quality of life. *Social Indicators Research, 48*(2), 125–157.

Patrick, D., Edwards, T., Topolski, T., & Walwick, J. (2002). Youth quality of life: A new measure incorporating the voices of adolescents. *QOL Newsletter, 28*, 7.

Singer, P. (2010). *The life you can save: How to do your part to end world poverty.* New York: Random House Incorporated.

Sirgy, M. J. (1998). Materialism and quality of life. *Social Indicators Research, 43*(3), 227–260.

Tonon, G. (2010). La utilización de indicadores de calidad de vida para la decisión de políticas públicas. *Polis Revista Latinoamericana, 9*(26), 361.

Ruskin, J. (1985). *Unto this last.* London: Penguin.

Suárez-Varela, M., Guardiola, J., & González-Gómez, F. (2016). Do pro-environmental behaviors and awareness contribute to improve subjective well-being? *Applied Research Quality Life, 11*, 429–444. https://doi.org/10.1007/s11482-014-9372-9.

World Commission on Environment and Development. (1987). *Our common future (the Brundtland Report).* Oxford: Oxford University Press.

Jorge Guardiola is Associate Professor at the Department of Applied Economics, and member of the Institute of Peace and Conflicts at the University of Granada, Spain. He holds a PhD in Economics from Universidad de Córdoba, Spain, and a Masters in Economics from the Université Catholique de Louvain-la-Neuve, Belgium. His research interests are subjective well-being, peace studies, sustainable development and human needs. He has field experience in Latin American countries, particularly Guatemala, Mexico, Ecuador and Honduras.

Chapter 11
Online Education and Quality of Life: Universidad de Palermo as a Model of Innovation in Latin America

Matías Popovsky

Live as if you were to die tomorrow. Learn as if you were to live forever.

Mahatma Gandhi

Context

At the beginning of the twenty-first century, Duderstadt (2001, p.2) argued:

> "Modern digital technologies such as computers, telecommunications and networks are reshaping both our society and our social institutions. These technologies have increased vastly our capacity to know and to do things and to communicate and collaborate with others".

We are undoubtedly experiencing a revolution in the world of education, in the way we teach and in understanding how students learn. However, what is a revolution? A revolution can be defined as a moment in time in which a radical and significant change occurs in the way things are done – a moment in which the inertia of doing the same thing in the same manner is no longer sufficient; it no longer permits progress or even subsistence. Previous revolutions were driven by the railway and the steam engine, by electricity and assembly lines, and by the advent of computers and digital technology in different areas of production and everyday life (Schwab 2016).

Technology is ubiquitous in everything we do today. What seemed to be science fiction in the past is now almost irritating when it is unavailable. Being able to make video calls and send and receive messages in real time with thousands of people has become so common that no-one remembers that, for instance, not so long ago it took months – if not years – in Argentina to have a landline installed. We can now access, download and read hundreds of thousands of books. We no longer need to

M. Popovsky (✉)
Education Lab, Universidad de Palermo, Buenos Aires, Argentina
e-mail: mpopov@palermo.edu

© Springer Nature Switzerland AG 2020
G. H. Tonon (ed.), *Teaching Quality of Life in Different Domains*, Social Indicators Research Series 79, https://doi.org/10.1007/978-3-030-21551-4_11

worry about book imports, about whether a book is too heavy for us to carry in a bag, or about taking good care of it and keeping it in good condition. Similarly, we can listen to all the music we want, when we want, in the order we want. Gone are the days when people had to spend hours on end listening to the radio waiting for their favourite song to be played in order to record it. We can watch all the films available when we want to, pause and watch them again. No more scratched DVDs, special plans to tune in TV programmes at the right time, or video club subscriptions.

Likewise, we no longer need large and costly equipment to capture special moments of our lives in photographs and videos. The industries of telecommunications, entertainment and music – to name a few – have been thoroughly shaken by a technological disruption like no other in history. Companies such as Amazon, Spotify, Netflix and others have transformed society's patterns of behaviour, as the pace of change and technological evolution accelerate and technology becomes more and more rapidly obsolete. How long did it take Kodak to fall from undisputed leadership to being almost swept away from the industry? And how long did it take Blackberry to slide from telecommunications innovator to irrelevant player? The first Blackberry was launched in 1999. By late 2007, Research in Motion, the company behind the device, had a market capitalisation of USD 60 billion. Only 10 years later it was worth USD 4 billion, the company's lack of innovation being the main reason for its spectacular collapse.

Today, the world's largest car transportation provider (Uber) owns no vehicles, the largest media company (Facebook) creates no content, the company with the highest advertising revenues (Google) is not a medium within the traditional meaning of the word, and the largest accommodation provider (Airbnb) owns no rooms. The evolution of the business world makes us rethink education so that it can be embedded in this new reality.

Automation and robotics pose a dichotomy that will need to be addressed by governments, international agencies, and public and private actors. Workers, companies and industries engaged in the Knowledge Economy will find a favourable environment to flourish and expand. This Fourth Industrial Revolution liberates talent and resources that can be used in higher impact jobs, in more and better work positions. According to recent surveys carried out by the World Economic Forum (2018) 38% of companies expect to expand their workforce in roles that improve productivity, and 25% expect automation to create new jobs in their organisations. However, at the same time, many jobs – particularly repetitive and low value added ones – will be lost. There will be a readjustment of employment and some workers will inevitably be marginalised. Along the same lines, based on the profiles of their current employees, nearly 50% of companies expect automation to reduce their workforce by 2022. Society must provide this "intermediate generation" with possibilities and opportunities to enter the new professional world, and it is here where education and its new paradigms become relevant.

Today's world combines an increasingly longer life expectancy (driven by advances in science and medicine and improvements in quality of life) with the existence of more and more competitive markets in which success depends on a constant update of knowledge. Nowadays it is absurd to conceive education as a model of discrete stages to be completed by certain groups at certain times. It can no longer be thought to be sufficient for students to attend school for 12 years, to then go on to pursue undergraduate and graduate studies and finally join the workforce until retirement, with no update of knowledge. The current pace of change requires education to be continuous. University programs must be expanded and adapted, and must incorporate the tools needed to satisfy the demands of an increasingly broader and more diverse demographic group. Students will not be of the same age, or at the same stage in their lives, nor will they seek to acquire the same skills. They will not have the same academic or professional background, and many of them will be based in different parts of the world. However, they will all have one feature in common: the need for knowledge, to connect with other people, to acquire tools that best interprets their needs. Some will want to prepare in the best possible way for the world of work with technical skills of their discipline. Others will seek to expand their areas of interest, in order to improve their general knowledge. Some people will want to send a signal to the market about their topics of interest or they might simply want to study for pleasure, to keep their senses and reasoning skills sharp. The reasons are, and will be, manifold; therefore, education must be flexible and higher education institutions must be sensitive to the current times.

Over the past few years there has been much discussion about the skills needed for the twenty-first century, and it still is an ongoing debate among faculty in higher education institutions. The perennial questions "what should we teach our students?" and "what abilities and skills should they have when they graduate?" are today more relevant than ever. For many years, education was almost entirely based on the transfer of information, which was an almost ritual act that allowed knowledge to be handed down from generation to generation, from parents to children, from teachers to students.

While this is still true and necessary, information today is no longer a distinguishing feature but virtually a commodity. Access to data in different formats is greater than ever, and the challenge that in the past was obtaining information has now become the ability to interpret it, to make sense out of it, to discern between fake news and quality information, to be able to validate a source, process data and different situations and analyse them critically.

In his book *21 Lessons for the twenty-first Century*, Harari (2018) highlights the importance for students to develop the four Cs: Creativity, Collaboration, Communication and Critical thinking. Developing a culture of innovation is critical to progress. Imagination is the human attribute par excellence; through it, we create a vision and carry it out. We will be increasingly more dependent upon imagination in the next few years. As once stated by Einstein (1931, p. 97), "imagination is more important than knowledge". Or why have some people with the same available resources been able to achieve extraordinary things, while others have not? Needless to say, multiple factors are involved; however, the path to great inventions begins in the sphere of imagination. How can we build a great skyscraper without first visualising it? Or how can we produce a masterpiece without first drawing it in our mind? All the letters of the alphabet were available for years and years, but the books written with them by the great authors were, first of all, great works of their imagination.

The iterative process of innovation is a trait of our species, and it is one of the factors that allow us to evolve. Education, as it is conceived in today's world, is a continuous process and a way of approaching life. Education is being open to the constant acquisition of knowledge.

One of the key factors the professionals of the future need to develop today is their ability to cope with change and constantly learn new skills, to learn and relearn, in a virtuous circle of adaptation to the environment and the challenges that lie ahead. They need to wonder: how do I solve problems, working in a team and in a collaborative manner? How do I communicate assertively, persuade and convince?.

The truth is, no-one knows for certain what inter-personal relationships will be like in 20- or 40-years' time, what businesses will be like, what our lifestyle or the traits that will make us more or less successful will be like. However, we can attempt to define the skills that are the most relevant today for students to better adapt and thrive in a context of permanent change. The World Economic Forum (2015) identifies 16 skills for the twenty-first century and divides them into three categories:

1. Foundational literacies: how students apply core skills to everyday tasks (literacy, numeracy, scientific literacy, ICT literacy, financial literacy, and cultural and civic literacy).
2. Competencies: how students deal with complex challenges (critical thinking / problem-solving, curiosity, creativity, initiative, communication, persistence, collaboration).
3. Character qualities: how students approach their changing environment (curiosity, initiative, persistence, adaptability, leadership, social and cultural awareness).

The other side of the question "what should we teach?" posed by university faculty members might well be the questions raised by many students in their senior years of high school: "What will I do when I am an adult?" and "What Degree will I pursue at the university?.

In response to these questions, students are usually advised to speak with different professionals and explore their everyday work, tasks and occupations, and their way of adding value to society with their jobs, so that students can picture themselves in that role. However, what is the appropriate way of addressing these questions today, when the evolution of work has rendered current examples unrepresentative of future scenarios and jobs?

Pink (2009) formulates the theory of intrinsic motivation. People perform better and are more productive when they enjoy their job, when the incentive to do their job comes from within rather than from an award and punishment structure. We could apply Pink's framework of autonomy, mastery and purpose to attempt to answer these questions.

Therefore, rather than letting students think what they will do or what they will study, we should push them to think about (1) (purpose) What problem do they wish to solve? What is the context of that problem, the long-term goal, the most important reason motivating them? What Degree brings them closer to solving that problem? (2) (autonomy) How do they want to solve it? Motivation through autonomy allows thinking creatively in less structured and ruled contexts, assuming responsibility for the results obtained, and (3) (mastery) What do they need to learn in order to do it? What are the skills that they will need to develop in their training and educational experience in order to successfully address those challenges? What Degree course best adapts to that path?

Universidad de Palermo (UP)

Universidad de Palermo is a young, innovative and entrepreneurial university located in Buenos Aires, Argentina. It is fascinating to describe the University due to the diversity of its academic groups (its more than 13,000 students are divided into six schools: Architecture, Business, Social Sciences, Law, Design and Communication, and Engineering), each group with its own culture and traits, its own set of traditions and views that enrich the University as a whole, and fundamentally, due to the faculty, who are recognised leaders in their professional fields and who push students to challenge their limits.

Universidad de Palermo has gained continuous international recognition in different university rankings as one of the most innovative and prestigious universities in Latin America. Moreover, its students have an outstanding performance in inter-university competitions, and its graduates are sought after by companies and institutions – both from Argentina and the region – that recognise in their talent and training an opportunity to achieve great things.

Based on the premise that universities must not only teach their students to innovate, but they must also be a driver of innovation and change in society, Universidad de Palermo is one of the main and most active catalysers of the latest advances in the science of learning. As such, it provides its academic community with access to world-class technology and an education for the future, preparing students to be successful professionals in a changing, diverse, and ever-competitive world, in which critical thinking, adaptation and continuous learning are essential. It is a university that prepares students to communicate, argue and convince; to develop their analysis and critical thinking skills; to have a significant level of general knowledge and express themselves fluently in writing; to work in teams in contexts of diversity; and to be able to adjust to change. And, fundamentally, it prepares students to continuously learn to relearn, adapt and reinvent themselves.

The Education Lab

The above-described scenario of disruption in the world of learning, coupled with the University's vision to continue to be at the forefront of education, was the foundation for the of the Education Lab, Universidad de Palermo's laboratory of innovation applied to education. A unique initiative in Latin America, the lab has allowed the University to consolidate its leadership in higher education in the region. Located in a dedicated building and comprised of an interdisciplinary team of professionals from different areas and academic backgrounds, the lab is tasked with the mission of reimagining education and reinventing the mode of teaching and learning, by taking advantage of the latest advances in the science of learning, using state-of-the-art technology and capitalising on the synergy of the different schools of the University. "Clearly, the digital age poses many challenges and presents many opportunities for the contemporary university" (Duderstadt 2001, p. 3).

In line with the above goals, the lab's first challenge was to design UP's online Degrees, Programs and courses. Following a period of best practices exploration in different universities from the US and Brazil —visits to their content production centres and audio-visual studios, and exchanging ideas with their leaders, the Education Lab developed a teaching model based on the University's pedagogical innovations and needs, with features and a style of its own.

UP's inclusion of online education followed a natural evolution. The path towards the convergence of online and on campus education is accelerating at a time when the knowledge economy is the main factor of growth, and the boundaries between both modes of study are becoming more and more blurred. The university's innovation tradition and the international profile of its students and graduates – along with the maturity of the educational technologies currently available – made the decision to offer online education not a difficult one. Quite on the contrary, it was a logical consequence in the organic growth of University of Palermo.

From the outset, the University's online learning initiative has been premised on a high standard of academic rigour and quality. This endorses the prestige of the other modalities of study at UP and meets the high expectations of students, who are accustomed to a rigorous, world-class educational experience at Universidad de Palermo.

The Education Lab comprises an interdisciplinary team of professionals with an academic background and professional expertise in areas so diverse as technology, education, humanities, design, philosophy, economics and psychology, to name but a few.

With the collaboration of the different schools and their academic authorities, an educational model was created that features the following characteristics:

Collaborative, highly interactive learning
State-of-the-art technology
Students' freedom to choose how to study
Faculty trained for online teaching
Study materials especially designed for online learning
Student connections
Participative teaching methodologies
Customization of learning
Education for the future

Collaborative, Highly Interactive Learning

The instructional design of the courses, the set-up of the groups, the development of the study materials and the faculty's teaching style all coalesce to promote collaborative learning, which allows students to learn both from their classmates and their professors. Students have a very high level of interaction, and courses are delivered in small groups in which professors really know their students, in interactive and participative classes. Each course has a tutor, who provides students with personalised guidance and support throughout each course. Focus is placed not only in the development of each student but also in the intelligence of the group as a whole.

State-of-the-Art Technology

Technology has an impact on everything we do, and this is an irreversible trend. Technology will continue to evolve, and we can safely say, almost on a note of future nostalgia, that today's state-of-the-art technology will be the worst our children will see in their lives.

At Universidad de Palermo technology is not conceived as an end in itself, but rather as a means to improve the quality of education, break the barriers of face-to-face learning and create a real-time communication infrastructure between professors and students.

Courses and programs delivered at UP use state-of-the-art technology for education. Available anywhere in any device, the online campus (both in its desktop and mobile app versions) gives students easy and intuitive access to materials and activities. The software used for synchronous video-classes integrates different tools for student's participation, strengthening bonds and providing more and better opportunities for interaction. Additionally, the University has interactive discussion tools and spaces. Different security measures are taken during examinations in order to confirm the identity of the students and ensure the integrity of evaluations.

Moreover, the online education team monitors students' academic performance using the information generated in different points of contact, and different data sources are integrated for feedback into an analytics proprietary system that provides an overall picture of each student which is highly useful to the work of professors and tutors.

Students' Freedom to Choose How to Study

The present and future of education is focused on the student – the person that studies and learns. Students at Universidad de Palermo can choose to take courses online, on campus, or to combine both alternatives. This helps foster autonomy, self-organisation and commitment, these being traits that contribute to academic development and professional growth.

Some students begin their studies in UP's urban campus in Buenos Aires, and then choose to take online classes. Others start studying online and then complete their degrees with on campus classes. And many choose to combine both modalities of study in each semester, selecting online and on campus classes in order to find their ideal mix. There are as many ways of studying as there are students' needs. Instead of students adapting to the university, the university adapts to them, and this is a very powerful concept.

Faculty Trained for Online Teaching

The faculty at Universidad de Palermo – experts and leaders in their fields – are especially trained for online teaching. They have vast experience in both teaching and professional practice. At the same time, tutors provide personalised guidance to students, help them adjust to online student life, offer strategies and reminders, connect students with available resources and assist them in achieving their academic goals. Both professors and tutors encourage students to learn and achieve, thus creating a challenging and, at the same time, collaborative learning environment.

Materials Especially Designed for Online Learning

Study materials are especially designed for online learning, following a rigorous content production process carried out by the pedagogic teams of the Education Lab, led by instructional designers and faculty members. The material includes cases and simulations, some prepared by the University and others published by internationally renowned universities.

Connections

Universidad de Palermo aims not only to develop the best educational contents and expand access to education, but also to create value in connecting students (Anand 2016), both inside and outside the (virtual) classroom. Through debate and argumentation, students learn from their classmates' contributions, and build a lifelong academic, social and professional network. Activities and academic work designed for individual study are combined with others especially tailored for teamwork.

The workload and demanding pace of studies of the University's distance education programs make the support of study groups critical, and create a teamwork experience that is highly valued by students and employers alike.

Participative Teaching Methodologies

Students at Universidad de Palermo engage in enquiry, reasoning, analysis and problem-solving throughout their studies, and use materials featuring real life problems and examples (Anand et al. 2015), so that they can later successfully address the situations they will come across in their professional life.

Students are exposed to different teaching styles and train their creativity and imagination to solve problems, thus creating original concepts, assessing and providing arguments for their decisions and reaching the highest levels of Bloom's (1964) taxonomy. For instance, Business students use cases and simulations for which they discuss and analyse business situations and gain experience in critical thinking and decision making with incomplete information, as is the case in the real world.

Customization of Learning

If individuals do not learn in the same way and they do not possess the same previous knowledge, why should they be taught in the same manner? Some need more practicing and activities; others, more time to internalise concepts. Some students benefit more from individual lessons, while others do better in group work. Some have an academic background in the topics covered whereas others are new to the discipline. Universidad de Palermo offers students different learning paths to attain the same knowledge objective. Adaptive learning is progressively being used in different courses in order to build a personalised educational experience using the University's world-class technology and specially developed materials tailored to each student's needs.

Education for the Future

Universidad de Palermo aims to train professionals with skills to adapt to a complex and evolving world, to prepare them to create employment and develop new industries, and to succeed in jobs that do not yet exist.

With these goals in mind, the University works on each course's hidden curriculum. Critical competencies to be developed by the students – aside from the skills specific to each subject – are defined and incorporated into the syllabi.

The Online Course on Quality of Life and Happiness

Graciela Tonon

The proposal of an online course on the study of quality of life is based precisely on the recognition of the relationship between quality of life and online learning since, as stated by Mercer (1994), quoted by Leung and Lee (2005, p. 162): "The quest for quality of life is a growing concern for individuals and communities seeking to find sustainable life satisfaction in a technologically changing world"[1].

The course is intended for advanced students of the different degree courses delivered by the University as well as for professionals and/or academics and/or researchers interested in the topic, whether they are graduates from the University or beyond.

The course is based on the following goals:

(a) To gain deeper knowledge of quality of life at the personal, community and social levels, taking account of different populational and cultural groups, as well as different geographic contexts.
(b) To gain deeper knowledge of happiness.
(c) To identify emerging fields in quality of life studies.

The course runs for 14 weeks and is organised into a first introductory module and 13 thematic modules, each of which focuses on a central theme, namely:

- Origin and evolution of the concept of quality of life
- Differences between the concepts of social welfare and personal well-being
- Community quality of life
- The socio-territorial space and quality of life
- Urban quality of life
- The use of quality of life measurements for public policy decision making
- Citizenship and quality of life
- The concept of happiness and innovative proposals for its measurement

---

[1] She is the designer and head lecturer of the course

- Children's quality of life
- Young people's quality of life
- Older adults' quality of life
- Culture and quality of life
- Physical activity and quality of life

During the course the following techniques were used:

Timeline
Discussion forum
Conceptual map
PowerPoint presentation
Argumentative texts
Collaborative mural
Computer graphics
Video forum
Social cartography exercise
Interview to expert
Professor's videos

These techniques allow students to learn each topic and consolidate their knowledge, and further facilitate the assessment of knowledge acquisition.

Conclusions

We consider that online education collaborate to improve student's quality of life reducing time and space barriers in relation with the different ways to learn, so the inclusion of a specific course dedicated to quality of life is a new enhancer of this first idea.

We are witnessing a fascinating paradigm shift in education, in which inertia and tradition clash with innovation, new technologies and the challenges posed by a new generation of students.

History will look back on our time as a turning point in the ways of teaching and learning. Those higher education institutions that do not take this opportunity to rethink their educational processes are bound to become obsolete, or worse still, irrelevant. Universidad de Palermo and its Education Lab work, today more than ever, to provide their academic community with another way of studying.

References

Anand, B. (2016). *The content trap. A strategist's guide to digital change*. New York: Random House, Penguin Random House.

Anand, B., Hammond, J., Narayanan, V.G. (2015). What harvard business school has learned about online collaboration From HBX. *Harvard Business Review. April 14, 2015.* Retrieved January 29, 2019, from https://hbr.org/2015/04/what-harvard-business-school-has-learned-about-online-collaboration-from-hbx.

Bloom, B. (1964). *Taxonomy of educational objectives: The classification of educational goals*. New York: D McKay Company.

Duderstadt, J. (2001, May 31) *The future of the university in the digital age*. The Glion Conference, Switzerland.

Einstein, A. (1931). *Cosmic religion and other opinions and aphorisms*. New York: Covici-Friede, Inc.

Harari, Y. (2018). *21 lessons for the 21st century*. New York: Spiegel & Grau/Random House, Penguin Random House.

Ko, S., & Rossen, S. (2008). *Teaching online. A practical guide*. New York: Routledge.

Leung, L., & Lee, P. (2005). Multiple determinants of life quality: The roles of Internet activities, use of new media, social support and leisure activities. *Telematics and Informatics, 22*, 161–180. Elsevier.

Pink, D. (2009). *Drive: The surprising truth about what motivates us*. New York: Riverhead Books, Penguin Group.

Schwab, K. (2016). Welcome to the fourth industrial revolution. *Rotman Management, 25*, 19–24.

World Economic Forum. (2018). *The future of jobs report*. Retrieved December 22, 2018, from https://www.weforum.org/reports/the-future-of-jobs-report-2018.

Matías Popovsky   Master in Business Administration The Wharton School at the University of Pennsylvania. Bachelor of Business Administration and Masters in Finance. Vice-Rector, Universidad de Palermo. Director, Education Lab. Universidad de Palermo, Argentina. His research interests include innovation in higher education, applied science of learning models, and higher education finance.

Chapter 12
Teaching and Learning Quality of Life in Urban Studies: A Mixed-Methods Approach with Walking Interviews

Javier Martinez

Introduction

This chapter presents an approach and a series of case studies related to the practice of teaching and learning Quality of Life (QoL) in the context of urban studies. This practice is embedded within an MSc program with a specialization in Urban Planning and Management (UPM). The nature and scope of the UPM specialization relates to the field of urban studies. In this chapter, urban studies is considered a transdisciplinary field (Ramadier 2004) related to various disciplines associated with the study of urban areas like urban geography, architecture and planning.

Urban studies is in many cases associated with quantitative studies. In particular, urban planning may be predominantly oriented towards rational and quantitative approaches. As Eizenberg and Shilon (2015 citing Gaber 1993: 140) note, if planners primarily focus on quantitative-orientated research they might miss "(1) The link between planning researchers and the people they plan for; (2) [Subjective aspects of] quality of life issues; and (3) Informal/illegal activity" in addition to conflicts and varied interests. The teaching and learning practice reflected in this chapter is aware of these constrains and hence incorporates perspectives that are derived from mixed-methods approaches and are context sensitive.

The aim of this chapter is to share an approach for teaching and learning QoL in the context of urban studies and to illustrate its possibilities with specific learning activities and outputs. This chapter starts with a brief theoretical discussion on how urban studies relates to the concept of QoL. It describes top-down as well as bottom-up people centred approaches and explain how they are incorporated within the UPM specialization. Both approaches can generate relevant knowledge about QoL

J. Martinez (✉)
Faculty of Geo-Information Science and Earth Observation,
Department of Urban and Regional Planning and Geo-Information Management,
University of Twente, Enschede, The Netherlands
e-mail: j.martinez@utwente.nl

© Springer Nature Switzerland AG 2020   209
G. H. Tonon (ed.), *Teaching Quality of Life in Different Domains*, Social
Indicators Research Series 79, https://doi.org/10.1007/978-3-030-21551-4_12

domains (objective and subjective) that are relevant to improve our understanding of the built living environment and its socio-economic context. To analyse and illustrate the foundations and challenges of these approaches, the chapter relies on the critical documentation of two courses carried out with a group of international MSc students in the last 10 years. Students following this approach were encouraged to define and operationalise spatial indicators to measure intra-urban QoL variations and to critically evaluate the use of several qualitative and quantitative methods. The teaching and learning described is grounded in the fields of planning, geography and critical cartography as well as mixed-methods. The chapter concludes with a discussion on the main challenges of this approach.

Quality of Life and Urban Studies

QoL is multidimensional in nature and relates to various domains of life such as housing, income, built and natural environment, health and the level of satisfaction that individuals have with those domains and the overall satisfaction with life (McCrea et al. 2006; Seik 2000; Sirgy et al. 2006; Tesfazghi et al. 2010). QoL studies distinguish between "objective" and "subjective" conditions. Objective QoL is usually measured by using indicators that represent observable and measurable conditions (e.g. durable housing, adequate water provision, availability of green areas, and accessibility to schools). It is usually considered as a relatively "objective" assessment done by experts. However, "objective" measures may require some sort of subjective judgment (for example, different standards may exist to consider a dwelling inadequate). Similarly, a "subjective" assessment is done by people when it is referred to subjective QoL.

In the UPM specialization, we follow a geographic and mixed-methods approach that facilitate the identification of both objective and subjective views as well as promote the integration of qualitative and quantitative data (Martínez 2009, 2016, 2018; Martínez et al. 2017), and more importantly, the integration of experts and people's views. The recognition of people's views and diversity of perspectives are also present in current co-production of knowledge, inclusive development and planning discourses (Feldman and Khademian 2007; Watson 2014). Eliciting people's views is also advocated by those who promote new pedagogical approaches in planning for the in-depth understanding of people's lived experiences (Eizenberg and Shilon 2015).

There is a long tradition in urban studies that explicitly engage with QoL (Smith 1973) in relation to human geography (Pacione 1982) and the social indicators movement (Wong 2006). The emergence of Geographic Information Systems (GIS) has also facilitated the integration of objective and subjective approaches as well as different forms of data sources (Marans and Stimson 2011). Marans and Stimson (2011) make use of the concept of quality of urban life (UQOL) which relates to objective conditions of the places in which people live and the different subjective judgments that people have on those conditions.

We can distinguish studies that incorporate top-down approaches aiming at urban and intra-urban comparisons (Baud et al. 2008) as well as bottom-up approaches that emphasize the context and the view of the residents. The social indicators tradition (Smith 1973), top- and bottom-up QoL studies as well as local government QoL reports[1] are integrated in the UPM teaching and learning practice. In particular, this UPM specialization emphasizes the relevance that QoL studies have to practice and policy by linking the need for a better understanding of QoL conditions with equity and social justice, the concepts of inclusive city and the just city (Fainstein 2010, 2014). In this manner, the concept of QoL (and variations of) can facilitate making inequalities more visible.

The Relevance of Empathic Forms of Quality of Life Mapping

In the UPM courses, we emphasize the importance of *empathic* forms of QoL mapping; these are forms of QoL analysis that make visible inequalities that negatively affect the ideal of a just and inclusive city. These empathic and sensitive forms of mapping require different forms of knowledge (not only the technical or scientific knowledge produced by experts) and the recognition of convergent and divergent views between different groups.

Our UPM students are trained in GIS, however we also encourage them to have a critical approach since maps cannot be considered neutral representations of reality, they are not value-free, but loaded with power and socially constructed (Harley 1989). We make our students aware of the implicit 'slants' that operationalization, validation, classification and spatial representation of information embody (Monmonier 1996). Informed by these critical cartography perspectives we explain to our students that cartographic representations of unequal QoL conditions (and other manifestations of inequalities) are shaped by three factors (Fig. 12.1). (1) the conceptualization of deprivations (e.g. theoretically driven), (2) the knowledge sources (e.g. census data and expert codified) and 3- the spatial representation (e.g. predefined census boundaries) (Martínez et al. 2016). All these factors are either shaped in top-down (by experts) or in a bottom-up (by people) fashion. Experts (e.g. urban planners) represent the external view -or in anthropological terms, the *etic view*- and peoples view represent the *emic views* (the internal view of the community) (Fig. 12.1).

Mapping only the etic or expert views (e.g. producing maps based only on objective QoL conditions) is probably not counting what counts for people. Therefore, in the UPM courses we combine the emic and the etic view: we combine objective QoL measured by experts and QoL derived from people's perceptions. QoL studies combining those views can determine divergent and convergent assessments of QoL conditions. One of the studies derived from the work of one of our UPM students

---

[1] See e.g. Bristol Quality of Life reports https://www.bristol.gov.uk/statistics-census-information/the-quality-of-life-in-bristol

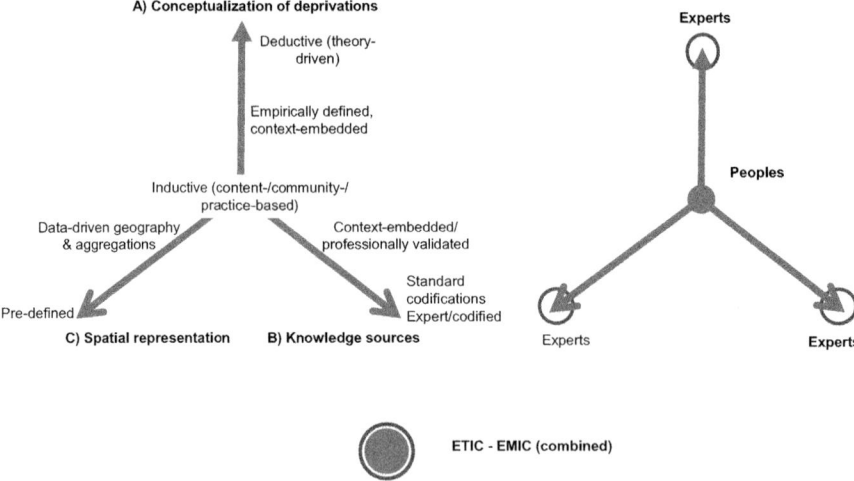

Fig. 12.1 Factors shaping cartographic representations, experts/peoples view, Etic-Emic. (Adapted from Martínez et al. 2016)

(Tesfazghi et al. 2010) illustrates how this combination allows four possible resulting states of QoL: well-being, deprivation, adaptation and dissonance (see Sect. 4).

The geographic dimension in this approach elicits spatial variations within and between neighbourhoods. This is of particular relevance for policy and planning because it maps the locations of deprived and well-being areas and places experiences and perceptions in their actual spatial context.

We make our UPM students aware of the risk of disciplinary bias when mapping QoL research only from an etic perspective. Rojas (2015, p. 340), while describing the risks of experts classifying people as being in a state of deprivation exclusively from their own constructs, writes:

> "It is a common complain of politicians that ordinary people do not show the same passion for wellbeing indicators as those who are constructing and using them show. In consequence, experts face the risk of classifying others based on their own disciplinary focus, rather than on people's own life focus" (Rojas 2015, p. 340)

The risks of a disciplinary bias can be reduced when both etic (expert) and emic (lay, peoples or communities) accounts are collected and when a multidisciplinary approach informs the QoL research. The two by two matrix in Fig. 12.2 reflects such an approach (Martínez et al. 2017).

In the following sections, we illustrate how this approach has been taught at the Faculty ITC, University of Twente (the Netherlands) within the Urban Planning and Management Specialization (UPM) of the 2-year Master's Geo-Information Science and Earth Observation.[2]

---

[2] The UPM specialization is run within the Department of Urban and Regional Planning and Geo-Information Management at Faculty ITC in Enschede (the Netherlands). The Faculty ITC was funded in 1950 and has accumulated extensive experience in capacity building and institutional

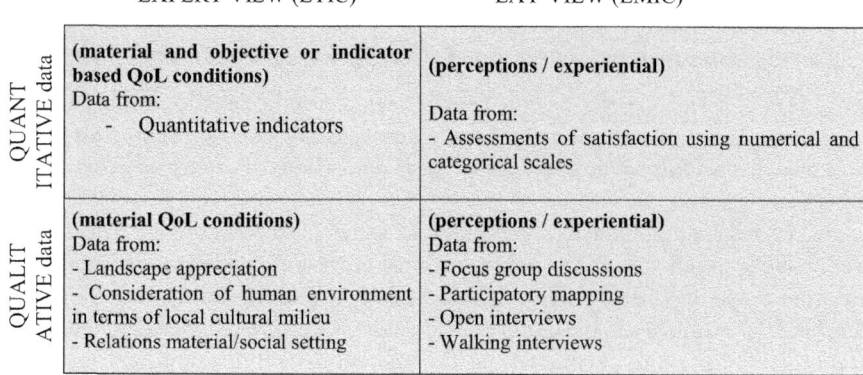

EXPERT VIEW (ETIC)	LAY VIEW (EMIC)
QUANTITATIVE data **(material and objective or indicator based QoL conditions)** Data from: - Quantitative indicators	**(perceptions / experiential)** Data from: - Assessments of satisfaction using numerical and categorical scales
QUALITATIVE data **(material QoL conditions)** Data from: - Landscape appreciation - Consideration of human environment in terms of local cultural milieu - Relations material/social setting	**(perceptions / experiential)** Data from: - Focus group discussions - Participatory mapping - Open interviews - Walking interviews

Fig. 12.2 Mixed methods approach to capture unequal QoL conditions and different ways it can be expressed

Teaching and Learning Quality of Life in an International Programme

For the last 10 years, I have been teaching in two UPM courses: *The Inclusive City* (5 ECTS[3] credits, compulsory) and *Analysis of Intra-Urban Socio-Spatial Patterns* (5 ECTS credits, elective). The Inclusive City course[4] relates to top-down city-wide approaches (predominantly etic views) while the Analysis of Intra-Urban Socio-Spatial Patterns course engages more within bottom-up, predominantly emic views and incorporates mixed methods and qualitative methods such as walking interviews and text analysis. The next sections describe in detail the learning objectives, content, methods, and (research) outputs derived from these two courses.

The Inclusive City Course. Social Indicators

In UPM course The Inclusive City, two learning objectives were designed to engage students with social justice perspectives and social indicators in urban studies. Upon completion of this course, the students are able to:

---

development of professional and academic organizations and individuals specifically from less-developed countries in the field of geo-information science and earth observation and its applications (See: www.itc.nl)

[3] ECTS corresponds to the European Credit Transfer and Accumulation System (ECTS) credits. According to this standard, one academic year corresponds to 60 ECTS credits. One ECTS is the equivalent to 28 h of total workload.

[4] The name of this course was initially called "Analyzing and Monitoring Urban Dynamics" and it was later changed to "The Inclusive City". Since September 2018, the course is called "the Inclusive and Competitive city".

- Explain the theoretical notions of equity, fairness and social justice and their relation to the inclusive city concept;
- Identify, construct and analyse spatial and non-spatial indicators of multiple deprivation.

Following Blooms taxonomy of learning objectives (Anderson et al. 2001) these two objectives relate to the cognitive process dimensions of comprehension, application and analysis.

A key teaching approach which prepares students to reflect and evaluate their methodological choices is the spiral learning process for indicators development (Martínez and Dopheide 2014). Martínez and Dopheide (2014) recognize that teaching the methods and the use of the indicators is a challenge, since it requires -in a short period of time- the practice of the different steps of the development of the indicators. The spiral learning process (Fig. 12.3) differentiates several steps: from counting, construction and operationalization of the indicators to steps related to

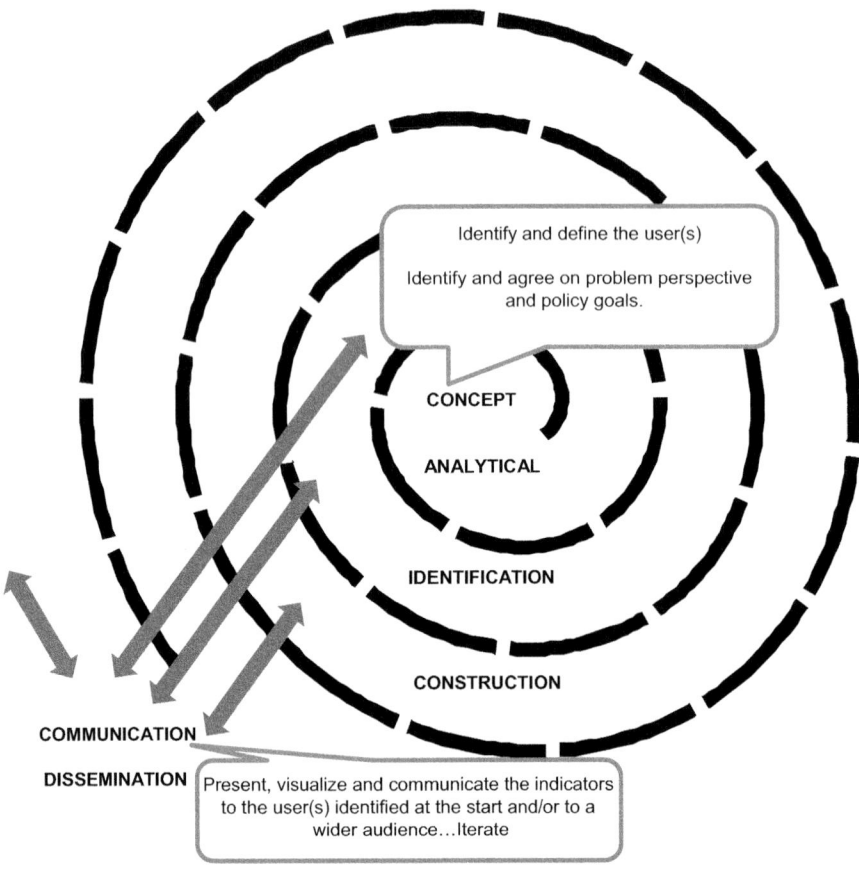

Fig. 12.3 Open spiral learning process for the indicators development (Martínez and Dopheide 2014). Steps adapted from Wong (2006, p. 106)

policy and learning that require a more critical, reflective process. Some of the steps are mechanistic while others require an iterative, reflective and metacognitive process.

In our teaching, we explain UPM students that indicators are qualitative or quantitative data that describe the characteristics of a given phenomenon and communicate an evaluation of the phenomenon in question. Furthermore, indicators should be explicitly selected for their relevance to policy issues and related to a specific time and place. With this definition, we want to emphasize the policy relevance of the indicators, particularly if they are used to inform planning. One of the strengths of indicators as a tool for urban planning is that they have the potential to communicate complex problems in a simple and understandable way. They help in the formulation of explicit objectives and in the development of a shared vision on relevant issues. They have the advantage of being objectively verifiable and can help monitor and evaluate progress. They are also a powerful communication tool that can inform the public, raise awareness about various topics of interest and encourage action and empowerment. In the context of governance and participation, it is worth noting that if indicators are properly developed they can promote transparency and accountability (Martínez and Dopheide 2014).

Our experience with teaching and researching on indicators shows that for a successful implementation and uptake of indicators some conditions are required. Key elements relate to stakeholders' participation, iterations and communication throughout all the steps of indicator development (Fig. 12.3), particularly in the identification of indicators and presentation (Martínez and Dopheide 2014). This spiral learning process pays explicit attention to the elements of communication, information sharing, collaboration, learning and empowerment.

This critical approach has been implemented in some of the MSc thesis of our students. For example, one of the first MSc studies resulting from this course was that of Trisusanti (2008) with a case study on multiple deprivation.[5] Using official (top-down) secondary data, this student showed how the resulting rank of deprived areas could vary just by altering the methods that synthesised the indicators into a final index (Fig. 12.4). In relation to transparency of methods, Trisusanti (2008) also stressed the need to evaluate and show the sensitivity of different techniques to policy and decision makers. This case shows how students can demonstrate how top-down "objective" measures are sensitive to experts' choice and are not neutral representations of reality. Despite that students are exposed to secondary (e.g. official census data) and predominantly etic views, we emphasize a critical perspective on indicators.

---

[5] The use of indices of multiple deprivations diffused from the United Kingdom experience towards cases in the Global South and other European countries. This is also replicated in research carried at Faculty ITC in relation to a critical analysis of the use of indicators to rank multiple deprived areas by the Dutch government (Dopheide and Martinez 2007).

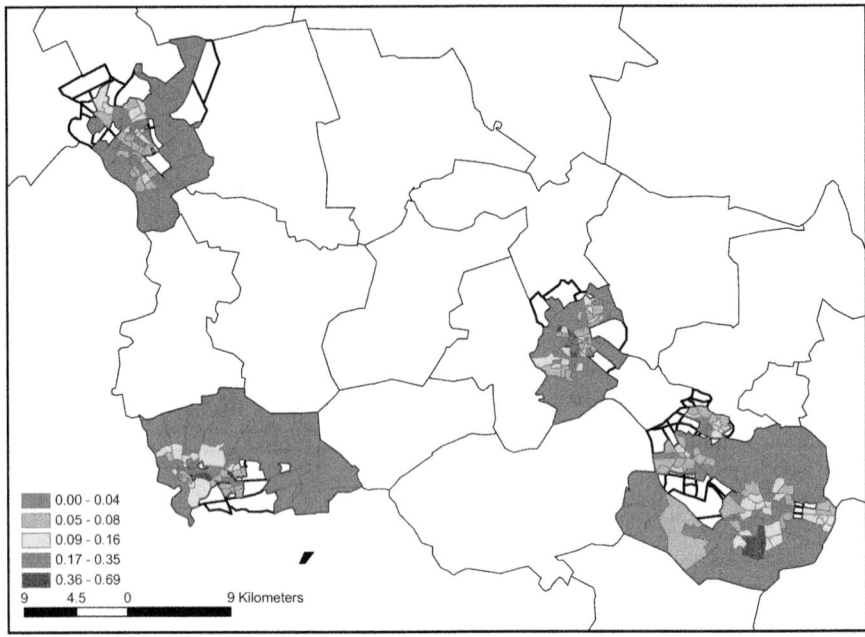

Fig. 12.4 Multiple deprivation across Overijssel. In read areas with high level of relative depriva-tion Trisusanti (2008)

Analysis of Intra-urban Socio-spatial Patterns Course. Mixed-Methods

In the UPM course Analysis of Intra-Urban Socio-Spatial Patterns, we explore issues of socio-spatial inequality, differentiation and fragmentation that have an impact on the urban environment and on the QoL of urban residents. The learning activities concentrate on capturing and understanding diverse forms of knowledge regarding intra-urban variations of QoL conditions and access to social infrastruc-ture (e.g. health and education services).

Many of the learning activities in the course include "hands-on experiences" such as walking interviews. Eizenberg and Shilon (2015, p. 1131) present "hands-on experiences" as one of the key pedagogical inputs for qualitative research meth-ods for planners as these methods require "stepping into the field and experiencing it". Eizenberg and Shilon (2015) claim that this approach is necessary because in this way students can develop a deep understanding of both the case study area (the spatial) and its users (the social). Some of the strengths relate to "engaging with the field and its users in their natural settings" and "Immersion in the users' point of view" (Eizenberg and Shilon 2015, p. 1131). One of the challenges the authors iden-tify is observed in this course and it relates to " the brief experience due to the scope limits of an academic course" (Eizenberg and Shilon 2015, p. 1131).

In the study guide that students receive before enrolling to this elective course we explain that "a better understanding of the resulting socio-spatial patterns is essential for targeting (multiple) deprived areas and implementing area-based and regeneration policies" In this way directly relate the concepts to practice and policy. Upon completion of this course, the student will be able to:

- Explain intra-urban socio-spatial patterns and the relation with current theoretical and empirical debates in urban studies;
- Explain the importance of intra-urban patterns and inequality analysis in planning;
- Apply a combination of qualitative, statistical and GIS-based spatial analytical methods to detect and analyse intra-urban variation patterns;
- Describe the relevance and validity of selected quantitative and qualitative methods in the context of urban studies;
- Examine and critically reflect on the methodological choice and the incorporation of both quantitative and qualitative data analysis;
- Interpret results and relate these both to theoretical debates as well as to policy implications.

Following Blooms taxonomy of learning objectives (Anderson et al. 2001) these objectives relate to the cognitive process dimensions of comprehension, application and analysis and metacognitive dimensions that require critical reflection and evaluation.

In different learning activities that include (guest) lectures and group presentations, students learn concepts related to Intra-Urban Socio-Spatial Patterns in Urban Studies; Spatial Justice; Spatial Inequality and Environmental Justice. QoL is presented together with the concepts Community Well-Being and Deprivation. Diverse forms of knowledge and etic and emic views are explained (Fig. 12.2).

This UPM course also introduces a mixed-methods approach. We present the concept of mixed-methods in the context of QoL (Tonon 2015). Through a combination of (guest) lectures, reading assignments, exercises, and a final group work assignment, students learn to combine quantitatively derived patterns and measures with urban residents' generated data and perceptions, and to interpret the complementary results acquired. Some of the quantitative tools learned are related to data reduction and factor analysis with examples in QoL (Pacione 2003a) and cluster analysis (K-means) as a form of neighbourhood analysis and targeting. Traditional quantitative GIS methods are taught to map intra-urban patterns and change as well a qualitative GIS.[6] In qualitative GIS we put emphasis on patterns of user generated data and qualitative data. A combination of these two methods allows students to distinguish between "objective" and "subjective" measures. Computer Aided Qualitative Data Analysis Software (CAQDAS) is taught to facilitate text analysis and geocode quotations.

---

[6] For a detailed discussion on GIS, geo-technologies and urban governance see (Pfeffer et al. 2015)

A key assignment during this course is a "hands-on experience" in the form of a group work that requires carrying out a walking interview. The following subsection, discusses in detail this assignment.

Walking Interview Assignment

A walking interview is a mobile method for interviewing. It has some similarities with transect walks and rapid appraisal methods. It involves the researcher and participant walking along specific streets. Depending on the interviewee familiarity with the area, the researcher might be guided by the participant. A structured route can be set by the researcher if there is a specific area that needs to be studied. Walking interviews are important for QoL studies because they explore the relationship between what people say and where they say it (Evans and Jones 2011), they capture people's understanding of a particular place or the whole neighbourhood.

The students that attend this UPM course are already familiar with traditional GIS software (i.e. ArcGIS™) which is designed for quantitative data analysis. The walking interview exercise allows students to experience the combination of qualitative data (text from the interviews) with GIS data (the track and location of the walk and points of interest mentioned by the interviewees). The importance of integrating qualitative data in a GIS is relevant in urban studies since people do not experience their lives in abstract Cartesian spaces but in places that have meaning and emotions. This has resulting in what is called qualitative GIS (Cope and Elwood 2009) and opened up as well the emergence of CAQDAS tools that integrate geocoding mechanisms (e.g. ATLAS.ti™). In order to analyse the walking interviews students learn with systematic instructions how to geocode data in a CAQDAS and perform basic analysis (i.e. coding and relations of codes in network diagram).

When we introduce these learning activities we explain to our students that there are several advantages associated to walking interviews (Clark and Emmel 2010; Evans and Jones 2011).

- They provide spatial context to the interview and allow to place events and experiences;
- They are useful to capture perceptions on QoL, built environment and how individuals perceive their neighbourhood;
- They provide policy makers with evidence on communities and individual perceptions, connections and identity with their neighbourhood.

In this UPM course, students practice walking interviews and learn to record the path or track they walk. For that purpose, they use a GPS or mobile GIS tools (e.g. Cybertracker, Locus, or a GPS-data logger device[7]). Voice and eventually video is recorded during the interview. Points of interests signalled by the interviewee are also photographed.

---

[7] For an example of the use of a GPS-data logger combined with walking interviews with older adults see (Zandieh et al. 2016)

The main objective for the walking the interviews is that students learn to collect, analyse and present geographic narratives. More specifically the student will be able to:

- Map the perception of the urban living environment / QoL of the city centre of Enschede (physical and social qualities). Identify patterns of negative and positive perception (e.g. across gender, age, country of origin)[8]
- Practice data collection via walking interviews
- Analyse the qualitative data with a CAQDAS software.

The outcomes of the walking interviews assignment includes: (1) a map indicating the location and extent of positive and negative hotspots as perceived by different students, (2) recorded interviews and geocoded photos of the visited areas, and (3) an analysis of the results in ATLAS.ti.

Before we introduce the topic students learn how some authors combine quantitative with qualitative data and how they show the variation of perceptions across different groups. For example the work of Pacione (2003b) where the author analysed gender-differentiated fear of crime at local level within the city of Glasgow. Pacione (2003b) collected information on perceived risk from criminal activities and perceived dangerous spaces by gender. Students also learn that qualitative GIS has been also used to analyse fear through geo-narratives (Kwan and Ding 2008). The work of Chawla (2002) and Alarasi et al. (2016) are used as an example to identify physical and social qualities of the local living environment focussing on children (Fig. 12.5).

The research of Alarasi et al. (2016) and Shumi et al. (2014) emerged from MSc theses. In both cases, the students had previously attended this UPM elective course and have learned to perform walking interviews. In turn, we also include their work in subsequent lectures to stimulate new student in the topic of QoL, qualitative GIS and mixed methods.

For the walking interviews assignment, students work in groups and exchange members in each round of interviews so that they interview each other. They interview four to six ITC students living in the city centre (at least two men and two women). The assignment consist of three parts: A- Preparation and concept consolidation, B- Walking interviews download, and C- Text analysis.

Part A: Preparation, concept consolidation and implementation

Before students go to the field, they discuss in a plenary the conceptualization of the urban living environment/QoL. We use the think-pair-share or snowballing

---

[8] In the first 2 years that we had run this course, during the walking interviews we had focused on the topic of perception of fear in the university campus and compared between gender and country of origin. Arranging the interviews with students living in the campus resulted in time-consuming efforts for the students therefore we opted for a topic that they could use to interview each other.

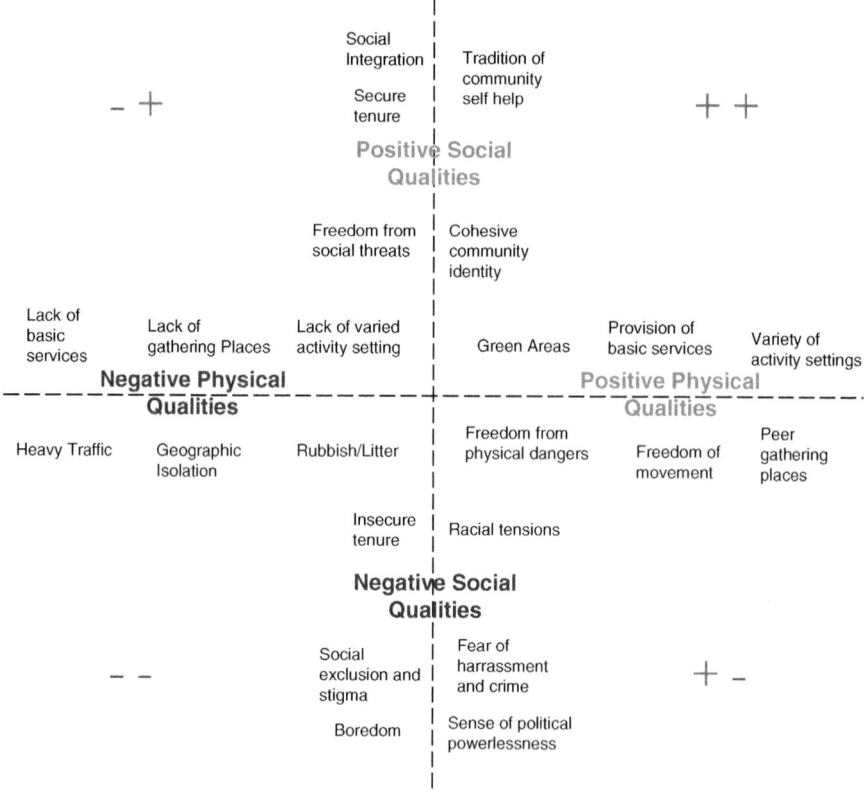

Fig. 12.5 Qualities of the living environment. (Adapted from Chawla 2001 by Al Arasi 2013)

approach so that students first reflect individually, then discuss in pairs and then in group the following points:

Firstly, how they would define the urban living environment and QoL. As a group, they need to agree on the same conceptualization (note that this also corresponds to the spiral learning of indicators step 1 in Fig. 12.3). They are encouraged to base the conceptualization on the literature as well as their own experience as residents of the city centre of Enschede (the students live at the same students' accommodation in the city centre). We suggest them to think about positive and negative social and physical elements and/or domains of life.

Secondly, students elaborate some hypothesis on the factors influencing the perception of quality of the urban living environment and possible variations across gender, age and country of origin, discipline and background of the interviewee.

Finally, we provide them with a draft interview guide with further instructions and we ask them to fine-tune the questions suggested for the walking interviews (Box 12.1). We ask them to revise the suggested questions based on their own conceptualization and hypothesis. We ask them to thing about items in the interview guide that they you should add or leave out.

Box 12.1: Walking Interview Guide
Note: For the walking interview, you need to carry with you:

- A paper map of the area (e.g. from Google Earth)
- A Tablet with GPS or Locus or OSM tracker app pre-installed
- A digital camera (with same time set as in the tablet GPS/app). Geocoded photos can also be taken with a tablet
- A digital recorder (note that to synchronise with the tablet GPS app you will need to turn on the recorder before the GPS app is open and verbally indicate when the GPS is on –add a verbal time stamp-)

At the starting point of the walking interview, you need to:
Explain briefly the aim of the activity.
Ask your interviewee if you could walk with him/her.

   Important: read issues of consent and confidentiality in Clark and Emmel 2010
   The interviewee decides the route. Options could be walking to: supermarket, square, shops, most visited place, etc.
   Explain that you will walk with them for a maximum of 30 min and stop at some points to take photos and notes on his/her perceptions and places they point at (in particular when they refer to positive and negative qualities).
   Begin the interview with the following (suggested) questions [add and discuss more questions before departing to the field]

Q1- Where have you been born?
Q2- How many months have you lived in Enschede?
Q3- Mark on this map the following:

   (a) *Where do you live?*
   (b) *Which areas do you frequently visit in the city centre?*
   (c) *Points and spaces where you observe positive and negative locations in the city centre. Why?*

Does your perception change during the night and during the day [Interviewer labels the points and areas in the map and distinguishes day and night]

Start the walking interview.

   Suggested open questions while walking:

As we walk around think about what do you like / and not like the area? What do you think about the quality of the public space? Why do you think that?
Ask also questions on key issues that you identified and based on how you defined in your group the urban living environment / quality of life.
E.g., *do you feel unsafe in any of the areas we walk by? Why?/Why not? Can you remember a time when you walked here and felt unsafe? Would you walk here anytime of the day? Why? Why did you choose this route?*

   Think in advance more questions

Currently we assign 4 h for this assignment but in our latest staff evaluation, we notice that this part (A) require more time (in the next year we expand the course from 5 to 7 ECTS).

Part B: Walking interviews download

Once students come back with the walking interviews, they follow instructions on how to download and analyse the data they collected during the walking interviews. They learn to import the track or transect, the audio, pictures and eventually video material. We remind them that they have to stick to the agreed conventions in terms of colour, symbol and type of object (point, line, and polygon). For each of the walking interviews: they digitize the perception of urban living qualities in ArcGIS or Google Earth (as points, lines and polygons).

If they worked with ArcGIS we asked them convert the map documents to a Google Earth file. They download the tracks, photos and audio in Google Earth and they compare the results of the different walking interviews. They save the result in a Google Earth file format (kmz) and share the file in the course Learning Management System (LMS). The results are discussed in a plenary session.

Students make use of a portfolio to present the results and discussion of this part. One of the outputs is a map indicating the location and extent of positive and negative hotspots as perceived by different interviewees. They are asked to briefly discuss the results in terms of geographic patterns, commonalities and differences across interviewees, unexpected results, etc.

Part C: Text analysis

In the last part of the assignment, students perform text analysis in ATLAS.ti. When students analyse the data that they collected during the walking interviews we ask them to experiment with the following points in text analysis while keeping the focus on urban living environment and QoL. They are asked to code a few relevant quotes and make links between them (networking diagrams).They also learn to add fieldwork notes with their observations and geocode the most relevant photos (e.g. of elements in the urban environment that are pointed at or referred to by the interviewees). The different transect walks of the walking interview places of positive and negative qualities could be added to the ATLAS.ti project and geocoded. Each member of the group codes separately and exports the work as project bundle.[9]

This part of the assignment is supported with online micro lectures (e.g. on 'Creating and Displaying Semantic Linkages') and specific online software tutorials. For instance, for organising and distributing the data analysis among the group members, students can have a look at the "How to Document 'Team Work with ATLAS.ti 8 Windows" tutorial.

Students make use of a portfolio to present the results and discussions of part C. One of the outputs is to present the three most relevant findings of the walking interview and ATLAS.ti analysis. They also have to critically reflect to what extent

---

[9]The bundle is something like an ATLAS.ti specific zip archive. It is used to merge the work of different group members.

the findings contribute to a better understanding of the patterns discussed in part B. Finally, they need to illustrate and support the findings with screenshots and photos of the walking interview, quotations, relevant parts of the codes and the semantic network.

Cases Resulting from the Teaching and Learning Approach

One of the first studies informed by this approach was that of Tesfazghi et al. (2010). It combines objective and subjective perspectives –the material and the experiential– determining divergent and convergent assessments of QoL conditions (Tesfazghi et al. 2010). GIS was used to visualize the four conditions of QoL in Kirkos sub-city (Fig. 12.6). Areas of *dissonance* are of particular interest since they show areas where the perception of QoL is worse than objective conditions.

Tesfazghi et al. (2010) mapped areas of *adaptation* and *dissonance* (where there was a mismatch between the etic and emic (experts and people's views on QoL). However, the quantitative methods used were insufficient to answer questions related to the reasons of divergence between the external (etic) and the internal view (emic). Henceforth, in subsequent studies the authors incorporated mixed methods,

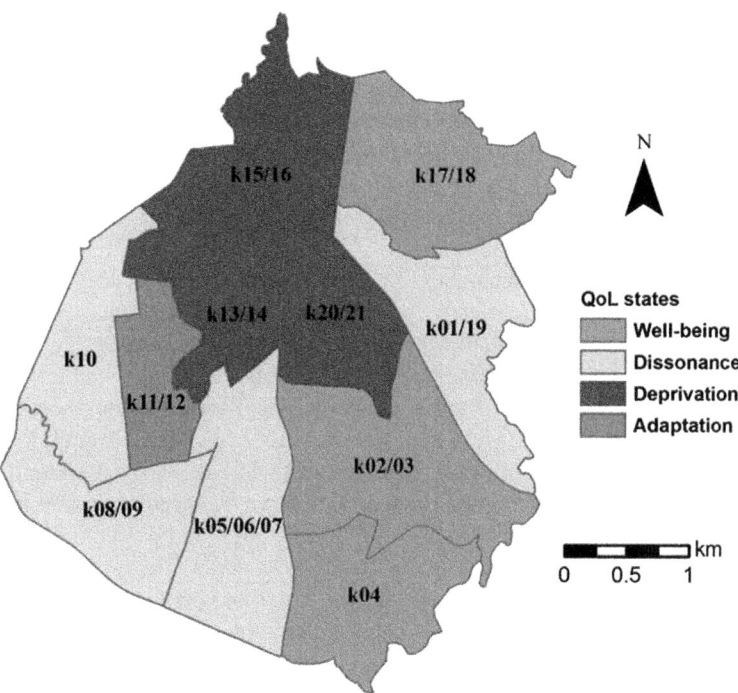

Fig. 12.6 Spatial variation of QoL states in Kirkos sub-city. (Source: Tesfazghi et al. 2010)

crossing the qualitative vs quantitative divide by looking for comprehensive, contextual, and explanatory accounts. Above all, it allows eliciting diversity of views: expert, lay and across residents. The authors incorporated walking interviews to bring a contextual explanation of *adaptation* and *dissonance*. The walking interviews helped identifying the reasons behind the divergence between emic and etic views (Berhe et al. 2014).

From the walking interviews, the authors found some explanations of *adaptation*:

> *we are only two even though the room is small it is enough for us. Even though it has no kitchen but I am satisfied. Getting a house is very difficult in this Ketena since it is located in the centre of the city.*

> *the house is small and it is not in a good condition but I am satisfied because I cannot pay more than what I am paying now for house rent if I do so my kids will starve.*

Explanations of *dissonance* were also sought in the QoL domain of education:

> *I am not satisfied because it is very expensive [access to education]. The other issue is most of the students in the school are from rich family and since they are teenagers there is high competition in dressing and school meals.*

While the etic view used GIS and considered access to social infrastructure (e.g. education) as an issue of proximity, the walking interviews with residents exposed other dimensions attached to accessibility such as affordability and safety (the school was located at the side of a busy road where children were exposed to traffic accidents).

Another student applied a mixed method approach to identify and compare the gendered (emic) QoL domains in a deprived and non-deprived neighbourhood in the city of Birmingham (Khaef 2013). Alongside the quantitative data obtained from an Index of Multiple Deprivation, open questionnaires and individual interviews were used to obtain residents' emic perceptions about QoL conditions in their neighbourhood.

Participatory mapping techniques allowed Khaef (2013) to identify the different perspectives and QoL concerns between men and women. The results also show that in deprived neighbourhoods both women and men mentioned similar QoL domains to be relevant for their community (access to facilities, street condition, safety, green space and social interaction). However, there were different emic views towards issues of safety, access to facilities and street condition. Overall, a qualitative analysis for the neighbourhoods revealed that while in deprived contexts many differences toward gendered perception of QoL have been found; in non-deprived areas respondents showed strong similarities in the perception of their neighbourhood.

One of the advantages of applying the mixed methods approach that we teach to our students is that it exposes many axis of differentiation that might be ignored if only an etic view or quantitative data is included. In particular, gender is one of the dimensions to be considered in the experience and perception of QoL in order to elicit emic views of vulnerable groups. In another study (Shumi et al. 2014), we used this mixed-method approach and elicited emic views to understand how the QoL of women garment workers in Dhaka (Bangladesh) was affected by the walking conditions of the routes the take from home to work. Next to gender we have also studied in the Global North (the city of Enschede, the Netherlands) children's perception (Alarasi et al. 2016) and ethnicity (Desriani 2011).

Conclusions

In this chapter, we presented an approach for teaching and learning QoL in the context of urban studies. In particular, we gave details on how we use a heuristic framework to critically look into expert and peoples view (Figs. 12.1 and 12.2), and how we frame indicators under an open spiral-learning process (Fig. 12.3). We give details on how this framework can be translated into a learning activity (the walking interview) and indicated the relevance of incorporating a mixed methods approaches.

We claim that the approach we use with our students facilitates a more sensitive and empathic form of QoL mapping. We illustrate this with some case studies that emerged from the work carried with our students. We showed how thanks to hands-on experiences our students learn how to elicit different forms of knowledge (not only from experts but also from residents) and the critical recognition of convergent and divergent views between different groups (Figs. 12.4, 12.5, 12.6, 12.7, and 12.8).

One of the main challenges identified in this approach relates to the group work characteristic of one of the assignments. The walking interview is performed as a group work assignment to facilitate hands-on-experience and learning from each other. Some of the advantages of group work are that students have the potential to maximize and share their skills with the rest of the group (Brewer and Klein 2006; Haigh and Gold 1993). However, during group work, cooperation is not always facilitated and motivated and it might be challenged when students have different cultural backgrounds, disciplines or skills (Hennebry and Fordyce 2018). From the different course evaluations, we know that our students appreciate the group work and the walking interviews. Nonetheless, some of the challenges of group work were observed, as students are required to share the interviews across members of the group and distribute labour intensive task such as transcription of the interviews in order to use them in a CAQDAS software. Furthermore, to be able to compare results among groups in the final presentation we ask them to collaborate with each other and agree on using the same mapping conventions and legends (e.g., how they mark things on the map -colours, symbols- and what kind of labels they will use). Under certain conditions, collaborative learning approaches can promote and facilitate among students each other's efforts to learn, resulting in *positive interdependence* (cooperation) (Brewer and Klein 2006), critical thinking (Cooper 1995) and students satisfaction (So and Brush 2008). In order to improve this teaching and learning approach we are currently studying a better implementation of the group assignment mediated by a Learning Management System (LMS). The main goal of

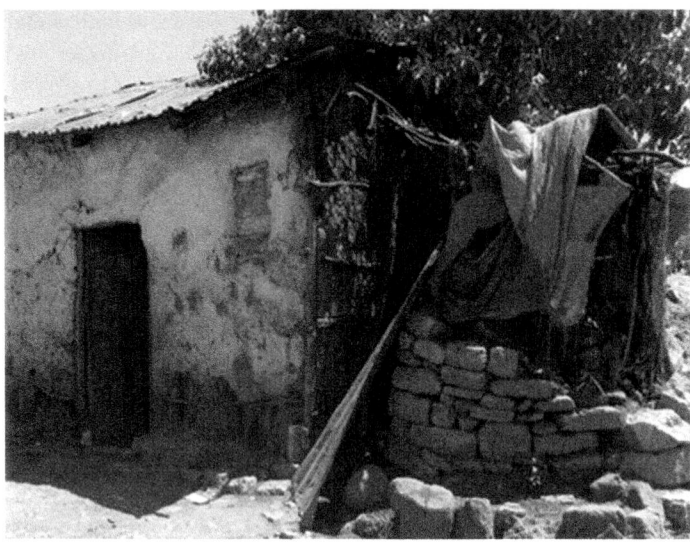

Fig. 12.7 Example of state of adaptation in QoL housing domain. Source: Berhe et al. (2014)

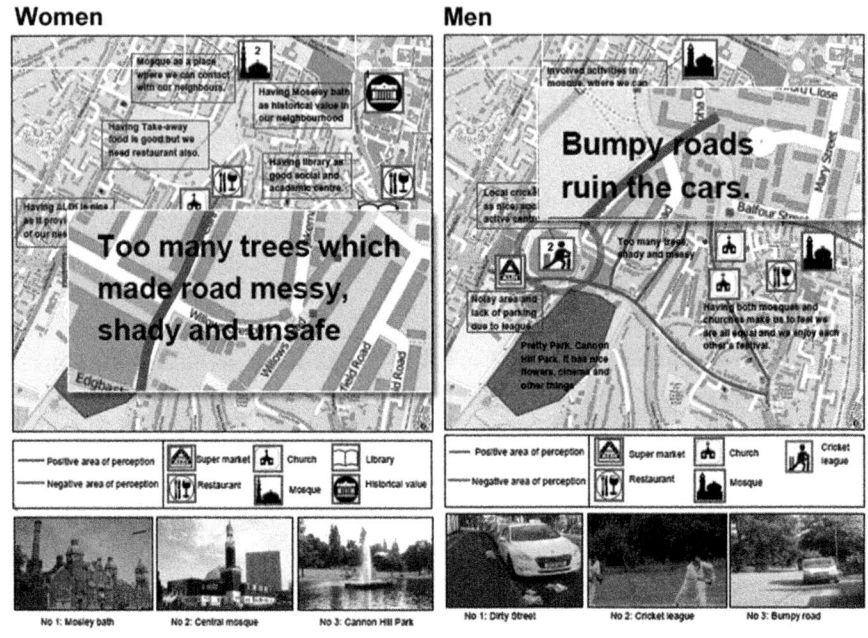

Fig. 12.8 Women and men perceptions. Source: Khaef (2013)

that research is to develop a (computer-supported) collaborative learning approach that promotes positive interdependence in this type of group assignments.

The main conclusion of this chapter is that teaching and learning QoL in urban studies can benefit by the combination of methods, critical approaches and empathic forms of QoL mapping. In the UPM courses, we emphasize the importance of forms of QoL mapping that make visible inequalities that negatively affect the ideal of a just and inclusive city. These empathic and sensitive forms of mapping require different forms of knowledge (not only the technical or scientific knowledge produced by experts) and the recognition of convergent and divergent views between different groups.

References

Al Arasi, H. A. (2013). *Study on children's perception of their local living environment*. Enschede: University of Twente Faculty of Geo-Information and Earth Observation (ITC). Retrieved from http://www.itc.nl/library/papers_2013/msc/upm/alarasi.pdf.

Alarasi, H., Martinez, J., & Amer, S. (2016). Children's perception of their city centre. A qualitative GIS methodological investigation in a Dutch city. *Children's Geographies, 14*(4), 437–452. https://doi.org/10.1080/14733285.2015.1103836.

Anderson, L. W., Krathwohl, D. R., & Bloom, B. S. (2001). *A taxonomy for learning, teaching, and assessing: A revision of Bloom's taxonomy of educational objectives* (Complete ed.). New York: Longman.

Baud, I., Sridharan, N., & Pfeffer, K. (2008). Mapping urban poverty for local governance in an Indian mega-city: The case of Delhi. *Urban Studies, 45*(7), 1385–1412. https://doi.org/10.1177/0042098008090679.

Berhe, R., Martínez, J. A., & Verplanke, J. (2014). Adaptation and dissonance in quality of life: A case study in Mekelle, Ethiopia. *Social Indicators Research, 118*(2), 535–554. https://doi.org/10.1007/s11205-013-0448-y.

Brewer, S., & Klein, J. D. (2006). Type of positive interdependence and affiliation motive in an asynchronous, collaborative learning environment. *Etr&D-Educational Technology Research and Development, 54*(4), 331–354. https://doi.org/10.1007/s11423-006-9603-3.

Chawla, L. (Ed.). (2002). *Growing up in an urbanising world*. London: UNESCO/Earthscan Publications Ltd.

Clark, A., & Emmel, N. (2010). *Using walking interviews. Realities Toolkit #13*. Manchester: ESRC.

Cooper, J. L. (1995). Cooperative learning and critical thinking. *Teaching of Psychology, 22*(1), 7–9. https://doi.org/10.1207/s15328023top2201_2.

Cope, M., & Elwood, S. (2009). *Qualitative GIS: A mixed methods approach* (1st ed.). Thousand Oaks: Sage.

Desriani, R. W. (2011). *Assessing residential segregation profiles for ethnic groups in Enschede, the Netherlands* (Master of science in geo-information science and earth observation). Enschede: University of Twente.

Dopheide, E. J. M., & Martinez, J. (2007). Hoe scoort mijn wijk? *Rooilijn, 40.*(2007(5), 338–343.

Eizenberg, E., & Shilon, M. (2015). Pedagogy for the new planner: Refining the qualitative toolbox. *Environment and Planning. B, Planning & Design, 43*(6), 1118–1135. https://doi.org/10.1177/0265813515604477.

Evans, J., & Jones, P. (2011). The walking interview: Methodology, mobility and place. *Applied Geography, 31*(2), 849–858.

Fainstein, S. S. (2010). *The just city*. Ithaca: Cornell University Press.

Fainstein, S. S. (2014). The just city. *International Journal of Urban Sciences, 18*(1), 1–18. https://doi.org/10.1080/12265934.2013.834643.

Feldman, M. S., & Khademian, A. M. (2007). The role of the public manager in inclusion: Creating communities of participation. *Governance-an International Journal of Policy and Administration, 20*(2), 305–324. https://doi.org/10.1111/j.1468-0491.2007.00358.x.

Haigh, M., & Gold, J. R. (1993). The problems with fieldwork – A group-based approach towards integrating fieldwork into the undergraduate geography curriculum. *Journal of Geography in Higher Education, 17*(1), 21–32. https://doi.org/10.1080/03098269308709203.

Harley, J. B. (1989). Deconstructing the map. *Cartographica: The International Journal for Geographic Information and Geovisualization, 26*(2), 1–20. https://doi.org/10.3138/E635-7827-1757-9T53.

Hennebry, M. L., & Fordyce, K. (2018). Cooperative learning on an international masters. *Higher Education Research and Development, 37*(2), 270–284. https://doi.org/10.1080/07294360.2017.1359150.

Khaef, S. (2013). *Perception of quality of life through a gendered lens: A case from the city of Brimingham*. Enschede: University of Twente Faculty of Geo-Information and Earth Observation (ITC).

Kwan, M. P., & Ding, G. X. (2008). Geo-narrative: Extending geographic information systems for narrative analysis in qualitative and mixed-method research. *The Professional Geographer, 60*(4), 443–465.

Marans, R. W., & Stimson, R. (2011). An overview of quality of urban life. In R. W. Marans & R. J. Stimson (Eds.), *Investigating quality of urban life: Theory, methods, and empirical research* (pp. 1–29). Dordrecht: Springer Netherlands.

Martínez, J. (2009). The use of GIS and indicators to monitor intra-urban inequalities. A case study in Rosario, Argentina. *Habitat International, 33*(4), 387–396. https://doi.org/10.1016/j.habitatint.2008.12.003.

Martínez, J. (2016). Mind the gap: Monitoring spatial inequalities in quality of life conditions (Case study of Rosario). In G. Tonon (Ed.), *Indicators of quality of life in Latin America* (pp. 151–172). Cham: Springer International Publishing.

Martínez, J. (2018). Mapping dynamic indicators of quality of life: A case in Rosario, Argentina. *Applied Research in Quality of Life*. https://doi.org/10.1007/s11482-018-9617-0.

Martínez, J., & Dopheide, E. (2014). Indicators: From counting to communicating. *Journal for Education in the Built Environment, 9*, 1–19. https://doi.org/10.11120/jebe.2014.00009.

Martínez, J., Pfeffer, K., & Baud, I. (2016). Factors shaping cartographic representations of inequalities. Maps as products and processes. *Habitat International, 51*, 90–102. https://doi.org/10.1016/j.habitatint.2015.10.010.

Martinez, J., Verplanke, J., & Miscione, G. (2017). A geographic and mixed methods approach to capture unequal quality-of-life conditions. In: Phillips R., Wong C. (Eds.), *Handbook of Community Well-Being Research. International Handbooks of Quality of-Life*. Dordrecht: Springer.

McCrea, R., Shyy, T.-K., & Stimson, R. (2006). What is the strength of the link between objective and subjective indicators of urban quality of life? *Applied Research in Quality of Life, 1*(1), 79–96. https://doi.org/10.1007/s11482-006-9002-2.

Monmonier, M. S. (1996). *How to lie with maps* (2nd ed.). Chicago: University of Chicago Press.

Pacione, M. (1982). The use of objective and subjective measures of life quality in human-geography. *Progress in Human Geography, 6*(4), 495–514.

Pacione, M. (2003a). Urban environmental quality and human wellbeing – A social geographical perspective. *Landscape and Urban Planning, 65*(1–2), 19–30. https://doi.org/10.1016/s0169-2046(02)00234-7.

Pacione, M. (2003b). Urban environmental quality and human wellbeing – A social geographical perspective. *Landscape and Urban Planning, 65*(1–2), 21–32.

Pfeffer, K., Martinez, J., O'Sullivan, D., & Scott, D. (2015). Geo-technologies for spatial knowledge: Challenges for inclusive and sustainable urban development. In J. Gupta, K. Pfeffer,

H. Verrest, & M. Ros-Tonen (Eds.), *Geographies of urban governance: Advanced theories, methods and practices* (pp. 147–173). Cham: Springer International Publishing.

Ramadier, T. (2004). Transdisciplinarity and its challenges: The case of urban studies. *Futures, 36*(4), 423–439. https://doi.org/10.1016/j.futures.2003.10.009.

Rojas, M. (2015). Poverty and people's wellbeing. In W. Glatzer, L. Camfield, V. Møller, & M. Rojas (Eds.), *Global handbook of quality of life* (pp. 317–350). Dordrecht: Springer.

Seik, F. T. (2000). Subjective assessment of urban quality of life in Singapore (1997–1998). *Habitat International, 24*(1), 31–49.

Shumi, S., Zuidgeest, M. H. P., Martínez, J. A., Efroymson, D., & van Maarseveen, M. F. A. M. (2014). Understanding the relationship between walkability and quality-of-life of women garment workers in Dhaka, Bangladesh. *Applied Research in Quality of Life*, 1–25. https://doi.org/10.1007/s11482-014-9312-8.

Sirgy, M. J., Michalos, A. C., Ferriss, A. L., Easterlin, R. A., Patrick, D., & Pavot, W. (2006). The quality-of-life (QOL) research movement: Past, present, and future. *Social Indicators Research, 76*(3), 343–466. https://doi.org/10.1007/s11205-005-2877-8.

Smith, D. M. (1973). *The geography of social well-being in the United States: An introduction to territorial social indicators*. New York: McGraw-Hill.

So, H. J., & Brush, T. A. (2008). Student perceptions of collaborative learning, social presence and satisfaction in a blended learning environment: Relationships and critical factors. *Computers & Education, 51*(1), 318–336. https://doi.org/10.1016/j.compedu.2007.05.009.

Tesfazghi, E., Martínez, J., & Verplanke, J. (2010). Variability of quality of life at small scales: Addis Ababa, Kirkos Sub-City. *Social Indicators Research, 98*(1), 73–88. https://doi.org/10.1007/s11205-009-9518-6.

Tonon, G. (2015). Integration of qualitative and quantitative methods in quality of life studies. In G. Tonon (Ed.), *Qualitative studies in quality of life* (Vol. 55, pp. 53–60). Cham: Springer.

Trisusanti, E. (2008). *Constructing indices of multiple deprivation for neighborhood ranking: A case study on five municipalicties in province of Overijssel*. Enschede: ITC.

Watson, V. (2014). Co-production and collaboration in planning – The difference. *Planning Theory and Practice, 15*(1), 62–76.

Wong, C. (2006). *Indicators for urban and regional planning: The interplay of policy and methods* (Vol. 11). London: Routledge:Taylor and Francis group.

Zandieh, R., Martinez, J., Flacke, J., Jones, P., & van Maarseveen, M. (2016). Older adults' outdoor walking: Inequalities in neighbourhood safety, pedestrian infrastructure and aesthetics. *International Journal of Environmental Research and Public Health, 13*(12), 1179.

Javier Martinez is Assistant Professor in the Department of Urban and Regional Planning and Geo-Information Management within the Faculty ITC, University of Twente, The Netherlands. He is also coordinator of the Urban Planning and Management specialization of the two-year master's degree in geo-information science and earth observation. PhD from the Faculty of Geosciences at Utrecht University. Arquitect. His research, publications and training experience are focused on the application of GIS, mixed methods and indicators for policy-making, urban poverty and quality-of-life and intra-urban inequalities. Since 2017, he has been a member of the board of directors of the International Society of Quality of Life Studies (ISQOLS).

Chapter 13
Teaching Quality of Life and Well-Being in Public Health

Chelsea Wesner, Diana Feldhacker, and Whitney Lucas Molitor

What Is Public Health?

Public health aims to improve the health, well-being, and equity of resources among populations and communities (American Public Health Association [APHA] n.d.). While clinicians respond to illness and injury through direct patient care, public health practitioners respond through interventions and policies that aim to prevent or reduce the risk of illness and injury (APHA n.d.). From the development of life-saving vaccines to responding to epidemics that range from infectious disease outbreaks to the effects of untreated mental illness, the dynamic field of public health draws professionals, researchers, and students from diverse academic backgrounds, cultures, and geographies.

Historical Overview

Public health has evolved over millennia, yet its mission to improve population health through preventive and protective measures remains unchanged. Some historians suggest the origins of public health began with Greco-Roman ideas of health and the four humors (Rosen 2015). During this era, the Romans developed one of

C. Wesner (✉)
Department of Public Health, University of South Dakota, Vermillion, SD, USA
e-mail: Chelsea.Wesner@usd.edu

D. Feldhacker
Department of Occupational Therapy, Creighton University, Omaha, NE, USA
e-mail: DianaFeldhacker@Creighton.edu

W. Lucas Molitor
Department of Occupational Therapy, University of South Dakota, Vermillion, SD, USA
e-mail: Whitney.LucasMolitor@usd.edu

© Springer Nature Switzerland AG 2020
G. H. Tonon (ed.), *Teaching Quality of Life in Different Domains*, Social
Indicators Research Series 79, https://doi.org/10.1007/978-3-030-21551-4_13

Table 13.1 Ten great public health achievements in the United States, twentieth and twenty-first centuries

1900–1999	2000–2010
Vaccination	Vaccine-preventable diseases
Motor vehicle safety	Prevention and control of infectious diseases
Safer workplaces	Tobacco control
Control of infectious diseases	Maternal and infant health
Decline in deaths from coronary heart disease and stroke	Motor vehicle safety
Safer and healthier foods	Cardiovascular disease prevention
Healthier mothers and babies	Occupational safety
Family planning	Cancer prevention
Fluoridation of drinking water	Childhood lead poisoning prevention
Recognition of tobacco use as a health hazard	Public health preparedness and response

CDC (1999, 2011)

the first public health systems when they engineered aqueducts to supply clean water and remove waste from the city of Rome. Effects of this work are estimated to have reached a population of one million in 1 CE (Morris 2010; Rosen 2015). During the Middle Ages, quarantine was used as a means to control plagues, while sanitation and hygiene were primary practices in the nineteenth century as a way to reduce communicable disease. In the latter part of nineteenth and early twentieth centuries, public health focused on the study of bacteria and the development of vaccines to protect against and eradicate preventable diseases (Rosen 2015).

Today, public health remains a critical aspect of protecting the livelihood and well-being of people and populations across the globe. As illustrated in Table 13.1, public health achievements in the United States during the twentieth century focused largely on recognizing and controlling diseases and environments as a way to improve health. This is in contrast to the gains during the first decade of the twenty-first century, which focused more on prevention as a means to improve health, sustain quality of life, and reduce preventable mortality and morbidity (Centers for Disease Control & Prevention [CDC] 1999, 2011). Despite this evolution of the profession, prevention remains a critical construct of public health efforts.

Twenty-First Century Challenges

Life expectancy and population health have improved throughout the world, largely due to enhanced public health systems and high quality medical care (CDC 1999, 2011; DeSalvo et al. 2017). However, as health and quality of life have improved, health inequalities have worsened (DeSalvo et al. 2017). During the past few decades, a growing body of research documents health disparities and inequities within and between populations, especially in lesser developed countries and among vulnerable, low income, minority, and marginalized populations (DeSalvo et al. 2017; Marmot 2015; Marmot and Bell 2012; Marmot et al. 2008). This social gradient of health and knowledge of how social, cultural, and behavioral factors influence health have emerged as two of the greatest public health challenges of the twenty-first century (Coreil 2010; Marmot 2015). With these challenges comes the need for interventions that use a social and ecological approach to health in order to target policy and structural changes, as well as social and behavioral factors that influence health (Coreil 2010; DeSalvo et al. 2017; Golden et al. 2015; McLeroy et al. 1988).

In 2008, the World Health Organization's (WHO) Commission on the Social Determinants of Health released a landmark report calling for global action on the social determinants of health, the conditions and characteristics in which we are born, live, work, play, and learn (Marmot et al. 2008). Following its release, the field of public health prioritized practice and research that address the inequities and root causes of poor health outcomes. This new era of public health seeks to address social determinants and improve quality of life through foci such as safe housing, early childhood education, employment, and access to healthy food. Initiatives work to generate collective impact from multiple sectors and communities (DeSalvo et al. 2017; Marmot 2015). In addition, complementary health science disciplines, especially occupational therapy, social work, nursing, and medicine, now emphasize teaching about the social determinants of health and incorporate these topics into practice and research, generating interprofessional scholarship and solutions on this critical topic.

Teaching About Quality of Life and Well-Being in Public Health

The core areas of public health traditionally include epidemiology, biostatistics, environmental and occupational health, health administration and policy, and social and behavioral sciences. Of these areas, social and behavioral sciences emerged as an important field in the 1950s when the WHO recognized psychosocial well-being as an important factor in health (Coreil 2010; WHO 1946). As the emphasis on improving social determinants and advancing health equity has grown in public health practice and research, topics of quality of life and well-being have become essential to teaching and empowering public health and health science students to work collaboratively with diverse communities and people. The following sections introduce conceptual frameworks for understanding quality of life and well-being in a population health context. Furthermore, this chapter demonstrates the application of an ecological model of health and a taxonomy of significant learning as a way to teach about quality of life and well-being across public health, health sciences, and medical professional curricula.

Quality of Life and Well-Being

Well-being, wellness, and health are often terms that are difficult to define, and a single agreed-upon definition of each does not exist. A reason for this is the complexity of the many associated terms: health education, disease management, safety, risk management, public health, population health, and health promotion, among others (Abbott and Baun 2015). While these definitions share in common an understanding that wellness, well-being, and health are not merely the absence of disease (WHO 1946), they also share the concept that each are multidimensional, encompassing a variety of areas including physical, mental, social, and spiritual components (Adams et al. 1998; Foster and Levitov 2012; Green 2016). These areas influence the ability to participate in meaningful activities, occupations, which are shown to prevent illness, disease, and disability (Pizzi and Richards 2017). The fields of occupational science and occupational therapy demonstrate that human wellness stems from the capability and opportunity to engage in the world, reflecting a clear link between occupation, health, and the environment (Pizzi and Richards 2017). In order to account for this complexity, a multifaceted approach to wellness is the recommended model for addressing and improving well-being and quality of life.

Six Dimensions of Wellness

In 1976 Dr. Bill Hettler, co-founder of the National Wellness Institute, created an interdependent model referred to as the six dimensions of wellness model. This holistic model captures the complexity of wellness and brings awareness to the interconnectedness of each of the six dimensions: occupational, physical, social, intellectual, spiritual, and emotional aspects of health, wellness, and well-being (Hettler 1976).

According to the six dimensions of wellness model (Table 13.2), occupational wellness is one's personal satisfaction and enrichment through life work (Hettler 1976). This specifically relates to attitudes about work and suggests that work should be personally meaningful and rewarding. Occupational wellness allows one's work to convey their values (Hettler 1976). The physical dimension regards a need for consistent physical activity and a nutritional diet. This dimension also relates to strength, flexibility, and endurance, as well as safety and ability to engage physically in self-care tasks. Overall, physical wellness relates to understanding one's body and how it performs (Hettler 1976). Social well-being reflects the interdependence between people and nature and communication with each, which is one's contribution to the environment and society, preserving beauty and balance with nature, friendships, and community (Hettler 1976). The fourth dimension of wellness, intellectual, is the ability to be creative and engage in mentally stimulating activities, including those requiring problem solving and learning. This involves striving to expand knowledge and skill and then sharing that knowledge and skill

Table 13.2 Six dimensions of wellness model

Dimension	Examples
Occupational	Satisfaction through work
	Meaningful and rewarding work that aligns with values
Physical	Regular physical activity, nutritious diet, and avoiding tobacco, drugs and alcohol
	Strength, flexibility, and endurance
Social	Contributing to environment and community
	Balance with nature and people
	Communication and friendships
Intellectual	Creativity, learning, and problem solving
	Expanding knowledge and sharing with others
Spiritual	Purpose and philosophy of life
Emotional	Awareness of feelings, expressing and managing effectively
	Forming respectful relationships
	Coping with stress and maintaining positivity

Hettler (1976)

with others (Hettler 1976). Spiritual wellness is the search for meaning and purpose in life. This includes a deep appreciation for the expanse of life and the universe; well-being in this dimension reflects peaceful harmony between internal feelings and emotions, especially when presented with rough challenges. Spiritual health is revealed in consistent beliefs and values and results in an ultimate "world view" or philosophy of life and conception of the world (Hettler 1976). The final facet of health in Hettler's (1976) model is emotional well-being. Stability and wellness in this facet include awareness and acceptance of feelings, managing and expressing emotions and behaviors, and coping with stress. Overall, feelings of positivity and enthusiasm about life, along with a realistic understanding of one's limitations, are indicative of emotional wellness. Emotional health allows forming of interdependent relationships, which are founded upon mutual respect and healthy conflict (Hettler 1976).

Several studies have expanded upon the six dimensions of wellness model to further account for the influences of perception, context, and meaningful activities. Adams et al. (1997) adapted Hettler's model to create a perceived wellness model, which describes the unique experience of wellness in that how one sees and encounters the world impacts their health. In following a systems theory and similar to Hettler (1976), Adams et al. (1997) discussed how the system of wellness is interdependent; one small change in an area of well-being impacts other areas and requires adaptability in order to maintain homeostasis. As such, they identified six areas of perceived wellness: physical, spiritual, psychological, social, emotional, and intellectual. Perception of well-being is a powerful predictor of health and quality of life. For example, perceived physical wellness is linked to an increase in physical activity; perceived spiritual wellness with improved self-esteem, social skills, and connectedness, as well as decreased loneliness; perceived social wellness with improved life satisfaction; and perceived emotional wellness with secure self-identity and positive self-regard (Adams et al. 1997).

Public Health and Wellness

Both the six dimensions of wellness model and the perceived wellness model focus on individual wellness; however, a public health perspective requires a broader approach. Beyond the individual is the need to create a wellness culture instead of a disease avoidance culture (Adams et al. 2000). Population perspectives account for the differences in dimensions that are influenced by context and include a social justice approach to wellness (Foster and Levitov 2012; Wilcox and Travis 2015). These everyday conditions of social, cultural, economic, educational, and occupational contexts as well as physical and mental environments shape public health (Dorner 2012). However, disparities within and across those determinants can lead to inequalities and reinforce the social gradient of health. Knowledge of the determinants of health from both an individual and population perspective is crucial for health planning and promotion (Dorner 2012; Rogerson et al. 2014).

Healthy People 2020 is a national initiative in the Unites States to improve the health of all Americans, with goals to enhance awareness and understanding of the determinants of health as a way to promote quality of life (Office of Disease Prevention and Health Promotion [ODPHP] 2010). Healthy People 2020 uses a place-based approach to highlight five key determinants of health: economic stability, education, social and community context, health and healthcare, and neighborhood and the built environment (Healthy People 2020 n.d.). Table 13.3 highlights key issues that underlie these social, economic, and physical determinants. In order to close health gaps and promote wellness and quality of life, Healthy People 2020 emphasizes the need to address each determinant at not only an individual level, but also at policy and population levels.

Table 13.3 Social determinants of health

Dimension	Examples
Economic stability	Employment, food security, housing instability, poverty
Education	Early childhood education and development, quality of education and job training, enrollment in higher education, high school graduation, language and literacy
Social and community context	Civic participation, discrimination, incarceration, social cohesion
Health and healthcare	Access to healthcare, access to primary care, health literacy
Neighborhood and built environment	Access to foods that support nutrition, crime and violence, environmental conditions, quality of housing, access to recreation and leisure activities, transportation options, access to mass media and emerging technologies

Retrieved from Healthy People 2020 (n.d.)

Health Education

Health education typically fails to equitably evaluate and promote all dimensions of health, often focusing on the physical and not accounting for other dimensions of health, the impact of social determinants, or the role of one's perception of health (Hawks et al. 2008). Health promotion is ineffective if not addressing all dimensions in an integrative fashion, spanning the social spectrum from individual to global populations and accounting for disparities. To be effective in improving and sustaining health and well-being, health promotion interventions must also address cultural and community perceptions of health. Good health, from a holistic perspective, allows for life meaningfulness and enables daily activities (Kaveh et al. 2016) which are context specific and culturally relevant. This perspective of occupation differs from Hettler (1976) in that it moves beyond work and instead aligns with that of occupational science and therapy, which define occupations as all life activities. Engagement in meaningful occupation is associated with improved well-being, life satisfaction, and physical and emotional health (American Occupational Therapy Association [AOTA] 2014; Gutman and Schindler 2007; Hilleras et al. 2001; Krause 2004; McIntyre and Howie 2002). These meaningful occupations, everyday life activities, influence overall health and include self-care, leisure and recreation, social participation, employment and work, and education (AOTA 2014; Hakansson et al. 2009). Similar to public health, occupational therapy promotes health of individuals and populations by connecting all dimensions of wellness in order to promote active engagement in living while also creating supportive environments that facilitate quality of life and well-being (Pizzi and Richards 2017). In combination, these complementary disciplines have the potential to strengthen interventions that promote health and well-being.

Overall, a public health approach expands dimensions of wellness by including social determinants and contexts that holistically address individual and population health, understand perceived health, and maintain the perspective of life meaningfulness and occupational participation. This approach leads to health, well-being, and quality of life across social and ecological systems. This relationship of the occupational health and wellness model as described by Feldhacker (unpublished) is illustrated in Fig. 13.1. The following section introduces a social ecology of health model to demonstrate how to teach about and develop interventions within public health and health science disciplines that aim to promote health and improve quality of life and well-being.

Social Ecological Model of Health

Ecological models in public health are frameworks to describe how physical, social, cultural, and political environments influence health behaviors (Golden et al. 2015; McLeroy et al. 1988; Stokols 1992). While earlier ecological models focused on

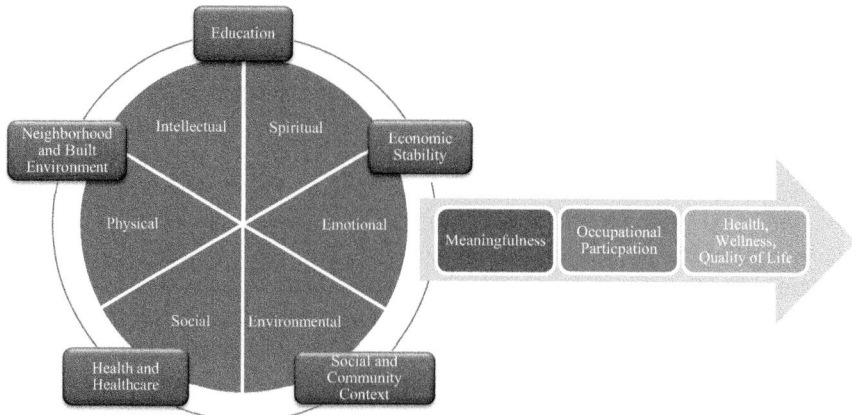

Fig. 13.1 The occupational health and wellness model: An approach to individual and population health, wellness, and quality of life that accounts for the impact of social determinants of health on the dimensions of wellness

understanding the factors that influence health behaviors, contemporary models inform the development of health promotion interventions (Sallis and Owen 2015). Unlike ecological models, most theories and behavioral models target one level of influence (e.g., individuals and/or their support network). As the focus of health behavior and health promotion has shifted from individuals to individuals *and* their environment, ecological models have evolved to show how a combination of individual, social, environmental, and policy-level interventions are necessary to positively influence and sustain health behaviors (Sallis and Owen 2015).

Strengths and Limitations

Ecological models serve as a framework for developing comprehensive, multi-level interventions that include policy and environmental changes (Sallis and Owen 2015). Instead of replacing existing health behavior theories, ecological models allow practitioners to combine multiple theories shown to target a specific health issue at different levels of influence. In addition, ecological models provide a framework to understand factors and determinants of particular health behaviors (Sallis and Owen 2015). In light of these benefits, a limitation of using ecological models is the difficulty in selection, as models range from those designed for specific health behaviors to others used across behaviors. Expense may also be a factor, as multi-level interventions can be costly and often require more planning and time to evaluate behavioral and environmental changes (Sallis and Owen 2015).

Ecological Model of Health Behavior

While a number of ecological models are used in public health, this chapter high-lights McLeroy et al.'s (1988) ecological model of health behavior, which was developed as a model for health promotion and inspired by Brofenbrenner's (1979) microsystem, mesosystem, and exosystem model. Table 13.4 outlines key factors in the ecological model of health behavior.

Intrapersonal At the individual level interventions and strategies include educa-tional programs, support groups, and peer counseling that aim to change individual behavior through improving knowledge, attitudes, and skills (McLeroy et al. 1988). For example, a breastfeeding support group may help a new mother gain skills and self-efficacy that increase the duration of breastfeeding during the first 6 months of her infant's life.

Interpersonal At the family and social level, interventions aim to change existing social relationships by targeting social norms and social influences (McLeroy et al. 1988). Building on the previous example, an interpersonal level intervention might include a family support program, peer support group, or the promotion of social norms that both normalize and promote breastfeeding at home and in public.

Institutional Institutional or organizational factors target environmental determi-nants of behavior change. At this level, the goal of organizational change is to create a supportive culture and environment, encouraging individuals to adopt and maintain

Table 13.4 Ecological model of health behavior

Level of influence	Key factors
Intrapersonal	Characteristics of an individual:
	Knowledge
	Attitudes
	Behavior
	Self-concept
	Skills
	Developmental history
Interpersonal	Formal and informal social network and social support systems:
	Family
	Work group
	Friendship network
Institutional	Social institutions with organizational characteristics and both formal and informal rules and regulations
Community	Relationships among organizations, institutions, and informal networks within defined boundaries
Public policy	Local, state, and national laws and policies

McLeroy et al. (1988)

healthy behaviors (McLeroy et al. 1988). For example, an intervention designed to promote and extend the duration of breastfeeding among mothers employed outside the home might encourage employers to adopt best practices in paid family leave and workplace breastfeeding policies.

Community According to McLeroy et al. (1988), community refers to (1) groups to which individuals belong (e.g., families, friendships, neighborhoods), (2) relationships among organizations and groups (e.g., nonprofits, local schools, health care providers), and (3) geographical and political entities with defined power structures. Interventions at this level might include coalitions that aim to increase community awareness and advocate for local policies around a common or shared issue. For example, maternal and child health representatives from different agencies might form a coalition to raise awareness of the benefits of extended breastfeeding and advocate for policies that support breastfeeding in hospitals, workplaces, child care centers, and community spaces.

Public Policy Policies are one of the most effective ways to improve population health (DeSalvo et al. 2017; Golden et al. 2015; McLeroy et al. 1988). Policy-level interventions protect and promote health through

- Restriction (prohibiting alcohol and tobacco sales among minors and smoke-free areas);
- Protection (seat belt and helmet use);
- Regulation (food quality);
- Behavioral incentives (taxation on tobacco products, alcohol, and sugar-sweetened beverages); and
- Allocation of funding and resources (health promotion programs and institutions within universities and state and tribal governments).

An example of a policy-level intervention to improve breastfeeding initiation rates is the Baby Friendly Hospital Initiative, which was established by the WHO and United Nations Children's Fund and recognizes hospitals and birthing centers that follow ten best practices set forth by the initiative (CDC 2013b).

Using the ecological model of health as an organizing framework for teaching about quality of life and well-being in public health requires thoughtful planning. Furthermore, learning how to apply the ecological model of health to improve well-being in low income, minority, and medically underserved communities calls for learning activities that inspire elements of caring, reflection, and systems thinking. The following section introduces a taxonomy of learning that values these elements as tenets of significant learning experiences.

Fink's Taxonomy of Significant Learning

Significant learning, a term that originated from the work of Fink (2013), is the product of a taxonomy for learning that emphasizes active learner engagement and integrated course design. This model incorporates six taxa: learning how to learn, foundational knowledge, application, integration, human dimension, and caring. The interaction between each of these six areas produces significant learning experiences. As public health is a dynamic field, incorporating this approach to teaching quality of life may produce learning experiences that are powerful, meaningful, and significant. Outlined below is a brief overview of the six taxa followed by specific examples of the relationship between each and the profession of public health. The chapter will culminate with an application of the taxonomy through examples of course objectives and active learning strategies that align with this approach.

Despite widespread application of Fink's (2013) taxonomy, its use in public health course design and teaching, particularly well-being and quality of life content, is not well documented. Regardless, the six taxa relate well to the constructs described above. In particular, emphasis on caring and the human dimension align well with public health. In addition, Fink's (2013) emphasis on active learner engagement aligns with contemporary pedagogy used increasingly by instructors to engage students, increase interaction, and, most importantly, link experiential aspects of courses to student learning as a means of promoting both applicability and retention.

Learning How to Learn

The notion that students pursuing a degree in higher education understand how to learn lacks sufficient support (Kirschner and van Merrienboer 2013). While students may be motivated to learn, they may not inherently possess skills that align with modern pedagogy. In fact, skills such as self-directed learning are often viewed differently between students and faculty (Fink 2013). In addition, the ability to critically reflect on the learning process may not come naturally to many students (Ryan 2013). For these reasons it is critical that courses begin with an overview of methods of learning versus diving directly into course content.

Fostering Reflective Learners Fink argues that in order for learning to be meaningful, students must possess the skills to reflect on the learning experience and relate it to both their personal and academic lives (Fink 2013). Reflection "encourage[s] students to draw connections between theoretical and practical knowledge and experiences," a process that is increasingly important in higher education (Barnes and Caprino 2016, p. 557). While formal and informal reflection are incorporated increasingly in the classroom, students may not be equipped to make modifications based upon feedback without training (Ryan 2013).

Foundational Knowledge

Fink (2013) describes foundational knowledge as providing "the basic understanding that is necessary for other kinds of learning" (p. 35). In public health, this includes an understanding of each pillar of the profession, including epidemiology, biostatistics, environmental and occupational health, health policy and administration, and health promotion sciences, as well interprofessional knowledge across the health sciences. As students gain a basic understanding of each area, this provides a foundation for future knowledge acquisition and broader application of such concepts, particularly in an interprofessional context.

Application

Research shows that comparison between students who have and have not taken a course often results in only minimal gains in knowledge among those who actually completed the course (Fink 2013). While surprising, the gap between a student's foundational knowledge and their retention of this information is in their ability to apply learning to real life situations. This process involves critical thinking, creativity, and practical application of skills (Fink 2013). As students apply knowledge gained as a foundational concept, they begin to develop a more in-depth awareness of how this information truly works. Within public health, application may include presenting information about a specific health issue or population and allowing students to create a solution to mitigate the issue. Despite the goal of enabling students to think multidimensionally (critically, creatively, and practically), this practice seldom links knowledge to actual application.

Integration

Despite application of knowledge involving critical thinking, a significant learning approach reaches farther and suggests students must learn to integrate ideas through drawing connection between concepts, courses, and real-world settings. Engaging this skill empowers learners and provides a means of making connections outside the classroom (Fink 2013). Through interprofessional collaboration and education, learning is linked among commonalities between individuals from one or more disciplines.

Human Dimension

Relating learning to real life, lived experiences occurs during the human dimension. In this taxa an appreciation for others, on a broader scale, occurs through realization of a globally connected and inter-related society. The process of self-discovery from the learner is the first step toward being capable of relating knowledge to others. The significance of linking learning to real life within public health curricula cannot be understated. This process may initiate with discovering oneself prior to branching out and learning about others. Personal competence includes self-awareness, self-regulation, and motivation towards goals (Goleman 1998, as quoted in Fink 2013). Next, learners are equipped to begin the process of social competence, a vital aspect to education in the fields of public health and health sciences which includes empathy and social skills. In doing so, awareness of others comes to light and can contribute to an appreciation for the differences among individuals, groups, communities, and populations leading to cultural humility, a lifelong process of recognizing and valuing differences (Tervalon and Murray-Garcia 1998). Finally, the human dimension enables the learner to be open to discovery of such differences and allows students to become better equipped to encounter multifactorial differences as professionals.

Emotional Intelligence Fink's (2013) concept of the human dimension is similar to emotional intelligence, which originated in 1998 with the work of Goleman (David 2014). This involves the interwoven relationship between oneself and inter-action with others through developing personal and social competence. Through both self and social awareness, students gain skills necessary for future work in the dynamic settings in which public health professionals work.

Caring

Fink (2013) describes how incorporating meaningful concepts serves to enhance learning. Caring includes both learner motivation to do well and establish goals along with an awareness of personal well-being, or a "commitment to live well" (Fink 2013, p. 41). Learners demonstrate caring as they gain an appreciation not only for curricular content, but also for seeking knowledge beyond the classroom.

In the following section, Fink's (2013) taxonomy is applied to teaching quality of life and well-being to public health students.

Applying Fink's Taxonomy to the Social Ecological Model of Health

Higher education is trending toward use active learning, yet specific methods of engaging students may not be well articulated, especially those that are most meaningful to students in a given discipline. For this reason, the following section includes a detailed description of in-class engagement activities designed specifically for public health students. Active learning involves engaged participation in the learning process along with reflection on actual learning (Fink 2013). Considering what students will do during class is a pivotal aspect of any course, yet advanced preparation is critical when implementing active learning. As described by Fink (2013), activities are grouped into five categories: receiving information and ideas, direct doing experiences, indirect doing experiences, observing, and reflection and the making of meaning. Each activity should be intricately linked to a course objective that aligns with one of the six taxa. Objectives, or learning goals, serve as one of the primary components in a strong course design (Fink 2013). Learning goals should align with course content rather than focusing on other taxa. Below, each level of the social ecological model includes examples of course objectives and active learning strategies that align with teaching quality of life and well-being to public health students.

Intrapersonal

Though it is well understood that individuals are embedded in a larger social system that influences health and well-being, professionals often design and deliver interventions at the individual level. At this level intrapersonal factors of health are addressed through lifestyle changes related to the attitudes, knowledge, beliefs, and skills of individuals (Golden and Earp 2012). Individuals, including their social, physical, economic, and cultural environments and behaviors, are complex; thus, interventions at the individual level must work to identify all areas of intrapersonal health and well-being.

Classroom activities for public health students must include building foundational knowledge of factors that influence individual health. When developing interventions at the individual level, students must be able to take this knowledge and incorporate it into programs and services. Teaching about the individual level should encourage students to gain appreciation for the content and to care about individual health risk and protective factors to a greater degree than before.

Course Objective: Foundational Knowledge Students will understand key social determinants and how these affect individual health including neighborhood and built environment, economic stability, education, health and healthcare, and social and community context.

Course Objective: Caring Students will be interested in understanding how different contexts influence health and demonstrate the desire to continue learning about individual social determinants of health.

Active Learning: Direct Doing Experience The following activity aims to build student foundational knowledge of social determinants and to encourage students to care about how each determinant influences individual health.

1. Students should be instructed to outline social factors that influence their health, creating an individual health diagram (see Fig. 13.2) using the following examples.

    (a) Neighborhood and built environment: safe housing, transportation, grocery stores, crime, access to mass media and technology
    (b) Economic stability: employment, food security, affordable housing, socioeconomic status
    (c) Education: quality of education (early childhood, high school, higher education), language, literacy
    (d) Health and healthcare: access to primary care, access to healthcare services, health literacy, health insurance
    (e) Social and community context: community events, friends, family, culture, social attitudes

2. Students will then divide into five groups.

    (a) Groups will be instructed to engage in discussion, comparing and contrasting social determinants in their community with sensitivity to differences and lived experiences.

Fig. 13.2 Individual health diagram. (Healthy People 2020 n.d.)

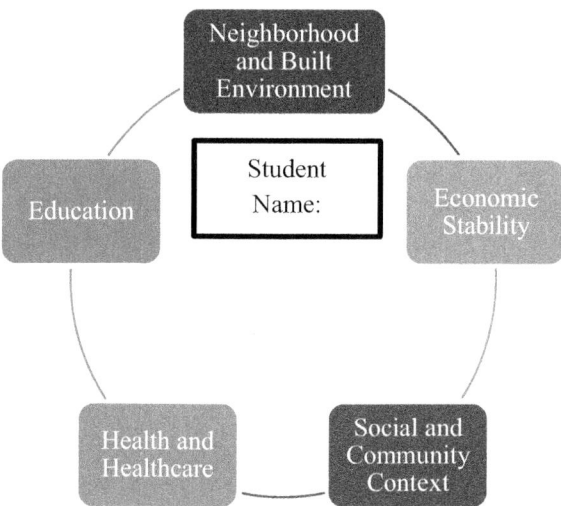

(b) Each group will then be given a variation to one social determinant. They will be asked to research and discuss with each other how the change would impact their individual health. Examples include

- Group 1: The closest grocery store closed, you do not have a cell phone, or your job requires you to move to a different zip code (neighborhood and built environment).
- Group 2: You have been laid off from your job, your insurance premiums doubled, or your landlord has increased rent by $500/month (economic stability).
- Group 3: English is not your primary language, schools in your area have poor ratings, or you cannot read (education).
- Group 4: You require specialized health services that are 2 h away, your employer cut health insurance benefits, or you do not understand what your doctor describes to you about your condition (health and healthcare).
- Group 5: Your closest family member lives 5 h away, there are no members of your cultural group nearby, or there are no centers for your spiritual practice (social and community context).

(c) Instructors will then ask groups to share and will guide reflection of the students, exploring how life events and simple changes in social factors can impact individual health.

Interpersonal

The family or interpersonal level regards how close relationships and social networks of family and friends influence individual behaviors. This level begins to account for how individuals and their identities and health are impacted by social influences and relationships. Contributing factors at this level include social support, social networks, associations, culture, peer influence, family environment, and emotional support (Max et al. 2015). When instructing public health students about interventions at this level, it is imperative that they connect and consider different perspectives.

Course Objective: Integration Students will think about health in an integrated way, rather than separated and compartmentalized, through their ability to identify the interaction between interpersonal influences and health.

Course Objective: Human Dimension Students will come to see themselves as leaders in advancing health equity by understanding other health science disciplines and taking pride in their role as public health professionals.

Active Learning: Indirect Doing Experience In order to address these learning objectives, students will engage in active learning, which will encourage them to analyze and critique issues related to interpersonal influences on health.

1. Students should watch videos of families and social groups with differing values, traditions, and cultural backgrounds. Students will then engage in dialogue to compare and contrast differences based upon the cases. Instructors will encourage students to integrate this information with that completed for the active learning of the individual level above, exploring how social influences impact health at a higher level.
2. Students will then explore resources to understand the role of public health in addressing family wellness. Students will share findings as a group and then apply those findings to the cases/videos reviewed.

Active Learning: Direct Doing Experience Using the cases and information gathered during the indirect learning experience, students will engage in direct learning to build interprofessional knowledge.

1. Students should identify at least two health professionals from different disciplines. With each professional, students will outline and describe the cases and interview them about the professional's role in addressing interpersonal influences of health.
2. Following the interview, the student will educate the health professional through sharing about their role as a public health professional.
3. This project will culminate with a paper comparing and contrasting the roles of varying health professionals in intervening to address health at the family level. Students should consider issues that arise from the cases and create new ideas about interprofessional collaboration in order to address these issues. Students will explore how they can be leaders in continuing to educate others in future practice.

Organizational

Organizations play a leading role in shaping and defining workplace, school, socio-cultural, political, and neighborhood environments (Sallis et al. 2006). Organizations are common institutions such as schools, universities, hospitals, clinics, local businesses, nonprofit organizations, faith-based organizations, libraries, grocery stores, banks, and civic organizations, all of which provide a shared space to address a common need, purpose, or affiliation. For example, developing an intervention that improves the food environment in an elementary school not only provides healthier options for individual students, but also changes social norms by creating an environment that supports and values healthful foods.

Learning opportunities that target the organizational-level should focus on building foundational knowledge about how to adapt or develop interventions for organizations such as schools, health systems, and food systems. Beyond building knowledge, having students partner with and serve in local organizations to address a public health issue builds a sense of caring and investment in the solution.

Course Objective: Foundational Knowledge Students will identify and critically evaluate social and behavioral interventions that target public health issues in organizations.

Course Objective: Caring Students will value the importance of creating health-supporting environments in institutions and organizations that serve the community.

Active Learning: Indirect Doing Experience To address the foundational knowledge objective, students will work in teams to develop a compendium of social and behavioral interventions that target a specific public health issue in an organizational setting (e.g., schools, health systems, nonprofit organizations, grocery stores, prisons, food pantries, or libraries).

1. Students will learn about social and behavioral theories and public health interventions through course readings and lectures.
2. Students will then have the opportunity to self-select teams based on shared interest in one of 10 pre-selected public health issues (e.g., mental health, nutrition, gun violence, or sexual and reproductive health). Teams will then identify and summarize a compendium of four interventions that aim to improve the public health issue in an organizational setting.
3. Teams will share findings with the class through brief face-to-face or recorded presentations.

Active Learning: Direct Doing Experience To address the caring objective, students will collaborate with a local organization and design a service learning project to address a local public health issue.

1. Student teams will identify a local organization that is actively addressing, or has the capacity to respond to, the public health issue defined in their compendium.
2. To begin the partnership, students will present their compendium and then work with the organization to address the public health issue through a service-learning project. During the project, students will have the opportunity to learn the importance and process of relationship building, as well as develop an appreciation for the complexity of addressing public health issues in a variety of organizations and institutions.

Community

Community constitutes a complex and rich environment. The term itself suggests an array of definitions with varying ideas of what the term means. Scaffa and Reitz (2014) eloquently discuss numerous explanations of community, which include people coming together to accomplish a shared goal, a celebration space, a social unit with resources and social norms, and an opportunity for a team to accomplish something that cannot be done alone. In relationship to the social ecological model, it is necessary to go beyond understanding what makes up a community in order to recognize how community-level interventions influence public health efforts. This includes population-based strategies, versus individual health interventions, that address cultural, political, environmental, social, and economic influences on health (Scaffa and Reitz 2014).

Community-level interventions are not designed in isolation. Instead, a participatory approach serves to engage and leverage local agencies, stakeholders, and community resources, all of which instill lasting influence and create community capacity for future change. Public health professionals alongside other health professionals from other disciplines may serve in a range of roles, including mentor, consultant, and community facilitator (Scaffa and Reitz 2014). Classroom activities designed for public health students must align with the complexities that coincide with community-level intervention.

Course Objective: Application Students will make decisions about well-being in relationship to social factors specific to a given community or population.

Course Objective: Human Dimension Students will understand others in terms of their occupational, cultural, and social influences on health and well-being in light of the role of public health professionals and community factors.

Active Learning: Indirect Doing Experience The following activity aligns with the application course objective listed above and can be utilized as a preface to direct community-level experiences. In this case application student teams address social determinants of health using a case vignette that is provided. Activities include

1. Using one of the case studies provided in class, students discuss the social determinants of health specific to the community and population identified.
2. Next, students create a map of social determinants depicting factors within the community or population.

    (a) Students identify determinants that relate to the location and community factors of the case.
    (b) Students should utilize resources to assist with details specific to the community (e.g., public health data or resource guides).
    (c) Students should then create a second map based on where they live or grew up.

3. In groups, students will discuss how the case relates to public health and make a determination regarding service and resource needs for the population based on all areas of public health. Students should consider

    (a) What social, cultural, economic, and environmental factors influence health in this community?
    (b) What services are available to address these health factors?
    (c) How might community health needs change throughout the year or across the lifespan?
    (d) What level(s) of intervention does this community require (primary, secondary, or tertiary)?
    (e) Are any other community resources or engagement of health systems needed? If so, which health systems, professionals, and services would benefit the community?
    (f) What differences in opportunities, occupational experiences, and health factors are unique to each community?

Active Learning: Direct Doing Experience For this activity, students will identify a specific community and conduct interviews with community members and public health professionals.

1. Based on this specific community, students will identify two individuals to interview, one community member and one public health professional that provides services within the community.
2. Once a community is identified, students should brainstorm information that they aim to gather through the interview. Students should begin by creating a list of interview questions. An overview of the interview should be included in the final assignment.
3. Next, students will interview the community member and public health professional to explore and understand their perspective of the health, quality of life, and well-being of the community or population. Physical, mental, and social factors should be considered.
4. Finally, students create a 5–7 min video clip (e.g., iMovie or voiced-over PowerPoint) that highlights this well-being profile of the individuals interviewed, specifically highlighting factors that impact quality of life and well-being based on community influences. Videos can be shared using an online learning platform or reviewed in class along with active discussion and reflection.

Policy

Policy development is a key strategy in addressing public health issues through structural and environmental changes (Golden et al. 2015). While policies have the ability to strengthen and promote health and well-being, they also have the ability to diminish health by creating environments and structures that are neither safe nor equitable across diverse populations. Examples of public policies that influence health and well-being include health insurance laws, motor vehicle safety standards and seat belt laws, public policies that determine eligibility for health and social service programs, minimum wage laws, and laws that regulate clean water and exposure to hazards (Golden et al. 2015). Beyond laws and public health codes, organizational level policies that support health and well-being include workplace safety policies, tobacco-free zones, breastfeeding policies, school immunization policies, infection control protocols in health facilities, and more.

Opportunities that target policy-level interventions should help students learn how to navigate the policy-making process. Beyond learning about the process of policy development, students will benefit from learning how to analyze, compare, and assess the public health impact of policies.

Course Objective: Learning How to Learn Students will know how to identify policies at the organizational, community, state, and national levels that aim to improve public health and well-being.

Course Objective: Integration Students will use a policy analysis framework to analyze and compare the impact, cost, and feasibility of policies that aim to improve health and well-being.

Active Learning: Indirect Doing Experience This activity provides an opportunity for students to explore health policies across multiple settings and levels of government. The project aligns with the first objective and aims to help students become self-directed learners and develop skills to use in practice and research.

1. Students will learn about the legislative process through course readings and a tutorial on how a bill or legislation becomes law. With this knowledge, students will select a public health issue of interest (e.g., maternal and child health, environmental health, or mental health). Given the focus area, students will identify and summarize two policies at each of the following levels: organizational, local, regional, and national.
2. The instructor will compile a master list of policies and develop a game-based quiz, in which students or teams match each policy to a specific setting or level of government.

Active Learning: Direct Doing Experience To address the integration objective, students will apply a policy analysis framework to legislation that has not yet become law.

1. Building on the previous activity, student teams will identify four bills at the national level that address a specific public health issue. Using an established framework, such as the CDC's Policy Analytical Framework (2013a), students then compare the public health impact, cost, and feasibility of the four bills.
2. Based on the comparison, teams will select the most promising bill and support their decision with data from the policy analysis process.
3. Optional activity for individual component: Students can write an opinion-editorial (op-ed) to promote awareness of their team's public health issue and advocate for the most promising bill to address the issue. This process connects the policy analysis process with advocacy.

Conclusion

To improve social determinants and advance health equity, the field of public health must strengthen and further develop interprofessional collaboration and education. Topics of quality of life and well-being are essential to teaching and empowering public health and health science students to work in partnership with communities and peoples that represent diverse cultures, environments, geographies, and socio-economic backgrounds. This chapter provides conceptual frameworks for understanding quality of life and well-being in a population health context. Furthermore, this chapter demonstrates the application of an ecological model of health and a taxonomy of significant learning as a way to teach about quality of life and well-being in public health, health sciences, and medical professional curricula.

References

Abbott, R. A., & Baun, W. B. (2015). The multi-dimensions of wellness: The vital role of terms and meanings. *American Journal of Health Promotion, 5*(29), 8–10.

Adams, T., Bezner, J., & Steinhardt, M. (1997). The conceptualization and measurement of perceived wellness: Integrating balance across and within dimensions. *American Journal of Health Promotion, 11*(3), 208–218.

Adams, T., Bezner, J., Garner, L., & Woodruff, S. (1998). Construct validation of the perceived wellness survey. *American Journal of Health Studies, 14*(4), 212–219.

Adams, T. B., Bezner, J. R., Drabbs, M. E., Zambarano, R. J., & Steinhardt, M. A. (2000). Conceptualization and measurement of the spiritual and psychological dimensions of wellness in a college population. *Journal of American College Health, 48*, 165–173.

American Occupational Therapy Association. (2014). Occupational therapy practice framework: Domain and process (3rd ed.). *American Journal of Occupational Therapy, 68*(Suppl. 1), S1–S48.

American Public Health Association. (n.d.). *What is public health?* Retrieved from: https://www.apha.org/what-is-public-health. Accessed 25 May 2018.

Barnes, M. E., & Caprino, K. (2016). Analyzing service-learning reflections through Fink's taxonomy. *Teaching in Higher Education, 21*(5), 557–575.

Brofenbrenner, U. (1979). *The ecology of human development*. Cambridge, MA: Harvard University Press.

Centers for Disease Control and Prevention. (1999). Ten great public health achievements – United States, 1900–1999. *Mortality and Morbidity Weekly Report (MMWR), 48*(12), 241.

Centers for Disease Control and Prevention. (2011). Ten great public health achievements – United States, 2001–2010. *Morbidity and Mortality Weekly Report, 60*(1), 619–623.

Centers for Disease Control and Prevention. (2013a). *CDC's policy analytical framework*. Atlanta: Centers for Disease Control and Prevention, U.S. Department of Health and Human Services.

Centers for Disease Control and Prevention. (2013b). *Strategies to prevent obesity and other chronic diseases: The CDC guide to strategies to support breastfeeding mothers and babies*. Atlanta: U.S. Department of Health and Human Services.

Coreil, J. (2010). Why study social and behavioral factors in public health? In J. Coreil (Ed.), *Social and behavioral foundations of public health* (pp. 3–21). Thousand Oaks: Sage.

David, L. (2014). *Emotional intelligence (Goleman) in learning theories*. Retrieved from https://www.learning-theories.com/emotional-intelligence-goleman.html

DeSalvo, K. B., Wang, Y. C., Harris, A., Auerbach, J., Koo, D., & O'Carroll, P. (2017). Public health 3.0: A call to action for public health to meet the challenges of the 21st century. *Preventing Chronic Disease, 14*, 170017.

Dorner, T. E. (2012). Public health. Social context and action. *International Journal of Integrated Care, 12*, 1–2.

Fink, L. D. (2013). *Creating significant learning experiences: An integrated approach to designing college courses*. San Francisco: Jossey-Bass.

Foster, T. W., & Levitov, J. E. (2012). Wellness during midlife and older adulthood: A different perception. *Adultspan Journal, 11*(2), 66–76.

Golden, S. D., & Earp, J. A. L. (2012). Social ecological approaches to individuals and their contexts: Twenty years of health education and behavior health promotion interventions. *Health Education & Behavior, 39*(3), 364–372.

Golden, S. D., McLeroy, K. R., Green, L. W., Earp, J. A. L., & Lieberman, L. D. (2015). Upending the social ecological model to guide health promotion efforts toward policy and environmental change. *Health Education & Behavior, 42*(15), 8S–14S.

Goleman, D. (1998). *Working with emotional intelligence*. New York: Random House, Inc.

Green, A. (2016). Seven dimensions of wellness: A holistic approach to health. *Alive*.

Gutman, S. A., & Schindler, V. P. (2007). The neurological basis of occupation. *Occupational Therapy International, 14*(2), 71–85. https://doi.org/10.1002/oti.225.

Hakansson, C., Lissner, L., Bjorkelund, C., & Sonn, U. (2009). Engagement in patterns of daily occupations and perceived health among women of working age. *Scandinavian Journal of Occupational Therapy, 16*, 110–117.

Hawks, S. R., Smith, T., Thomas, H. G., Christley, H. S., Meinzer, N., & Pyne, A. (2008). The forgotten dimensions of health education research. *Health Education Research, 23*(2), 319–324. https://doi.org/10.1093/her/cym035.

Healthy People 2020. (n.d.). *Social determinants of health*. Retrieved from https://www.healthypeople.gov/2020/topics-objectives/topic/social-determinants-of-health

Hettler, B. (1976). *The six dimensions of wellness model*. National Wellness Institute. Retrieved from https://cdn.ymaws.com/www.nationalwellness.org/resource/resmgr/pdfs/SixDimensionsFactSheet.pdf

Hilleras, P. K., Jorm, A. F., Herlitz, A., & Winblad, B. (2001). Life satisfaction among very old: A survey on a cognitively intact sample of aged 90 years or above. *International Journal of Aging and Human Development, 52*(1), 71–90.

Kaveh, M. H., Ostovarfar, J., Keshavarzi, S., & Ghahremani, L. (2016). Validation of perceived wellness survey (PWS) in a sample of Iranian population. *Malaysian Journal of Medical Science, 23*(4), 46–53. https://doi.org/10.21315/mjms2016.23.4.6.

Kirschner, P. A., & van Merriënboer, J. J. (2013). Do learners really know best? Urban legends in education. *Educational Psychologist, 48*(3), 169–183.

Krause, N. (2004). Stressors arising in highly valued roles, meaning in life, and the physical health status of older adults. *Journal of Gerontology, 59*(5), S287–S297.

Marmot, M. (2015). *The health gap: The challenge of an unequal world.* New York: Bloomsbury Press.

Marmot, M., & Bell, R. (2012). Fair society, healthy lives. *Public Health, 126,* S4–S10.

Marmot, M., Friel, S., Bell, R., Houweling, T. A., Taylor, S., & Commission on Social Determinants of Health. (2008). Closing the gap in a generation: Health equity through action on the social determinants of health. *The Lancet, 372*(9650), 1661–1669.

Max, J. L., Sedivy, V., & Garrido, M. (2015). *Increasing our impact by using a social-ecological approach.* Washington, DC: Administration on Children, Youth and Families, Family and Youth Services Bureau.

McIntyre, G., & Howie, L. (2002). Adapting to widowhood through meaningful occupations: A case study. *Scandinavian Journal of Occupational Therapy, 9,* 54–62.

McLeroy, K. R., Bibeau, D., Steckler, A., & Glanz, K. (1988). An ecological perspective on health promotion programs. *Health Education Quarterly, 15*(4), 351–377.

Morris, I. (2010). *Why the west rules-for now: The patterns of history and what they reveal about the future.* London: Profile Books.

Office of Disease Prevention and Health Promotion. (2010). *Healthy People 2020.* Retrieved from https://www.healthypeople.gov/sites/default/files/HP2020_brochure_with_LHI_508_FNL.pdf

Pizzi, M. A., & Richards, L. G. (2017). Promoting health, well-being, and quality of life in occupational therapy: A commitment to a paradigm shift for the next 100 years. *American Journal of Occupational Therapy, 71*(4), 170010p1–170010p15. https://doi.org/10.5014/ajot.2017.028456.

Rogerson, B., Lindberg, R., Givens, M., & Wernham, A. (2014). A simplified framework for incorporating health into community development initiatives. *Health Affairs, 33*(11), 1939–1947. https://doi.org/10.1377/hlthaff.2014.0632.

Rosen, G. (2015). *A history of public health.* Baltimore: Johns Hopkins University Press.

Ryan, M. (2013). The pedagogical balancing act: Teaching reflection in higher education. *Teaching in Higher Education, 18*(2), 144–155. https://doi.org/10.1080/13562517.2012.694104.

Sallis, J. F., & Owen, N. (2015). Ecological models of health behavior. *Health Behavior: Theory, Research, and Practice, 5,* 43–64.

Sallis, J. F., Cervero, R. B., Ascher, W., Henderson, K. A., Kraft, M. K., & Kerr, J. (2006). An ecological approach to creating active living communities. *Annual Review of Public Health, 27,* 297–322.

Scaffa, M. E., & Reitz, S. M. (2014). *Occupational therapy in community-based practice settings* (2nd ed.). Philadelphia: F.A. Davis.

Stokols, D. (1992). Establishing and maintaining healthy environments: Toward a social ecology of health promotion. *American Psychologist, 47*(1), 6–22.

Tervalon, M., & Murray-Garcia, J. (1998). Cultural humility versus cultural competence: A critical distinction in defining physician training outcomes in multicultural education. *Journal of Health Care for the Poor and Underserved, 9*(2), 117–125.

Wilcox, D. A., & Travis, J. W. (2015). How culture interacts with the concept of wellness: The role wellness plays in a global environment. *American Journal of Health Promotion, 5*(29), 6–8.

World Health Organization. (1946). *The Constitution.* Retrieved from http://apps.who.int/gb/bd/PDF/bd47/EN/constitution-en.pdf?ua=1

Chelsea Wesner, MPH, MSW, CSW, is Instructor and Program Coordinator of Public Health at the University of South Dakota, USA. She teaches social and behavioral sciences, health policy, and indigenous public health. Her interests include maternal and child health, food security, and food sovereignty in American Indian and Alaska Native communities.

Diana Feldhacker, OTD, OTR/L, BCPR is Assistant Professor of Occupational Therapy at Creighton University in Omaha, Nebraska, USA. She teaches physical rehabilitation and neuro-occupation. Her research interests include health promotion, vision rehabilitation, and effective teaching

Whitney Lucas Molitor, OTD, MS, OTR/L, BCG is Assistant Professor of Occupational Therapy at the University of South Dakota, USA. She teaches adult physical rehabilitation, home modifications, and health promotion along with foundational coursework in research and occupational performance of adulthood. Her research interests include productive aging, health promotion, visual performance, and contextually meaningful service provision in occupational therapy.

Chapter 14
Teaching Well-Being Within the Context of Sport: The What, Why, How and for Whom!

Diane E. Mack, Philip M. Wilson, Caitlin Kelley, and Jennifer Mooradian

> *...science must begin with myths and with the criticism of myths.*
>
> Sir Karl Popper (1963, p.26)

Myth

Athletes exhibit superior psychological health than non-athletes. This myth may stem from an overall inclination to idealize athletes, their physical attributes, and accomplishments. Similarly, psychological disorders among athletes have historically been stigmatized therefore may be underreported (Bar and Markser 2013). The widely held belief that 'only mentally strong athletes can be successful' (Markser 2011) may not reflect the reality of sport. Other than understanding the prevalence of, and risk factors for, eating disorders (e.g., Joy et al. 2016), a paucity of research has been conducted examining issues linked to ill- and well-being in athletes. As a result, sport governing bodies have generally been slow in responding to issues dealing with psychological health in athletes (Reardon and Factor 2010).

The purpose of this chapter is to detail pedagogical content tailored to teaching well-being within the context of sport. Organized around four central questions – What? Why? How? and For Whom? – recent developments in our understanding of well-being reported by athletes are highlighted. The chapter ends with select resources that could be implemented in any university-based course focused on teaching well-being in sport.

D. E. Mack (✉) · P. M. Wilson · C. Kelley · J. Mooradian
Behavioural Health Sciences Research Lab, Department of Kinesiology, Faculty of Applied Health Sciences, Brock University, St. Catharines, ON, Canada
e-mail: dmack@brocku.ca

© Springer Nature Switzerland AG 2020
G. H. Tonon (ed.), *Teaching Quality of Life in Different Domains*, Social Indicators Research Series 79, https://doi.org/10.1007/978-3-030-21551-4_14

What?

What is well-being? Although a widely used concept in the psychological sciences, 'well-being' has proven challenging to define and understand (Michalos et al. 2011). The World Health Organization (WHO 2004) defined health as "a state of well-being in which the individual realizes his or her own abilities, can cope with the normal stresses of life, can work productively and fruitfully, and is able to make a contribution to his or her community" (p. 12). Health therefore was defined as the presence of a positive state of functioning, and not simply the absence of psychological disorders (i.e., ill-being). Extending to psychological health, Keyes (2005) suggested a two continuum model whereby ill- and well-being are distinct but related dimensions that exist on separate continua. The first spans the presence/absence of ill-being, whereas the second is anchored by the presence/absence of well-being. From this perspective, several profiles could emerge. For example, an athlete could simultaneously have both high levels of ill- and well-being, an athlete could report low levels of ill-being while still not being well, etc. Evidence is to support Keyes (2005) model has been forthcoming in the literature (e.g., Suldo and Shaffer 2008). Given the focus of this chapter on well-being, attention to ill-being in sport is given limited attention.

Historically, our understanding of well-being in psychology has focused predominantly on symptom reduction (Huppert 2014). The sport literature is no different in this regard (e.g., Noon et al. 2015). The term health-related quality of life (HRQoL) was advanced to include subjective perceptions people's thoughts, feelings, and reactions to life circumstances that stem in part from condition diagnosis and subsequent treatment (Diener 2005). Huppert and So (2013) suggested that HRQoL may be of limited utility to describe positive aspects of well-being given their focus on physical functioning, limitations, and negative feelings. Yet, the inclusion of quality of life in sport holds meaning for teaching well-being in sport given its (1) historical grounding and (2) prominence in the medical/rehabilitation literature.

Extending beyond HRQoL, contemporary views link well-being with optimal functioning (Ryan and Deci 2001), with hedonic and eudaimonic traditions comprising essential components. Hedonic, or subjective well-being, is an individual's evaluation of his/her life measured by the relative balance of high positive and low negative affect, as well as, the cognitive evaluation of life satisfaction (Diener and Suh 1997). The eudaimonic tradition is most often linked with Ryff (1989), who introduced six dimensions that define human potential and flourishing. These dimensions include: (a) Autonomy, (b) Environmental Mastery, (c) Personal Growth, (d) Positive Relationships, (e) Purpose in Life and (f) Self-Acceptance. Recognizing the importance of considering both traditions, Huppert and So (2013) identified three core well-being components each comprised of multiple dimensions:

- Psychological characteristics: This dimension includes emotional stability, vitality, optimism, resilience, positive emotions, and self- esteem.

- Psychological functioning: This dimension is comprised of engagement, competence, meaning, and positive relationships.
- Positive appraisal: This dimension consists of life satisfaction and positive emotions.

Measuring Well-Being

The unresolved debate surrounding the conceptualization of well-being has spill-over effects in term of the optimal approach to measuring this psychological construct. The result of this challenge has been a proliferation of instruments available for use by researchers (Lindert et al. 2015; Linton et al. 2016). Adding to the confusion, sport-based researchers have at times, purported to measure well-being through the use instruments which in point of fact were designed to measure ill-being (e.g., Schuring et al. 2017). In such cases, the absence of ill-being should not be equated to high the presence of higher levels of well-being (Huppert and So 2013; Keyes 2005).

To measure well-being, researchers should adopt instruments that adequately capture positive experiences within the item content. Stated differently, items should focus on positive functioning or adaptive features if an instrument is measuring well-being. Single items focused on well-being such as "Taking all things together, how happy would you say you are?" (Downward and Rasciute 2011) are often used to measure well-being in population studies. Single items have the advantage of being simple, direct and brief. Conversely, single-item instruments are plagued by concerns over content relevance and representation, sensitivity and the challenges of estimating score reliability using conventional approaches (Cooke et al. 2016).

Multi-item instruments may tap into one (e.g., the Subjective Vitality Scale [SVS], Ryan and Fredrick 1997) or multiple dimensions (e.g., Scales of Psychological Well-being, Ryff 1989) of well-being. Common instruments used by sport-based researchers have been the Positive and Negative Affect Schedule (Watson et al. 1988) and the SVS (e.g., Mack et al. 2011) linked with the hedonic and eudaimonic traditions respectively. These instruments are often used to measure global well-being or have been modified to the sporting context. Calls have emanated for the development of sport specific instruments to represent the breadth of well-being as a psychological entity consistent with its multi-dimensional nature and defining characteristics (e.g., Foster and Chow 2018; Sarkar and Fletcher 2013).

Scientific advancement does not require the universal adoption of a solitary instrument to measure well-being. The key consideration for researchers when selecting an instrument to measure well-being is the intended purpose of the study. The instrument of choice should have a theoretical basis and contain the full complement of well-being domains expected to be influenced by sport or the unique characteristics of the athletes being sampled. Researchers at the University of Cambridge have recently developed an interactive tool to guide researcher's when selecting an instrument to measure well-being (http://webmat.micsti.at/what-is-webmat/)

Why?

Why study well-being in athletes? Well-being has been deemed a fundamental human goal (Huppert 2014). As recognition of the importance and value of understanding well-being in sport grows, it behooves all with a vested interest in optimizing athlete development to investigate the individual and contextual characteristics that drive well-being. If as Popper (1963) asserts that science includes the "criticism of myths" (p. 26), it behooves researchers to revisit the following question: Are athletes more psychologically healthy compared to non-athletes?   A   clear shift to understanding ill-being in athletes has begun (Rice et al. 2016). Elite athletes are at comparable risk of both depression and anxiety compared to the general population (Gulliver et al. 2015; Schaal et al. 2011). In response to this growing understanding, sport psychiatry has become an emerging field of study (Bar and Markser 2013) with government agencies (UK Government 2018) and the European Federation of Sport Psychology (Moesch et al. 2018) responding to urgent calls to address ill-being in sport.

What evidence attests to quality of life and well-being? Elite adapted sport athletes reported higher quality of life compared to non-sport counterparts (Yazicioglu et al. 2012) and comparable quality of life compared to those without mobility limitations (Côté-Leclerc et al. 2017). Vella et al. (2014) investigated whether HRQoL differed across four sport participation classifications over a 2-year period in children ranging in age from 8 to 10 years. Parent perceptions of their children's HRQoL was significantly higher for those who had maintained sport participation over the 2 years compared to those who had never participated, those who had dropped out, or those who had commenced sport participation after the age of 8 years. While conclusions speak to the possible benefits of on-going sport participation to well-being, skepticism is warranted given the effect sizes reported by Vella et al. (2014) were negligible. To investigate the long-term benefits of sport participation, the National Collegiate Athletic Association (NCAA) undertook a survey to examine whether former student athletes differed on quality of life from students who were not athletes (NCAA 2014). In total, 9% of former student athletes were found to be high in quality of life across all 5 domains compared to 8% of those who did not compete in NCAA sport. When examined individually, former student athletes reported greater social, community and physical health in comparison to their non-athlete counterparts.

In adults, sport participation has predicted greater happiness especially if the sport included social interaction when compared to non-participants (Downward and Rasciute 2011). Former student athletes reported a greater sense of purpose than former students who were not athletes (NCAA 2014). Adapted sport athletes reported higher satisfaction with life compared to non-sport participants (Yazicioglu et al. 2012). No differences in self-esteem were reported between active and retired Paralympic athletes (Marin-Urquiza et al. 2018).

In summary, the literature is inconclusive as to whether athletes differ from non-athletes in terms of reported well-being, or whether sport participation holds protective long-term effects for psychological health. Many factors likely impact this conclusion including, but not limited to, characteristics of the sample, study design, the domain of quality of life or well-being that is of interest to the researcher, and the choice of instrument.

How?

How can well-being be nutured? Understanding how to nurture well-being, and the factors linked to thwarting an athletes' well-being, is a relatively new area of research focus within the sport literature. Keyes' (2005) model implies that the promotion of athletes' well-being cannot be grounded in strategies directed toward the reduction and prevention of ill-being. This next section introduces select interpersonal and contextual areas of intervention that hold promise to enhancing well-being in athletes.

Resilience

Why do some individuals seem more capable in their ability to 'bounce back' from (or thrive) despite encountering hardships? This question marks the foundation for the study of resilience. While resilience is identified as a marker of well-being (Huppert and So 2013), Fletcher and Sarkar (2013) also defined resilience as a process through which "the role of mental processes and behavior in promoting personal assets and protecting an individual from the potential negative effect of stressors" (p.16) is examined. Understanding resilience within a sport context is necessary as, in addition to being exposed inadvertently to stressors, (e.g. death of a loved one); athletes purposely seek out challenges to overcome (e.g., balancing sport and life; Sarkar and Fletcher 2014).

Tamminen et al. (2013) investigation of elite female athletes highlights the potential for athletes to experience growth following adversity (e.g., desire to help others, realizations of strength, gaining perspective). Olympic athletes have also identified how adversity was seen as a determinant for their later athletic triumphs as these stressors were used as motivation to persevere, improve and grow (Sarkar et al. 2015). Olympic athletes also viewed themselves as resilient by actively engaging with the challenges they faced (Fletcher and Sarkar, 2012). Therefore, experiencing some adversity has the potential to facilitate positive outcomes via resilience.

Interventions designed to facilitate resilience focus on training athletes to positively adapt to stressors and adversities that may be experienced (Fletcher and Sarkar 2016). The intervention first targets an athletes' dispositional characteristics (e.g., extraversion, motivation, attributional style, etc.) and psychological skills such as imagery or goal-setting that protect an individual from negative consequences. Second, the athlete is exposed to environments which foster challenge in a supportive manner through increasing exposure to pressure. Finally, the intervention emphasizes how to productively evaluate and interpret various pressures that may be encountered by the athlete. In their attempt to augment resilience the main objective of Fletcher and Sarkar (2016) intervention was to maintain functioning and performance under pressure.

Self-Compassion

How would you treat a teammate who is experiencing difficulties? Even when your teammate is partly responsible for these difficulties? Now, place yourself in that same circumstance! Would you treat yourself in the same way you would your teammate? This is the essence of self-compassion. Self-compassion is defined as a positive and caring attitude of an individual toward themselves in the face of failure and shortcomings (Neff 2003). Being self-compassionate refers to the combination of three mutually interacting components (Neff 2003). First, self-kindness involves treating oneself with kindness as opposed to harsh self-criticism or judgment. Common humanity, the second component, acknowledges that going through difficulties is a common human experience. The third component, mindfulness, involves accepting difficulties while holding it in balanced awareness as opposed to over-identifying with experience. In their meta-analysis, Zessin et al. (2015) found an average effect size of .47 between self-compassion and well-being. Specific to the sporting context, Ferguson et al. (2014, 2015) reported that self-compassion is positively linked with several markers of eudaimonic well-being in athletes.

Self-compassion is adaptive and most relevant during times of difficulty (Ferguson et al. 2015; Neff 2003). In their interviews with six women athletes, Sutherland et al. (2014) detailed experiences of self-compassion including the acceptance of injuries as a reality of sport beyond personal control and common humanity in their experiences of failure and injury through sharing their experiences with others around them. In light of these findings, increasing self-compassion in athletes may be a valuable skill to help circumvent negative events in sport. In one of the only sport-based self-compassion interventions to date, Mosewich et al. (2013) asked athletes to recant personal negative experiences and frame the experience consistent with self-compassion. Compared to those in the attention control condition, athletes in the intervention group were found to adopt a self-compassionate frame of mind to their negative experience over the course of a month.

Mindfulness

Being mindful has been used to describe a psychological trait, a state of awareness, and a psychological process (Germer et al. 2005). The three main components of contemporary mindfulness-based models are: (1) nonjudgmental awareness of the moment (2) placing attentional focus on external in lieu of internal processes and (3) commitment to action that is aligned with one's values and desires (Gardner and Moore 2012). In essence, being mindful equates to being aware of what is happening in the present moment. Dispositional mindfulness in athletes has been linked with positive affect (Chang et al. 2018) and eudaimonic well-being (Nolte et al. 2016).

While mindfulness approaches have been used to facilitate sport performance, Gardner and Moore (2017) called for sport psychologists to extend their focus towards other areas through which mindfulness would positively shape an athlete's well-being. Mindfulness-based interventions differ from psychological skills training (e.g., goal setting, self-talk, etc.) typically adopted in the literature to facilitate optimal performance. Psychological skills training uses control of the internal state as its core premise (e.g., changing one's thought patterns, or modifying emotional states). Mindfulness-based interventions allow for the acceptance of thoughts and emotions and discourage efforts to alter them. Yet, few researchers have accepted Gardner and Moore's (2017) challenge to include well-being as a focal outcome. One exception to this trend is a study by Thompson et al. (2011) whereby athletes retrospectively indicated their satisfaction with life was higher 1-year following a mindfulness-based workshop.

Basic Psychological Needs Theory

Under the rubric of Basic Psychological Needs Theory (BPNT), Ryan and Deci (2017) posit that social contexts which fulfill the basic psychological needs for competence, autonomy and relatedness in an on-going and authentic manner promote integration, adaptation and well-being. In contrast, social contexts perceived to thwart psychological needs will likely engender ill-being and a fragmented sense of self (Ryan and Deci 2017). The psychological need for competence refers to individual's natural desire to explore, manipulate, and feel proficient when mastering optimal challenges within the environment (White 1959). Autonomy concerns feeling self-governing in that behavior is engaged in volitionally and stems from an internal locus of causality (deCharms 1968). Behaviour is engaged in autonomously when consistent with personal interests, preferences, and choices. Relatedness reflects the psychological need to establish and maintain satisfying and supportive social relationships and feel emotionally connected to others (Baumeister and Leary 1995). The fulfillment of relatedness extends beyond simply being in a relationship (e.g., coach-athlete), but being in a relationship whereby one feels valued and significant.

According to Ryan and Deci (2017), psychological need fulfillment represent essential foundations that exert unique and 'direct' effects on well-being. Support for the key tenets of BPNT (Ryan and Deci 2017) have emerged from research studies using cross-sectional (Mack et al. 2011) and longitudinal designs (Reinboth and Duda 2006). Similarly, when psychological needs are thwarted (or frustrated), lower levels of vitality and positive affect have been reported by athletes (Bartholomew et al. 2011).

Interpersonal Supports: Understanding the Role of the Social Context in Psychological Need Fulfillment

A recent newspaper article (Donaldson 2018) chronicled the changing sport culture in New Zealand suggesting there has been a systemic failure to adapt to the changing dynamic between coach and athlete. Exemplars highlighted in the article speak to the traditional 'command and control' culture whereby coaches impose practices without discussion or consultation, give vague or irrelevant feedback, discourage alternate opinions and, appear cold and distant. A shift in the sporting culture is recommended whereby the fulfillment of athlete psychological needs is the focus of coach-athlete interactions.

Interpersonal styles focused on perceptions of autonomy support, structure, and involvement can provide a framework to understand coach-athlete interactions in sport (Wilson et al. 2010). Autonomy supportive coaches provide the athletes with choice, opportunities to initiate and control their behaviours, while minimizing controlling statements, pressures, and demands (Ryan and Deci 2017). Coaches who provide structure, communicate their expectations clearly and provide the necessary information to understand what to do and how to do it in sport through feedback, learning strategies, standards, challenges, plans, and schedules (Ryan and Deci 2017). Involved coaches offer emotional resources (e.g., sympathy), show genuine interest in the athlete as a person, acknowledge their feelings, and spend time with them (Ryan and Deci 2017). Desirable consequences such as greater psychological need fulfillment, greater persistence, sustained engagement, and well-being are apparent in individuals when they experience greater autonomy support, structure, and involvement from coaches (e.g., Pope and Wilson 2014; Ryan and Deci 2017).

Adopting a coaching style consistent with being interpersonally supportive (Ryan and Deci 2017) may not come naturally to all. Training opportunities for coaches (Mahoney et al. 2017) and physiotherapists (Lonsdale et al. 2017) have been implemented to educate those who work closely with athletes. Murray et al. (2018) developed an observational tool designed to evaluate practitioner/coach use of interpersonal supports which can further be used as training tools in the field.

For Whom?

The following section focuses on well-being in select groups of athletes (i.e., For Whom). Although not exhaustive, the focus of this section will be on athletes living with a physical or intellectual disability and common transitional periods in an athletes' life.

Disability

It is estimated that 15.6% of people 15 years of age and older are living with a disability (WHO 2011). Using the International Classification of Functioning, Disability and Health (WHO 2001), disability is defined as an umbrella term for impairments, activity limitations, and participation restrictions. Impairments are problems with body function or structure. Activity limitations are difficulties encountered in executing a task or action. Finally, participation restrictions are problems that may be experienced across engagement in life situations. Disability therefore is a dynamic interplay between features of a person's body (e.g., the challenges of living with cerebral palsy) and those of the society (e.g., negative attitudes, transportation limitations). For those living with a disability, the natural imbalance of needs/potentialities and environment makes it even more urgent to pursue the enhancement of psychological well-being (Puce et al. 2017).

People, regardless of disability status, benefit from participation in activities and settings that provide an appropriate level of challenge, social engagement, belonging, and autonomy (Ryan and Deci 2017). However, both children (Tonkin et al. 2014) and adults (Jaarsma et al. 2014) with disabilities experience significant restrictions to participating in physical activity. Efforts to promote well-being in those living with disabilities through participation in recreational sports was first recorded in 1948, followed by the Paralympics in 1960, and the establishment of the Special Olympics in 1968 (Wilson 2002). The focus of the next two sections will be on two sub-categories of disability, namely those living with physical or intellectual disabilities.

Physical Disability

Persons living with a physical disability experience physiological, mobility or dexterity limitations. In spite of such limitations, people living with physical disabilities typically report quality of life ranging from 'good' to 'excellent' (Martin 2017). When compared to those without activity limitations, adapted sport athletes have reported comparable levels of quality of life (Côté-Leclerc et al. 2017) and greater eudaimonic well-being (Fiorilli et al. 2013). In their review, Macdougall et al. (2015) noted the availability of studies testing differences in well-being between

Paralympic and Olympic sport athletes is limited. Building on this, Macdougall and colleagues (2017) reported no differences between Paralympic and Olympic sport athletes across psychological domains of HRQoL and hedonic/eudaimonic well-being. Differences were found for measures of HRQoL linked to physical functioning (e.g., bodily pain). Therefore, based on the available research, adapted sport athletes show comparable levels of well-being compared to non-athletes and athletes alike. Increased self-esteem, accomplishment and a sense of belonging to a group were reasons identified by adapted sport athletes as contributors to their overall well-being (Côté-Leclerc et al. 2017). The extent to which these (or other) contributors differ between adapted and non-adapted sport athletes is unclear.

Examples of organizations that understand the benefits sport can provide to persons with physical disabilities include SCI Action Canada (http://sciactioncanada.ca/) and Invictus Games (https://invictusgamesfoundation.org/). Both organizations serve niche populations, namely persons with spinal cord injury (SCI) and veterans disabled during military service in hopes of education, inspiration and advocacy on behalf of those living with a physical disability.

Intellectual Disability

People living with intellectual disabilities demonstrate significant limitations in cognitive functioning and adaptive behaviour (conceptual, social and practical skills; Schalock et al. 2011). The Special Olympics is the main provider of sport programming for people living with intellectual disabilities regardless of level of ability. Through organizational programming, individuals living with an intellectual disability can compete alongside those with, or without, intellectual disabilities (i.e., Unified sport activities).

Individuals living with intellectual disabilities have reported more positive emotions when participating in sport as opposed to not (Glidden et al. 2011). Researchers have increasingly used visual media to further understand the sporting experiences of people living with intellectual disabilities. As an example, Weiss et al. (2017) used photovoice methodology to capture the experiences of Special Olympic participants. One of the main themes emanating from their work was the sense of connectedness to others that resulted from sport participation. Although not unequivocal, evidence for positive psychological, emotional and social outcomes has been reported from participation in Special Olympics programming (Tint et al. 2017).

Injury Rehabilitation

Injury is an inherent risk linked to involvement in sport regardless of level of participation. Being injured is often linked with time lost from practice or competition, reductions in activity and the need for medical attention (Patel et al. 2017). Athletic therapy often focuses on physical rehabilitation of the injured athlete, yet attention to the psychological toll of sport injurywarrants consideration.

Understanding the athlete's response to sport injury has typically been examined through (a) response to the injury, (b) psychological factors linked to treatment compliance and (c) readiness to return to sport. Common psychological responses to an injury include frustration, depression, anger, feelings of isolation, and anxiety (Brewer 2017). Less frequently considered has been the effects of injury on an athletes' well-being. In their review, Houston et al. (2016) reported that HRQoL was lower in injured athletes than non-injured athletes. Yet, athletes have reported injury-related benefits including opportunities for personal growth and competence based physical/technical development (Udry et al. 1997). Positive affect was not associated with treatment compliance (Lu and Hsu 2013) yet has been linked with fewer concerns about returning to sport (Podlog et al. 2010). Collectively this line of research reinforces the need for clinicians working with injured athletes to consider both physical and psychological health during the rehabilitation process. The minimal consideration afforded well-being in injured athletes warrants greater consideration by researchers to understand athlete responses to injury that subsequently can inform clinicians facilitating their transition through the rehabilitation process and (ideally) return to sport.

Transitioning out of Sport

Exploring retirement from sport has been a subject of interest in sport psychology from pioneering work in the late 1960s (e.g., Mihovilovic 1968) to current times (e.g., Knights et al. 2016). The transition from sport may be an anticipated (e.g., from active engagement to discontinuation) or unanticipated (e.g., injury, being cut from a team) event and can occur at any developmental level. The predictability of anticipated transitions affords some opportunity to prepare athletes to cope in comparison to the lower predictability of unanticipated transitions. Understanding how to successfully transition out of sport now focuses on a "whole person" lifespan perceptive that should include attention to retirement planning, coping strategies, the availability of social support and the larger sport system (Stambulova et al. 2009). Lavallee (2005) found that athletes engaged in an intervention prior to retirement from sport experienced a more positive transition. This has led sports organizations including the International Olympic Committee (2018) and the NCAA (2018) to develop resources to facilitate career transition for athletes as they move out of sport.

Only recently have researchers highlighted the need to focus on the well-being of athletes as they transition out of sport. In their review, Knights and colleagues (2016) noted that athletes who voluntarily transitioned out of sport, those who developed a broad range of life skills, and those who perceived they accomplished their sporting goals were more likely to report higher well-being upon transitioning. Yet there is still much to understand specific to athlete well-being as they transition out of sport. Consistent with Keyes (2005) two continua model, a focus on ill-being during the transition from sport should not be equated with the absence of well-being. Assessing dynamic fluctuations in well-being during other transitional periods including from lower to higher competitive levels, or movement from one team to another, all represent areas ripe for additional investigation.

Teaching Well-Being in Sport

The promotion of well-being in athletes has become an emerging area of importance for researchers, coaches, sport science professionals and sport organizations. This burgeoning interest renders the delivery of a course on well-being in sport appealing to academics and students. Student interest may extend beyond kinesiology majors, to those studying in the psychological sciences, sport administration, etc. This chapter offers insight into topics that could be covered in such a course within the curriculum (see Table 14.1 for an illustrative outline of topics and readings). For academics who have longer teaching semesters, or who want to offer a full-year course, topics such as heredity and well-being, predictors of well-being, other theories (Broaden and Build; Fredrickson 2004) and interventions (e.g., gratitude) could be included as content. The focal instructional content of this course permits academics the opportunity to deliver novel material such has engaging students in mindfulness exercises, comparing different well-being instruments, shared personal experiences, and the opportunity to invite guest speakers (e.g., athletes who have transitioned out of sport). The accessible documents supporting athlete's well-being from organizations such as the IOC and NCAA could also be examined for relevant content. Finally, the content of this course lends itself to flexible delivery formats spanning traditional lectures, blended learning, and/or synchronous or asynchronous online delivery options.

Table 14.1 Resources to facilitate the delivery of teaching well-being in sport

Week 1: What is well-being
Reading:
Lundqvist (2011). Well-being in competitive sports—The feel-good factor? A review of conceptual considerations of well-being. *International Review of Sport & Exercise Psychology, 4,* 109–127
Week 2: Measuring well-being
Website:
The measurement of Well-being advisory tool: http://webmat.micsti.at/method/
Week 3: Why study well-being
Reading:
UK Government (2018). Mental health and elite sport action plan. https://assets.publishing.service.gov.uk/government/uploads/system/uploads/attachment_data/file/691770/180320_FINAL_Mental_Health_and_Elite_Sport_Action_Plan.pdf
Week 4: Resilience
Reading:
Sarkar, M., & Fletcher, D. (2014). Psychological resilience in sport performers: A review of stressors and protective factors. *Journal of Sports Sciences, 32,* 1419–1434

(continued)

Table 14.1 (continued)

Podcast:

Bridging the gap: http://bridgingthegappodcast.libsyn.com/
adversity-in-elite-sport-and-resilience-in-the-workplace

Week 5: Self-compassion

Reading:

Ferguson, L., C. Kowalski, K., Mack, D., & Sabiston, C. (2015). Self-compassion and
eudaimonic well-being during emotionally difficult times in sport. *Journal of Happiness
Studies, 16*. doi.org/10.1007/s10902-014-9558-8

Week 6: Mindfulness

Reading:

Gardner, F. L., & Moore, Z. E. (2017). Mindfulness-based and acceptance-based interventions
in sport and performance contexts. *Current Opinion in Psychology, 16,* 180–184

Podcast:

Bridging the gap: http://bridgingthegappodcast.libsyn.com/
an-empirical-examination-comparing-the-mindfulness-acceptance-commitment-approach-
and-psychological-skills-training-for-the-mental-health-and-sport-performance-of-female-
student-athletes

Week 7: Basic psychological needs theory

Reading:

Orr, K., Tamminen, K. A., Sweet, S. N., Tomasone, J. R., & Arbour-Nicitopoulos, K. P.
(2018). "I've had bad experiences with team sport": Sport participation, peer need-thwarting,
and need-supporting behaviors among youth identifying with physical disability. *Adapted
Physical Activity Quarterly, 35,* 36–56

Week 8: Interpersonal supports

Reading:

Wilson, P. M., J. P. Gregson, & Mack, D. E. (2010). The importance of interpersonal style in
competitive sport: A self-determination theory approach. *Sport psychology: Coping,
performance, and anxiety* (pp. 259–276). Nova Publishers: Hauppauge NY

Week 9: Athletes living with physical disabilities

Reading:

Martin, J. (2017). Persons with disabilities and quality of life: The role of physical activity. In
Mitchell (Ed), *Physical Disabilities: Perspectives, Risk Factors and Quality of Life (p, 1–15).*
Nova science publishers: Hauppage *NY*

Organization:

Invictus Games https://invictusgamesfoundation.org/

Week 10: Athletes living with intellectual disabilities

Tint, A., Thomson, K., & Weiss, J. A. (2017). A systematic review of the physical and
psychosocial correlates of Special Olympics participation among individuals with intellectual
disability. *Journal of Intellectual Disabilities, 61,* 301–324

Organization:

Special Olympics: http://www.specialolympics.ca/

Week 11: Athletic injury

Reading:

Brewer, B. (2017). *Psychological responses to sport injury.* Oxford Research Encyclopedia of
Psychology

http://psychology.oxfordre.com/view/10.1093/acrefore/9780190236557.001.0001/
acrefore-9780190236557-e-172

(continued)

Table 14.1 (continued)

Week 12: Transitioning out of sport
Reading:
Stambulova, N., Alfermann, D., Statler, T., & Côté, J. (2009). ISSP Position stand: career development and transitions of athletes. *International Journal of Sport and Exercise Psychology, 7*, 395–412
IOC athlete career transition programs https://www.olympic.org/athlete-career-programme

References

Bar, J.-J., & Markser, V. Z. (2013). Sport specificity of mental disorders. The issue of sport psychiatry. *European Archives of Psychiatry & Clinical Neuroscience, 263*, s205–s210.

Bartholomew, K. J., Ntoumanis, N., Ryan, R. M., Bosch, J., & Thøgersen-Ntoumani, C. (2011). Self-determination theory and diminished functioning: The role of interpersonal control and psychological need thwarting. *Personality & Social Psychology Bulletin, 37*, 1459–1473.

Baumeister, R. F., & Leary, M. R. (1995). The need to belong: Desire for interpersonal attachments as a fundamental human motivation. *Psychological Bulletin, 117*, 497–529.

Brewer, B. (2017). Psychological responses to sport injury. *Oxford Research Encyclopedia of Psychology*. Retrieved June 21, 2018, from http://psychology.oxfordre.com/view/10.1093/acrefore/9780190236557.001.0001/acrefore-9780190236557-e-172

Chang, W. H., Chang, J.-H., & Chen, L. H. (2018). Mindfulness enhances change in athletes' Well-being: The mediating role of basic psychological needs fulfillment. *Mindfulness, 9*, 815–823.

Cooke, P. J., Melchert, T. P., & Connor, K. (2016). Measuring well-being: A review of instruments. *The Counseling Psychologist, 44*, 730–757.

Côté-Leclerc, F., Boileau Duchesne, G., Bolduc, P., Gélinas-Lafrenière, A., Santerre, C., Desrosiers, J., & Levasseur, M. (2017). How does playing adapted sports affect quality of life of people with mobility limitations? Results from a mixed-method sequential explanatory study. *Health and Quality of Life Outcomes, 15*, 22. https://doi.org/10.1186/s12955-017-0597-9.

deCharms, R. (1968). *Personal causation: The internal affective determinants of behavior.* New York: Academic.

Diener, E. (2005). Guidelines for national indicators of subjective Well-being and ill-being. *Journal of Happiness Studies, 7*, 397–404.

Diener, E., & Suh, E. (1997). Measuring quality of life: Economic, social, and subjective indicators. *Social Indicators Research, 40*, 189–216.

Donaldson, M. (2018). *In wake of Pedan and Heraf controversies it seems New Zealand sport model is now 'outdated'.* New Zealand Herald, https://www.nzherald.co.nz/sport/news/article.cfm?c_id=4&objectid=12076611. Accessed 24 June 2018.

Downward, P., & Rasciute, S. (2011). Does sport make you happy? An analysis of the well-being derived from sports participation. *International Review of Applied Economics, 25*, 331–348.

Ferguson, L. J., Kowalski, K. C., Mack, D. E., & Sabiston, C. M. (2014). Exploring self-compassion and eudaimonic well-being in young women athletes. *Journal of Sport & Exercise Psychology, 36*, 203–216.

Ferguson, L., Kowalski, K. C., Mack, D., & Sabiston, C. (2015). Self-compassion and eudaimonic well-being during emotionally difficult times in sport. *Journal of Happiness Studies, 16*, 1263. https://doi.org/10.1007/s10902-014-9558-8.

Fiorilli, G., Iuliano, E., Aquino, G., Battaglia, C., Giombini, A., Calcagno, G., & di Cagno, A. (2013). Mental health and social participation skills of wheelchair basketball players: A controlled study. *Research in Developmental Disabilities, 34*, 3679–3685.

Fletcher, D., & Sarkar, M. (2012). A grounded theory of psychological resilience in Olympic champions. *Psychology of Sport and Exercise, 13*, 669–678.

Fletcher, D., & Sarkar, M. (2013). Psychological resilience: A review and critique of definitions, concepts, and theory. *European Psychologist, 18*, 12–23.

Fletcher, D., & Sarkar, M. (2016). Mental fortitude training: An evidence-based approach to developing psychological resilience for sustained success. *Journal of Sport Psychology in Action, 7*, 135–157.

Foster, B. J., & Chow, G. M. (2018). Development of the sport mental health continuum – short form (sport MHC-SF). *Journal of Clinical Sport Psychiatry.* https://doi.org/10.1123/jcsp.2017-0057.

Fredrickson, B. L. (2004). The broaden-and-build theory of positive emotions. *Philosophical Transactions of the Royal Society of Londone (Series B), 359*, 1367–1377.

Gardner, F., L., & Moore, Z. E., (2012). Mindfulness and acceptance models in sport psychology: A decade of basic and applied scientific advancements. Canadian Psychology/Psychologie Canadienne, 53, 309–318.

Gardner, F. L., & Moore, Z. E. (2017). Mindfulness-based and acceptance-based interventions in sport and performance contexts. *Current Opinion in Psychology, 16*, 180–184.

Germer, C. K., Siegel, R. D., & Fulton, P. R. (2005). *Mindfulness and psychotherapy.* New York: Guilford Press.

Glidden, L. M., Bamberger, K. T., Draheim, A. R., & Kersh, J. (2011). Parent and athlete perceptions of Special Olympics participation: Utility and danger of proxy responding. *Intellectual & Developmental Disabilities, 49*, 37–45.

Gulliver, A., Griffiths, K. M., Mackinnon, A., Batterham, P. J., & Stanimirovic, R. (2015). The mental health of Australian elite athletes. *Journal of Science and Medicine in Sport, 18*, 255–261.

Houston, M. N., Hoch, M. C., & Hoch, J. M. (2016). Health-related quality of life in athletes: A systematic review with meta-analysis. *Journal of Athletic Training, 51*, 442–453.

Huppert, F. A. (2014). The state of wellbeing science: Concepts, measures, interventions and policies. In F. A. Huppert & C. L. Cooper (Eds.), *Wellbeing: A complete reference guide* (Vol. IV, pp. 1–50). Oxford: Wiley.

Huppert, F. A., & So, T. T. C. (2013). Flourishing across Europe: Application of a new conceptual framework for defining wellbeing. *Social Indicators Research, 110*, 837–861.

International Olympic Committee. (2018). *Athlete365 Career+.* Accessed at: https://www.olympic.org/athlete365career-plus

Jaarsma, E. A., Dijkstra, P. U., Geertzen, J. H. B., & Dekker, R. (2014). Barriers to and facilitators of sports participation for people with physical disabilities: A systematic review. *Scandivivian Journal of Medicine and Science in Sport, 24*, 871–888.

Joy, E., Kussman, A., & Nattiv, A. (2016). 2016 update on eating disorders in athletes: A comprehensive narrative review with a focus on clinical assessment and management. *British Journal of Sports Medicine, 50*, 154–162.

Keyes, C. L. M. (2005). Mental illness and/or mental health? Investigating axioms of the complete state model of health. *Journal of Consulting & Clinical Psychology, 73*, 539–548.

Knights, S., Sherry, E., & Ruddock-Hudson, M. (2016). Investigating elite end-of-athletic-career transition: A systematic review. *Journal of Applied Sport Psychology, 28*, 291–308.

Lavallee, D. (2005). The effect of a life development intervention on sports career transition adjustment. *The Sport Psychologist, 19*, 193–202.

Lindert, J., Bain, P. A., Kubzansky, L. D., & Stein, C. (2015). Well-being measurement and the WHO health policy health 2010: Systematic review of measurement scales. *European Journal of Public Health, 25*, 731–740.

Linton, M.-J., Pieppe, P., & Medina-Lara, A. (2016). Review of 99 self-report measures for assessing wellbeing in adults: Exploring dimensions of well-being and developments over time. *BMJ Open, 6*, e010641. https://doi.org/10.1136/bmjopen-2015-01064.

Lonsdale, C., Hall, A., Murray, A., Williams, G. C., McDonough, S. M., Ntoumanis, N. (2017). Communication skills training for practitioners to increase patient adherence to home-based rehabilitation for chronic low back pain: Results of a cluster randomized controlled trial. *Archives of Physical Medicine and Rehabilitation, 98*, 1732–1743.

Lu, F. J. H., & Hsu, Y. (2013). Injured athletes' rehabilitation beliefs and subjective well-being: The contribution of hope and social support. *Journal of Athletic Training, 48*, 92–98.

Mack, D. E., Wilson, P. M., Oster, K. G., Kowalski, K. C., Crocker, P. R. E., & Sylvester, B. D. (2011). Well-being in volleyball players: Examining the contributions of independent and balanced psychological need satisfaction. *Psychology of Sport & Exercise, 12*, 533–539.

Mahoney, J. W., Gucciardi, D. F., Gordon, S., & Ntoumanis, N. (2017). Psychological needs support training for coaches: An avenue for nurturing mental toughness. In S. T. Cotterill, G. Breslin, & N. Weston (Eds.), *Sport and exercise psychology: Practitioner cases* (pp. 193–213). London: Wiley.

Marin-Urquiza, A., Ferreira, J. P., & Van Biesen, D. (2018). Athletic identity and self-esteem among active and retired Paralympic athletes. *European Journal of Sport Sciences, 18*, 861–871.

Martin, J. (2017). Persons with disabilities and quality of life: The role of physical activity. In Mitchell (Ed.), *Physical disabilities: Perspectives, risk factors and quality of life* (pp. 1–15). Hauppage: Nova Science Publishers.

Markser, V. Z. (2011). Sport psychiatry and psychotherapy. Mental strains and disorders in professional sports. Challenge and answer to societal changes. *European Archives of Psychiatry & Clinical Neuroscience, 261*, 182. https://doi.org/10.1007/s00406-011-0239-x.

McDougall, H., O'Halloran, P., Shields, N., & Sherry, E. (2015). Comparing the well-being of Para and Olympic sport athletes: A systematic review. *Adapted Physical Activity Quarterly, 32*, 256–276.

McDougall, H., O'Halloran, P., Shields, N., & Sherry, E. (2017). Putting the athlete first: A comprehensive assessment of elite Para-athlete well-being. *Journal of Well-Being Assessment, 1*, 35–47.

Michalos, A.C., Smale, B., Labonté, R., Muharjarine, N., Scott, K., Moore, K., Hyman, I. (2011). *The Canadian index of wellbeing.* Technical Report 1.0. Waterloo, ON.

Mihovilovic, M. (1968). The status of former sportsmen. International Review of Sport Psychology, 3, 73–93.

Moesch, K., Kentta, G., Kleinert, J., Quignon-Fleuret, C., Cecil, S., & Bertollo, M. (2018). FEPSAC position statement: Mental health disorders in elite athletes and models of service provision. *Psychology of Sport & Exercise, 38*, 61–71.

Mosewich, A. D., Crocker, P., E, R., Kowalski, K. C., & Delongis, A. (2013). Applying self-compassion in sport: An intervention with women athletes. *Journal of Sport & Exercise Psychology, 35*, 514–524.

Murray A., Hall A., Matthews, J., Williams G. C., McDonough S. M., Ntoumanis, N … Lonsdale C. (2018). Assessing clinicians' communication skills for promoting patient autonomy for self-management: Development and evaluation of the Communication Evaluation in Rehabilitation Tool. *Disability and Rehabilitation, 27*, 1–7.

NCAA. (2014). *Understanding life outcomes of former NCAA student-athletes.* The Gallup-Purdue Index Report. https://www.ncaa.org/about/resources/media-center/news/gallup-study-measures-long-term-life-outcomes-former-student-athletes. Accessed 10 July 2018

NCAA. (2018). *After the game: Former student athlete experience.* Accessed at: http://www.ncaa.org/student-athletes/former-student-student-athlete

Neff, K. (2003). Self-compassion: An alternative conceptualization of a healthy attitude toward oneself. *Self & Identity, 2*, 85–101.

Nolte, K., Steyn, B. J. M., Krüger, P. E., & Fletcher, L. (2016). Mindfulness, psychological well-being and doping in talented young high-school athletes. *South African Journal for Research in Sport, Physical Education & Recreation, 38*, 153–165.

Noon, M. R., Hames, R. S., Clarke, N. D., Akubat, I., & Thake, C. D. (2015). Perceptions of well-being and physical performance in English elite youth footballers across a season. *Journal of Sport Sciences, 33*, 2016–2115.

Patel, D. R., Yamasaki, A., & Brown, K. (2017). Epidemiology of sports-related musculoskeletal injuries in young athletes in United States. *Translational Pediatrics, 6*, 160–166.

Podlog, L., Lochbaum, M., & Stevens, T. (2010). Need satisfaction, well-being, and perceived return-to-sport outcomes among injured athletes. *Journal of Applied Sport Psychology, 22,* 167–182.

Pope, J. P., & Wilson, P. M. (2014). Testing a sequence of relationships from interpersonal coaching styles to rugby performance, guided by the coach–athlete motivation model. *International Journal of Sport and Exercise Psychology, 13,* 1–15.

Popper, K. (1963). *Conjectures and refutations: The growth of scientific knowledge.* London: Routledge.

Puce, L., Marinelli, L., Mori, L., Pallecchi, I., & Trompetto, C. (2017). Protocol for the study of self-perceived psychological and emotional well-being of young Paralympic athletes. *Health & Quality of Life Outcomes, 15,* 219. https://doi.org/10.1186/s12955-017-0798-2.

Reardon, C. L., & Factor, R. M. (2010). Sport psychiatry: A systematic review of diagnosis and medical treatment of mental illness in athletes. *Sports Medicine, 40,* 961–980.

Reinboth, M., & Duda, J. L. (2006). Perceived motivational climate, need satisfaction and indices of well-being in team sports: A longitudinal perspective. *Psychology of Sport & Exercise, 7,* 269–286.

Rice, S. M., Purcell, R., De Silva, S., Mawren, D., McGorry, P. D., & Parker, A. G. (2016). The mental health of elite athletes: A narrative systematic review. *Sports Medicine, 46,* 1333–1353.

Ryan, R. M., & Deci, E. L. (2001). On happiness and human potentials: A review of research on hedonic and eudaimonic well-being. *Annual Review of Psychology, 52,* 141–166.

Ryan, R. M., & Deci, E. L. (2017). *Self-determination theory: Basic psychological needs in motivation, development, and wellness.* New York: Guilford Publishing.

Ryan, R. M., & Frederick, C. M. (1997). On energy, personality and health: Subjective vitality as a dynamic reflection of well-being. *Journal of Personality, 65,* 529–565.

Ryff, C. D. (1989). Happiness is everything, or is it? Explorations on the meaning of psychological well-being. *Journal of Personality and Social Psychology, 57,* 1069–1081.

Sarkar, M., & Fletcher, D. (2013). How should we measure psychological resilience in sport performers? *Measurement in Physical Education & Exercise Science, 17,* 264–280.

Sarkar, M., & Fletcher, D. (2014). Psychological resilience in sport performers: A review of stressors and protective factors. *Journal of Sports Sciences, 32,* 1419–1434.

Sarkar, M., Fletcher, D., & Brown, D. J. (2015). What doesn't kill me…: Adversity-related experiences are vital in the development of superior Olympic performance. *Journal of Science and Medicine in Sport, 18,* 475–479.

Schaal, K., Tafflet, M., Nassif, H., Thibault, V., Pichard, C., Alcotte, M., Guillet, T., El Helou, N., Berthelot, G., Simon, S., & Toussaint, J.-F. (2011). Psychological balance in high level athletes: Gender-based differences and sport-specific patterns. *PLoS One, 6,* e19007. https://doi.org/10.1371/journal.pone.0019007.

Schalock, R. L., Borthwick-Duffy, S. A., Bradley, V. J., Buntinx, W. H. E., Coulter, D. L., Craig, E. M. (2011). *Intellectual disability: Definition, classification, and systems of supports* (11th ed.). Washington, DC: American Association on Intellectual and Developmental Disabilities.

Schuring, N., Kerkhoffs, G., Gray, J., & Goutbearge, V. (2017). The mental wellbeing of current and retired professional cricketers: An observational prospective cohort study. *Physician & Sportsmedicine, 45,* 463–469.

SCI Action Canada. (2018). *Spinal cord injury and physical activity.* http://sciactioncanada.ca/

Stambulova, N., Alfermann, D., Statler, T., & Côté, J. (2009). ISSP position stand: Career development and transitions of athletes. *International Journal of Sport and Exercise Psychology, 7,* 395–412.

Suldo, S. M., & Shaffer, E. J. (2008). Looking beyond psychopathology: The dual-factor model of mental health in youth. *School Psychology Review, 37,* 52–68.

Sutherland, L. M., Kowalski, K. C., Ferguson, L. J., Sabiston, C. M., Sedgwick, W. A., & Crocker, P. R. E. (2014). Narratives of young women athletes' experiences of emotional pain and self-compassion. *Qualitative Research in Sport, Exercise & Health, 6,* 499–516.

Tamminen, K., Holt, N., & Neely, K. (2013). Exploring adversity and the potential for growth among elite female athletes. *Psychology of Sport and Exercise, 14*, 28–36.

Thompson, R. W., Kaufman, K. A., De Petrillo, L. A., Glass, C. R., & Arnkoff, D. B. (2011). One year follow-up of mindful sport performance enhancement (MSPE) with archers, golfers, and runners. *Journal of Clinical Sport Psychology, 5*, 99–116.

Tint, A., Thomson, K., & Weiss, J. A. (2017). A systematic review of the physical and psychosocial correlates of Special Olympics participation among individuals with intellectual disability. *Journal of Intellectual Disabilities, 61*, 301–324.

Tonkin, B. L., Ogilvie, B. D., Greenwood, S. A., Law, M. C., & Anaby, D. R. (2014). The participation of children and youth with disabilities in activities outside of school: A scoping review. *Canadian Journal of Occupational Therapy, 81*, 226–236.

Udry, E., Gould, D., Bridges, D., & Beck, L. (1997). Down but not out: Athlete responses to season-endng injuries. *Journal of Sport & Exercise Psychology, 19*, 229–248.

UK Government. (2018). *Mental health and elite sport action plan.* Accessed at: https://www.gov.uk/government/publications/mental-health-and-elite-sport-actionplan

Vella, S. A., Cliff, D. P., Magee, C. A., & Okely, A. D. (2014). Sports participation and parent-reported health-related quality of life in children. Longitudinal associations. *Journal of Pediatrics, 164*, 1469–1474.

Watson, D., Clark, L. A., & Tellegen, A. (1988). Development and validation of brief measures of positive and negative affect: The PANAS scales. *Journal of Personality & Social Psychology, 54*, 1063–1070.

Weiss, J. A., Burnham Riosa, P., Robinson, S., Ryan, S., Tint, A., Viecili, M., MacMullin, J., & Shine, R. (2017). Understanding special olympics experiences from the athlete perspectives using photo-elicitation: A qualitative study. *Journal of Applied Research in Intellectual Disabilities, 30*, 936–945.

White, R. W. (1959). Motivation reconsidered: The concept of competence. *Psychological Review, 66*, 297–333.

Wilson, P. E. (2002). Exercise and sports for children who have disabilities. *Physical Medicine & Rehabilitation Clinics of North America, 13*, 907–923.

Wilson, P. M., Gregson, J. P., & Mack, D. E. (2010). *The importance of interpersonal style in competitive sport: A self-determination theory approach* (Sport psychology: Coping, performance, and anxiety) (pp. 259–276). Hauppauge: Nova Publishers.

World Health Organization. (2001). *The international classification of functioning. Disability and health.* Geneva: World Health Organization.

World Health Organization. (2004). *Promoting mental health: Concepts, emerging evidence, practice (summary report).* Geneva: World Health Organization.

World Health Organization. (2011). *World report on disability.* Retrieved from http://www.who.int/disabilities/world_report/2011/report/en/

Yazicioglu, K., Yavuz, F., Goktepe, A. S., & Tan, A. K. (2012). Influence of adapted sports on quality of life and life satisfaction in sport participants and non-sport participants with physical disabilities. *Disability & Health Journal, 5*, 249–253.

Zessin, U., Dickhäuser, O., & Garbade, S. (2015). The relationship between self-compassion and well-being: A meta-analysis. *Applied Psychology: Health & Well-Being, 7*, 340–364.

Diane E. Mack, PhD is a professor in the Department of Kinesiology at Brock University, Canada. Dr. Mack co-directs the Behaviour Health Sciences Research Lab with Dr. Philip M. Wilson. The research that fuels her curiosity is grounded in the promotion of well-being, particularly eudaimonic well-being, through physical activity. Best times are spent with two- (Phil) and four-legged family members that fuel her well-being in all its forms.

Philip M. Wilson, Phd is a professor in the Department of Kinesiology at Brock University, Canada. His research program is focused on addressing the following questions: (1) What motivates people to exercise? and (b) How could we measure psychological concepts integral to understanding exercise participation? In his spare time, Dr. Wilson can be found enjoying active living with Diane (and Portia) while finding time to follow his favourite teams (Liverpool F.C. and England) and spoiling a good walk by 'trying' (and failing) to play golf!

Caitlin Kelley joined the Behaviour Health Sciences Research Lab in pursuit of her MA in Applied Health Sciences at Brock University, Canada, under supervision of Dr. Mack. Prior to this, she attained an undergraduate in psychology at McGill University. She is primarily interested the relationship between physical activity in the natural outdoor environment and well-being. An avid hiker, Caitlin can typically be found planning her next trip to the backcountry. Off the trail, she pursues creative writing and dance.

Jennifer Mooradian, BA, BHSc, is a graduate of the midwifery education programme at McMaster University and retired registered midwife. She is currently pursuing her Master's degree in Community Health at Brock University, St. Catharines, Ontario, Canada. Her research interests include physical activity and persons with intellectual disability.

Chapter 15
Training Emerging Researchers in Constrained Contexts: Conducting Quality of Life Research with Children in South Africa

Sabirah Adams, Shazly Savahl, Maria Florence, Kyle Jackson, Donnay Manuel, Mulalo Mpilo, and Deborah Isobell

The extent of Quality of Life Research on Children in South Africa

The emergence of QoL research in South Africa can be traced back to the work of Lawrence Schlemmer and Valerie Møller in the early 1980s (Møller 2013a). Their work developed within the oppressive context of apartheid and challenged the status quo of governance at the time. Among the seminal studies on QoL conducted in South Africa during this period, the first focused on a comparative analysis of attitudes toward beach integration of 'Black' and 'White' individuals in Durban (Møller and Schlemmer 1982), and the second on developing an instrument to determine national QoL (Møller and Schlemmer 1983). The instrument included both subjective indicators ("Overall subjective satisfaction and happiness, Concern-specific satisfaction items, Mood and affect indicators") and objective indicators ("Assessments of gratification of basic needs and objective assessments of income, material possessions, savings capability, access to key goods and services, living conditions etc.") (Møller and Schlemmer 1989, p. 281). One of the key projects initiated by Schlemmer during this tumultuous period of inequality and disenfranchisement of the majority of the population was *Indicator South Africa* (see Møller 2013a). *Indicator South Africa* provided an exploration of both objective and

S. Adams
Language Development Group, Centre for Higher Education Development,
University of Cape Town, Cape Town, South Africa

S. Savahl (✉) · M. Florence · K. Jackson · D. Manuel · M. Mpilo · D. Isobell
Child and Family Studies Faculty of Community and Health Sciences,
University of the Western Cape, Cape Town, South Africa
e-mail: ssavahl@uwc.ac.za; mflorence@uwc.ac.za; 3165160@myuwc.ac.za;
3688375@myuwc.ac.za; 2636988@myuwc.ac.za

© Springer Nature Switzerland AG 2020
G. H. Tonon (ed.), *Teaching Quality of Life in Different Domains*, Social
Indicators Research Series 79, https://doi.org/10.1007/978-3-030-21551-4_15

subjective indicators of QoL (Møller 2013b). The seminal work of Møller and Schlemmer (see Møller and Schlemmer 1982, 1983; Møller 1997, 2013a; Møller and Roberts 2014) has contributed to shaping the state of QoL literature in South Africa with adults, and understanding the contextual realities influencing people's lives.

Another key contribution to the QoL literature by Møller (2013b) and Møller and Roberts (2014) was The South African Quality of Life Trends study (SAQoL) which assessed the subjective well-being (SWB) of South African adults across three decades (1980–2010); from apartheid to democracy. As Møller (2013b, p.915) notes, the findings indicated that:

> Subjective well-being peaked in the month following the first open elections in April 1994 when Black and White South Africans were equally satisfied and happy at levels found in other democratic societies. But post-election euphoria was short-lived and levels of well-being dropped the following year and racial inequalities in evaluations of life re-emerged. The tenth and latest wave in the study was conducted a few months after South Africa's successful hosting of the Soccer World Cup. In 2010, the proportions of all South Africans expressing satisfaction, happiness and optimism was among the highest since the coming of democracy – just over half stated they were satisfied, close on two-thirds were happy, and half felt life was getting better. Nonetheless, while the standard of living has increased for a minority of formerly disadvantaged South Africans and a small black middle class has emerged, there are still huge disparities in both material and subjective well-being. In 1997 and 2010, South Africans were asked what would make them happier in future. In 2010, the majority of citizens still hoped for basic necessities, income and employment, to enhance their quality of life.

While 25 years later the socio-political landscape in South Africa has changed substantially with the advent of democracy, the country still faces an array of challenges infringing on individuals' QoL. These range from having one of the highest levels of (income and social) inequality in the world, to having among the highest rates of crime and violence, particularly among vulnerable groups such as children and women (see Savahl et al. 2015c). Over the last two decades, the importance of understanding children's QoL has become a key point on the governmental agenda. This point has been reinforced with significant legislation enacted in South Africa, protecting and advancing the rights of children (such as Section 28 of the Bill of Rights, the South African Constitution; the Children's Act [No. 38 of 2005], the Children's Amendment Act [No. 41 of 2007], and the Child Justice Act [2008]), and the ratification of the United Nations Convention on the Rights of the Child (UNCRC) in 1995. Furthermore, through the Social Security Agency Act of 2004, the government has ensured that children are the beneficiaries of social grants to mitigate against vulnerability and poverty. Acceding to these legal contracts has entrenched the rights and needs of children in the development strategies of the government, as well as guaranteeing children's socio-economic rights and protection from abuse, exploitation, and neglect. Co-ordinated by the Office on the Rights of the Child (ORC), the National Programme of Action (NPAC) was put in place to provide "an holistic framework for the integration of all policies and plans developed by government departments and civil society to promote the well-being of children" (https://www.gov.za/documents/national-programme-action-children-framework). With children now being elevated to the legal status of rights holders, with the government ultimately accountable as the principal duty bearer, children's well-being and QoL is ostensibly afforded the highest priority within government.

Over the past two decades, the South African government has also made significant progress in developing strategies to measure the state and well-being of its children. These initiatives highlighted the development and collection of objective indicators, that refer to observable measures that assess a range of pre-determined objective standards of living. Research on children's QoL is generally accessible and made possible via administrative data such as general household surveys and census data; and a range of population-based surveys such as the National Income Dynamics Survey, National Demographic and Health Survey, Trends in International Mathematics and Science Study, and the Progressive International Reading Literacy Study. The data from these studies provide a comprehensive set of QoL indicators across a range of dimensions of well-being. Annual reports, such as the South African Child Gauge published by the Children's Institute (www.ci.uct.ac.za) provides aggregated data on a range of different themes related to children using these administrative datasets. Other national population-based surveys conducted by independent research institutes have also contributed to QoL data on children. These include the Optimus Study on Sexual Violence against Children (www.optimus-study.org), The National School Violence Study (Burton and Leoschut 2013) and the Birth to Twenty Plus (bt20+) cohort Study (Richter et al. 2018).

Several participatory research studies have been conducted in South Africa within the past decade that foreground the subjective voices and perspectives of children on the key aspects of their lives. Research by Savahl and colleagues (Adams and Savahl 2015, 2017a, 2018; Benninger and Savahl 2016; Savahl 2010; Savahl et al. 2015a, b, c; September and Savahl 2009) has explored children's perspectives of their well-being and QoL across various contexts in South Africa, and has contributed to the literature on children's understandings from the developing South. These studies engaged children in research using a child participation framework and focused on understanding children's subjective perceptions of their well-being. Acknowledging the epistemological standpoint that children are knowledgeable experts on matters affecting their lives, Benninger and Savahl (2016) put forward the Children's Delphi, a technique developed to engage children in the research process on aspects affecting their well-being. Through the use of photovoice, community mapping, focus group interviews, the Children's Delphi and children participating as co-researchers and co-constructors of knowledge in these studies, it ultimately advances their right to participation and to be heard on the matters that affect them.

However, after 25 years of democracy and despite the legislative advancements, the QoL of South Africa's children remains compromised (Savahl et al. 2015c). This is reflective of the high levels of social inequality in South Africa, which is regarded as an important indicator of children's well-being. Notwithstanding the fundamental premise of equality in the South African Constitution, inequality remains pervasive in the country. With a Gini Index of 0.69 (World Bank 2018), considered to be one of the highest in the world (in terms of wealth and income), it demonstrates a great discrepancy of both wealth and income between the privileged and the disadvantaged. Although this inequality is experienced by the majority of the population, the burdens of these multiple overlapping layers of inequality are often endured by children who necessitate care and supervision from adults for both safety and basic tenets of their well-being (Hall et al. 2012).

The South African Context

South Africa is a constitutional democracy inhabited by approximately 57.73 million people (Statistics South Africa 2018), including a diversity of ethnic and cultural groups. Its diversity is reflected in the constitution, whereby 11 official languages are recognised. The diverse languages are further evinced by the different 'racial groups'[1] in the country, namely 'Black African' (80.9%), 'Coloured' (8.8%), 'Indian/Asian' (2.5%), and 'White' (7.8%). During Apartheid, the different population groups were segregated according to racial categories to reinforce a segregated society. Based on a philosophy of segregation and exclusion, the apartheid legislative framework characterised the socio-political landscape of South Africa for nearly five decades. It was characterised by systematic oppression and domination of one group over another. These policies resulted in a significant proportion of the population being disenfranchised, denied access to resources, land, education opportunities and basic human rights, while promoting the affluence and privilege of a favoured minority. The current extreme levels of social inequality experienced by the majority of the population are among the most devastating legacies of apartheid.

Despite South Africa's notable constitutional advancement, inequality is widespread, reflected in the Human Development Index (HDI) of 0.69 and ranked 113 of 189 countries (United Nations Development Programme, 2018). In the country, disadvantaged communities are characterised by low educational attainment and income, high rates of substance use, unemployment, crime, and violence (Savahl, Adams et al. 2015), and a lack of access to resources. These burdens are often endured by children who are dependent on adults for safety and care (Hall et al. 2012). In terms of health, the under-five mortality rate is reported at 42.4, an infant mortality rate of 32.8, and a neonate mortality rate of 12.4, per 1000 respectively (Statistics South Africa 2017). Regarding nutritional health, 29% of children in

---

[1] The racial groups, that is 'Coloured', 'Black African', and 'Indian/Asian', were employed as racial categories within the Apartheid era to reinforce a segregated society, and refer to those who were not afforded the same benefits as 'Whites' in this era. These terms are used here solely for descriptive purposes, and does not imply acknowledgement of these terms by the authors.

South Africa are reported to be living below the food poverty line, 13% of households have reported child hunger, and 77% of children aged six to 23 months being fed inadequate diets (Jamieson et al. 2017a). Additionally, when considering housing, 12% of children live in informal housing, and 59% live in overcrowded conditions (Jamieson et al. 2017a).

Furthermore, violence against children is a ubiquitous problem in South Africa, with many children having witnessed and experienced some form of violence (Matthews and Benvenuti 2014). Specifically, cases reported to the South African Police Services SAPS between January and March 2017, demonstrate that children experienced various forms of violence such as rape (4028 cases), sexual assault (704 cases), grievous bodily harm (2248 cases), common assaults (2742 cases), attempted murder (40 cases), and child homicide (196 cases) (South African Police Services [SAPS 2017]). It should be noted that the SAPS statistics report the number of reported cases only, which means that many more may go unreported. And therefore are not reflected in these statistics. Violence against children under the age of five includes abandonment at birth, blunt force injuries, and strangulation/asphyxiation deaths (Mathews and Martin 2016). Corporal punishment, cruel and humiliating forms of psychological punishment, sexual and gender-based violence, and bullying have also been identified as forms of violence children experience. Furthermore, while violence transcends boundaries of class and socio-economic status (SES), children in impoverished communities experience higher levels of violence as they are exposed to violence on a daily basis. Research shows that children who experience first-hand violence may develop an array of psychological and health consequences including post-traumatic stress disorder, depression, and anxiety (Jamieson et al. 2017b).

In terms of education, children from higher SES backgrounds are more likely to complete secondary school, while those from disadvantaged backgrounds are three times less likely to do so (Statistics South Africa 2017). South Africa's language in education policy states that mother-tongue instruction is advanced for grades 1 to 3, with a switch to English or Afrikaans in grade four. Given the 11 official languages in the country, this poses particular challenges (Department of Basic Education 2016). However, many children struggle with this transition as they are not fluent in English, which influences their academic performance. According to the Progress in International Reading Literacy Study (Howie et al. 2017), grade five learners in South Africa had the lowest scores in comparison to grade four learners in the 39 participating countries. The inherited inequities in the education system further reflects disparities in the quality of education offered by schools, and the opportunities offered to children in low SES communities (Hall et al. 2012). Although the government has aimed to provide opportunities for those from disadvantaged, contexts, many schools lack necessary resources such as qualified teachers, textbooks, stationery, educational aids, and office equipment, hindering children as recipients of quality education.

Key Considerations for Training Emerging QoL Researchers

Preparing and training young and emerging researchers for conducting QoL research with children and adolescents requires a focused investment in student training and development. This development extends beyond academic training and includes conscientising students around the contextual and socio-historical realities influencing children's lives. The context of South Africa, characterised by high levels of social inequality, poverty, and crime, creates a unique and challenging environment. This is intensified by the diversity of cultures and language groups. In this section we put forward a potential syllabus that could be followed to capacitate emerging researchers.

Given the focus of the chapter on training emerging researchers on children's SWB and QoL within the South African context, a proposed syllabus would encompass the following key content areas, discussed below:

1. Contextualising children and childhood in South Africa
2. Children's QoL and inequalities
3. Theories of children's SWB
4. Methodological considerations
5. Children's rights and SWB

The following section is not an exhaustive syllabus of key readings and theories for teaching QoL and SWB, but is intended as an initial reading about the field.

Contextualising Children and Childhood in South Africa

In training emerging researchers on QoL and SWB it is foremost critical that they have a comprehensive understanding of the contextual realities of children and adolescents in South Africa. Here, the status and diversity of children's lives and childhoods is significant. Essentially, by contextualising the realities of children in South Africa it would enhance the understanding of a situated overview of SWB and QoL. One of the key aspects which should be addressed is the way SES shapes the lives of children in South Africa. A number of studies exploring children's SWB in South Africa (see Adams and Savahl 2015; Adams et al. 2017a; Savahl et al. 2015c; Savahl et al. 2017) have found SES to be a determining factor in children's subjective perceptions of their lives. Given the history of apartheid and oppression within South Africa, emerging researchers should be aware and informed of the deleterious, lingering effects on children in the country. It should be highlighted that the historical, social, and political consequences of this still encumbers the majority of the population of 57.73 million people (Statistics South Africa 2018), of which over 18 million are children. While the focus is on SWB and QoL, which are essentially subjective evaluations, the importance of being knowledgeable about the most recent context-specific objective indicators of well-being is necessary. The high levels of inequality and exclusion in the country should be emphasised, such as the Gini coefficient and the HDI. In addition to the pervasive inequality in the country, it is requisite to foreground the excessively high levels of violence against children, as well as the aetiology of violence. These high levels of violence are most likely to be perpetrated by an adult familiar to the child. While the country has progressive legislation to protect children against violence, the monitoring and implementation thereof is less than superlative. Further, although there have been renewed efforts to protect children, rates of violence against children continue to increase. Of great concern is the child homicide rate in the country, double the global average, with most victims younger than 5 years old (see Mathews and Benvenuti 2014). The key take-home message regarding violence should be that these statistics are not just numbers, but rather that each number contributing to the proportion represents an individual child whose rights and dignity have been violated. The corollary of the various forms of violence and abuse that many children experience may be damaging, particularly given the lack of access to appropriate psychological and health services within communities. Among the key statistics which should be presented are the under-five mortality rate, and the infant and neonatal mortality rates (see Statistics South Africa 2017). Further, the rates of stunting should be indicated (Jamieson et al. 2017a). Finally, the fact that 62% of children in the country live below the upper bound of the poverty line, while 13% live in extreme poverty should further be indicated to demonstrate the daily challenges children face. Other key objective indicators that demonstrate the widespread lack of access to education, access to healthcare, civic participation, and the various forms of increased levels of bullying (see Savahl et al. 2018) should be explicated. Against this contextual backdrop, emerging researchers will begin to be cognisant of the varying aspects and factors affecting children's lives. However, it should be accentuated that while the objective indicators provide useful information for understanding the influences on children's lives, they only provide a partial viewpoint. It is important to highlight the intergenerational transmission and cycle of poverty, evident in among half of the population receiving social grants, a substantial proportion are children. Thus, asking children directly about what the key aspects are that influence their well-being is essential, ideally with population-based samples.

Children's QOL and Inequalities

When considering objective standards of children's QoL in South Africa in training emerging researchers, it is incumbent to acknowledge the historical 'situatedness' of childhood which has resulted in a plurality of childhood experiences. This 'plurality' is best understood if the objective indicators are examined from the position of social inequality whereby unequal social backgrounds in general have reinforced unequal conditions (Dawes et al. 2007). Regardless of the fundamental premise of the South African Constitution, high levels of social inequality remain prevalent, with a great discrepancy in wealth and income between the privileged and the disadvantaged communities (Savahl et al. 2015c). Further, access to basic resources such as water and sanitation, electricity, formal housing, food and nutrition and health care are also limited. The direct impact of this on children's development trajectories should be noted. As Diener and Scollon (2014 p.4) indicate:

> When are people happy, and when are they unhappy? One answer, of course, is that people tend to be happy when good things happen to them and unhappy when bad things happen to them. But it turns out that this answer is overly simple. For one thing, people tend to adapt to events and circumstances, so that they become accustomed to good and bad things, and these circumstances thereafter exert a lot less influence on their SWB. For this reason, the predictors of long-term SWB are not always the same as the factors that make a person's moods swing up and down over the course of a day or a week.

Once the tensions around the theoretical traditions and considerations of QoL are explored, along with definitions of QoL and SWB and contextual aspects in children's SWB in South Africa, the topic of indicators and domains of SWB should be explicated. UNICEF's Report Card 7 and systematic reviews by Cummins (1996) and Pollard and Lee (2003) should be used as a basis for discussing the key indicators of children's QoL and well-being. Firstly, UNICEF's Report Card 7 proposed six main dimensions, that is: material well-being, health and safety; education; peer and family relationships; behaviours and risks; and young people's own subjective perceptions of their well-being (UNICEF Office of Research 2007). While it is apparent that these dimensions of well-being span across a range of aspects concerning child development, there is no clear differentiation between the subdimensions of underlying well-being, and no temporal developmental distinctions. Therefore, indices relating to different 'stages' of childhood are grouped together devoid of consideration given to the timing of measurements and the importance of the prenatal period and the first few years of a child's life (Conti and Heckman 2012). Secondly, the reviews by Cummins (1996) and Pollard and Lee (2003) identified seven categories: economic and material well-being; health; safety; productive activity; place in community; intimacy; and emotional well-being. Research from the South African context (September and Savahl 2009) identified five domains of SWB: protection and safety; basic needs and material resources; psycho-social well-being; social relationships; community resources and infrastructure.

Research on SWB has also shown that akin to results with adults, children have a propensity toward an 'optimism bias' (Casas 2011; Gilman and Huebner 2003; Savahl et al. 2015a), whereby they assess their lives positively; and is particularly manifest between the ages of 12 and 13 years (Casas et al. 2012). In terms of the trend of an 'optimism bias' in children's SWB, Casas (2016, p.12) argues that "When the tendency to give positive answers becomes "constant" for many participants, as is the case with many items in children's samples, we face a serious methodological problem: extreme answers distort the mean and decrease the variance, raising problems for statistical calculations and interpretations." While some recommend deleting these cases from the dataset (International Wellbeing Group 2006), Casas (2016) indicates that an alternative is to deem these extreme positive scores as valid. He therefore suggests that "Children giving extreme positive answers to all satisfaction items have been deleted and those only giving extreme positive answers on psychometric scales have not, because they are considered reliable enough" (Casas 2016, p. 12).

Theories of Children's SWB

There are numerous theories of SWB which have been put forward, within the hedonic and eudaimonic traditions. While there are limited child-specific theories on SWB the following theories are significant: the Structural Model of Child Well-being (Minkkinen 2013); Factors contributing to child well-being: A conceptual framework to situate place in context (McKendrick 2014); the Two Source Theory of Child Well-Being (Raghavan and Alexandrova 2015), the Capability Approach (CA) (Fegter and Richter 2014), and Child Standpoint Theory (Fattore et al. 2017). Several hedonic theories include: the Adaptation Level Theory of Well-being (Brickman and Campbell 1971), Diener et al.'s (2006) Revision to the original Treadmill Theory, Cummins' Homeostasis Theory of Subjective Well-being (1995, 2003, 2010, 2014), and the 3P Model (Durayappah 2011). Eudaimonic theories include Self-determination Theory (Deci and Ryan 1985, 2008a, b), and recently Flourishing Theory (Seligman 2011). Emerging researchers should be well-versed in theories on children's SWB as this serves a twofold significance of enabling them to understand, and apply the theory to research conceptualisation and findings.

Although the field was developed on the perspectives of adult populations, the focus on the significance of children's SWB was advocated with early efforts to elevate the status of children's self-reported well-being. A key role-player in the paradigm shift from a focus on pathogenesis to salutogenesis was the World Health Organisation (1946) with their definition of health which emphasised not only the absence of ill-health but also the physical, mental, and social components related to an individual's health. The influence of this shift was evident across numerous disciplines, which resulted in a changing focus of research and theory. Additionally, the ratification of the UNCRC (1989) and the 'sociology of childhood' (James and Prout 1990) provided further momentum in promoting the rights of children. Considerations of children's lives across an array of domains were no longer sought from adults (such as parents, teachers or guardians) as proxies for children, but rather research was being conducted with children as social actors and no longer as subjects (Ben-Arieh 2009, 2010).

The Structural Model of Child Well-being (SMCW) (Minkkinen 2013) and the Two Source Theory (Raghavan and Alexandrova 2015) are recent child well-being theories. The SMCW (Minkkinen 2013) argues that children are influenced by their own culture, and contribute to and replicate culture, referred to as interpretive reproduction (see Corsaro 1992). The CA has been developed over the past two decades by Sen (1985, 1993, 2005, 2007) and Nussbaum (1988, 2000), and focuses on participation, human well-being, and freedom as core components of development; merging ethics and economics (Comim et al. 2011). The emphasis of the CA is on the QoL that individuals are capable of achieving. The key closely-related concepts which the framework proposes are functionings, capabilities, freedom, and agency (Dang 2014). Handbooks and edited book series such as Children and the good life: New challenges for research on children (2010, edited by Sabine Andresen et al.), Children and the Capability Approach (2011, edited by Mario Biggeri et al.), Handbook of Child Well-Being: Theories, methods and policies in global perspective (2014; edited by Asher Ben-Arieh et al.) and Children's rights and the Capability Approach: Challenges and prospects (2014, edited by Daniel Stoecklin and Jean-Michel Bovin) evince this growing focus on children's capabilities. Biggeri et al. (2011) argue that children's development cannot be synonymous with reducing poverty and impoverishment as well-being cannot solely consider material components of well-being. More recently, building on seminal qualitative research methods and theoretical considerations (see Fattore et al. 2007), Fattore et al. (2017) put forward Child Standpoint Theory wherein childhood is conceptualised as a structural phenomenon, which needs to be understood within the complexities of adult-child relations.

Cummins' Homeostasis Theory of SWB (1995, 2003, 2010, 2014) builds on the Adaptation Level Theory, in its notion of maintaining a 'normal' sense of well-being. Cummins (2014) indicated that the theory should be used with children from 12-years old as they possess the cognitive maturity for self-report. He posits further that data obtained when assessing children's well-being in the specified age cohort, when understood within SWB homeostasis, can illuminate the difficulties and supports they experience during this period in their lives. This can be used as a basis from which to tailor interventions for children. McKendrick's (2014) conceptual model, Factors contributing to child well-being: A conceptual framework to situate place in context, shows how children's neighbourhoods play a pertinent role in their well-being. Key considerations include adequate resources, equal opportunities for all children, and children's active participation, and more broadly family aspects (SES, parenting, and dynamics of family life); advancing the 'geographies of well-being for children', and ultimately 'good places' which enhance children's QoL. Given the high levels of inequality and violence in South Africa and its influence on children's lives, this framework is important to consider. Similar to the Adaptation Level and Homeostasis Theories, the 3P Model (Durayappah 2011) shows that current life events influence happiness, however, the extent of this is escalated in the 3P Model which affirms that the memories of our experiences govern our feelings of SWB in temporal states (present, the past, and the prospect). In summary, it is crucial for emerging researchers to note the contention by Savahl et al. (2019, p.17) that "While some theories have been applied and specifically developed for children, there is the necessity to test the applicability of these theories with children in diverse contexts, with more research required in developing countries, and further cross-national comparison studies. Contextually relevant theoretical frameworks, should however, go beyond a consideration of space and an acknowledgement of diversity, to include a cautionary consideration to not reproduce western narratives of childhood and well-being (Fattore et al. 2018)." A final point to note is the shift toward a comprehensive understanding of QoL that includes both eduaimonic and hedonic components, conceptualised under the broad heading of flourishing (see Seligman 2011). It is recommended that emerging researchers be encouraged to actively with these theoretical advancements.

Methodological Considerations

As Savahl et al. (2019) note, among the key considerations in children's SWB in terms of method is the delineation of population-based survey research using random samples, as well as authentic participatory research. In South Africa there are overarching considerations that researchers should be acutely aware of given the diverse context. Among the key considerations are language and dialect, cultural understandings, adaptations of research instruments, and geographical location. Appended to this, within impoverished communities in South Africa are aspects such as illiteracy, children with undiagnosed learning disorders given a lack of access to healthcare (often due to Fetal Alcohol Spectrum Disorders), and teachers who do not have the required qualifications. Moreover, the state of the education system in the country has a direct influence on children's ability to achieve.

Given the complexity of the construct of SWB and QoL, measuring SWB has received a substantial focus in research with children. It is important to discuss the dichotomy identified by Fattore et al. (2012) in relation to two approaches to researching SWB and subjective QoL, of which the distinction lies in their epistemological frameworks. The first is premised on objectivist notions and is used more widely and aligns to the employment of standardised quantitative data collection methods, using Diener's (1984, 2000) definition of SWB. The second approach is founded on the 'sociology of childhood' which foregrounds the "acknowledgement of children as valid informants and participants in the research process, and the subsequent shift towards soliciting their knowledge, opinions, attitudes and perceptions on matters that affect them." (Savahl et al. 2015c, p. 750). It should be noted that Fattore et al. (2012) caution against using the objectivist approach without critical reflection; and assert that despite the distinction in these approaches, both are consistent in children's active participation. In training emerging researchers on measuring children's SWB, the use of the two methodological frameworks aligned to the two approaches noted above should be underscored. In terms of developing and conceptualising a quantitative study on children's SWB and QoL, the use of randomly selected population-based samples is ideal, particularly to create normed data.

Within South Africa, the participation in the Children's Worlds study which explores children's subjective perceptions of their well-being across various domains and three waves of study, is a good example. The project is the largest international study on children's well-being, with Wave I including over 34,500 children from 14 countries, Wave II including over 56,000 children from 15 countries, and Wave III currently underway, including over 100,000 children from 43 countries. The study aims to collect information about children's perceptions and evaluations of their SWB, time use, and daily activities, across three age cohorts (8, 10, and 12 years) (see www.isciweb.org). South Africa's contribution to the study for Wave III is a sample of approximately 7400 based on a proportionate nationally representative stratified random sample of children from all nine provinces. In this regard Diener and Scollon (2014, p.3) note that: "*Another reason for students to study SWB is that national accounts of SWB are on the horizon. Diener (2000) proposed that nations track SWB to help shed light on various policy debates, much as they track economic indicators such as employment rate and gross domestic product (GDP).*" It is also important to highlight to students the significance of working with 'population level data'. Rees and Main (2015) further emphasise the importance of the use of weighted data which enables the consideration of systematic errors in the dataset. In weighting variables, the potential bias in age, gender, and region dispersions within the sample can be corrected. Explicit guidelines on the method of weighting and calculations employed should be outlined for those who will be working with the dataset. In terms of data analysis for large-scale quantitative studies, the use of basic and advanced statistical techniques is necessary. Data modelling is often used to this end, such as confirmatory factor analysis and structural equation modelling. It is therefore necessary for senior researchers to be appropriately skilled to be able to train and capacitate students in using advanced data modelling which has the advantage of further providing them with unique skills and experience.

Drawing on the work of Savahl et al. (2019), and aligned to the 'sociology of childhood' is training students in the development and conceptualisation of qualitative methodological studies, using participatory methods such as: the Children's mosaic approach (Clark and Moss 2012), photovoice (Wang and Burris 1994, 1997), community mapping (Amsden and VanWynsberghe 2005), and the Children's Delphi (Benninger and Savahl 2017b), discussed in the following section. A significant project to present to emerging researchers in this regard is the Multinational Study on Children's Understandings of Well-Being – Global and Local contexts (CUWB) which uses "an ethnographic component documenting the fieldwork setting, and completion of two fieldwork stages each with core and optional modules" (Fattore et al. 2018, p.14). The aim of the study is to understand children's perceptions of their well-being and daily lives, ages 11–14 years, using a qualitative perspective. The study currently includes 27 countries from across the world and uses a participatory approach, with children as agents and co-constructors of knowledge. The CUWB study employs the use of interviews, community mapping, photovoice, and digital storytelling (short films) with participants involved in creating, editing, and finalising the short films reporting on their perspectives of their lives and well-being. The study uses a modular approach: the first is centred on the thematic analysis of interviews conducted providing a basis for synthesising themes and posing subsequent questions to be explored; the second explicates children's subjective perceptions and experiences on domains of well-being; and the third includes the development of short films that highlight the key aspects of their lifeworlds to share with children in other parts of the world (see Savahl et al. 2019).

Participatory Techniques: Children's Mosaic Approach, Photovoice, Community Mapping, and the Children's Delphi

Advancing the key premise of the 'sociology of childhood' of children as co-constructors of knowledge, the *Children's Mosaic Approach* is noteworthy. The Children's Mosaic Approach (Clark and Moss 2012) encompasses various participatory data collection techniques such as focus group interviews, community mapping, photovoice, and walking interviews. Each participatory technique employed forms part of the mosaic. Espousing a framework of 'listening', the central characteristic of the approach is a multi-method participatory approach that is reflexive, adaptable, and is embedded into practice (Clark 2005). The CUWB has incorporated a version of the Children's Mosaic Approach (Clark 2005), which is evident in the work of Savahl and colleagues exploring children's well-being in South Africa (Adams and Savahl, 2017a, b; Adams et al. 2017; Benninger and Savahl 2017a). A study by Benninger and Savahl (2016) sought to explore children's constructions of the self across two urban communities in Cape Town, South Africa, using photovoice and community mapping. Similarly, a study by Malone (2016) explored children's encounters with place in La Paz, Bolivia, using the photovoice method. Additionally, a study by Adams et al. (2017) used the photovoice and community mapping methodology to explore children's representations and perceptions of natural spaces. A key finding of the study was the influence of SES on children's understandings of well-being and concerns around safety.

The second participatory technique which should be explored with students is photovoice (Wang and Burris 1994, 1997). Through this participatory research method, children are considered as collaborators who possess agency, and are given a platform to present photo journeys of neighbourhood experiences. It is evident from the literature that photovoice as a participatory method has been increasingly employed with children across diverse contexts (see Adams et al. 2017; Benninger and Savahl, 2016; Kopnina 2011; Malone 2016; Sancar and Severcan 2010; Strack et al. 2004; Zuch et al. 2013).

Community mapping is the third technique that could be used in a participatory study. It is a visual data collection technique that affords unique representations of children's worlds. Amsden and VanWynsberghe (2005) note that community mapping may be utilised to document significant spaces and places, and abstract data elicit rich narratives in the accompanying discussions. Community mapping is premised on the validation of the participants experiences (Amsden and VanWynsberghe 2005). Additionally, given the participatory nature of this technique, it is considered to address the issue of power dynamics and inequities present in the researcher-participant relationship. The use of community mapping is explicated in two participatory studies in the South African context with children exploring their perceptions of the 'self' and well-being (Benninger and Savahl 2017a) and of natural spaces and their SWB (Adams and Savahl, 2017a; Adams et al. 2017). This data collection technique is often complemented by photovoice and focus group interviews in research studies.

Finally, a recently developed novel technique is the Children's Delphi (Benninger and Savahl 2016) which places the child participants as experts in the Delphi process. Benninger and Savahl (2017b) developed the Children's Delphi technique and used it in a study that aimed to explore children's perceptions of the nature and content of intervention programmes aimed at improving children's self-concept within two impoverished communities of the Western Cape, South Africa. The Children's Delphi technique was conducted with a group of ten children between the ages of 10 and 12 years. The child experts' participation in the Delphi process allowed them to represent a population (children in poverty) who are often excluded from decision-making processes. The final Delphi outcome was an agreed upon list of suggestions for intervention programmes which aimed to support the self-concept of children. This included a focus on safety, the provision of social support, the creation of opportunities for learning and play, and the provision of basic material needs. It is recommended that research investigating issues related to children's well-being consider including the Children's Delphi into the compendium of methods of data collection with children and young people. It is a research method aligned to the UNCRC and the 'sociology of childhood', which encourages researchers to listen to children's viewpoints and to view children as experts in their own lives (Langhout and Thomas 2010). It advances the notion that children are the authentic knowers and authoritative experts of their lives and offers a structured framework for the meaningful inclusion of children's views in research.

Alongside the goal of providing emerging researchers with comprehensive knowledge and understanding of these participatory techniques, training in data collection and preparation for fieldwork is vital. This should include discussions around language and levels of literacy among the child population with whom research will be conducted; familiarisation with the data collection instrument; and most importantly, building rapport with child participants. Savahl et al. (2019, p.11) thus state that:

> Considering the fledging nature of research into children's SWB (Bradshaw 2015), it is axiomatic that a greater investment in empirical research is required. Calls for large-scale population-based surveys are apposite and would allow much needed standardised data. However, the challenges related to cross-cultural measurement is heightened in the multicultural context of South Africa. Epistemological advancements and legislation foregrounding the children's participation has fostered a greater interest in developing participatory methodologies.
>
> Not with standing the differential and significant contribution of each methodological approach to QoL research, it is recommended that researchers consider using mixed-methods or multiple methods research designs. This would advance a more comprehensive understanding of QoL in diverse contexts and with diverse populations.

Children's Rights and SWB

Aligning to the Social Indicators and Child Indicators movement, the field of children's SWB espouses children's rights to participation by enabling children's voices to be heard (see Hart 1984, 1994). In capacitating emerging researchers about children's rights and QoL, it is essential to include a discussion of seminal child rights legislation applicable to the South African context, as well as research ethics. An important consideration is noted by Casas (2016, p. 10) in the following:

> In addressing child well-being and quality of life, we must not forget that by definition, quality of life includes the perceptions, evaluations, and aspirations of everyone involved, and those of children and adolescents are therefore essential. In other words, we must not confuse child well-being with adult opinions of child well-being. Both are important, but they are not the same, and both are a part of the complex social reality we call child well-being. Therefore, we face the challenge of filling the large information gap concerning the younger population's point of view of the social reality that affects humanity.

The first legislation that students should be familiarised with is the UNCRC adopted by the UN General Assembly in 1989, and considered the most comprehensive international treaty which foregrounds the human rights of children (those younger than 18-years of age). The UNCRC advances children's rights in all aspects of their lives (54 articles), and holds States Parties liable to ensure that all children have the opportunity to be heard in matters that affect their lives (such as economic, social, and cultural rights). Among the guiding principles of the UNCRC are: Non-discrimination; adherence to the best interests of the child; the right to life, survival, and development; and the right to participate. The monitoring of the UNCRC is assessed by the UN Committee on the Rights of the Child. As of January 2019, the UNCRC has 197 country signatories bound to it by international law – excluding the United States of America. Governments are then bound in international law to put children first and develop legislation and policies to ensure that the rights enshrined in the convention are actioned. In South Africa, the UNCRC was ratified in 1995, with the government acceding to undertake the obligations of the Convention by committing to protect and guarantee the rights of every child. In addition to ratifying the UNCRC, South Africa enacted a range of legislations reflecting the commitment to children's rights, evident in the Bill of Rights in the Constitution, the Children's Act of 2005 and the Child Justice Act of 2010. It is noted that a key endeavour toward "genuine realization of the Convention's goals is the education and training of people who work with children…" (Hammaberg 1995, p. viii).

Considering current global advocacy for children's rights, particularly in countries that have adopted the UNCRC (United Nations General Assembly, 1989), there is a growing consensus among scholars engaging in research with children that societies' responsibility to advocate and guard children's rights to survival, protection, and development warrants special precedence in developmental initiatives and human rights work (Ben-Arieh 2008; Lloyd and Emerson 2017; Chawla 2007; Green 2015; Himes 1993; Savahl et al. 2015c). For this reason, Hart (1992) has emphasised the need for children to be part of meaningful projects with adults, as it is "unrealistic to expect them to all of a sudden become mature, participating adult citizens at the age of 16, 18, or 21 devoid of previous exposure to the skills and responsibilities involved" (p. 5). Weinstein and Ryan (2010) assert further that when children feel competent, autonomous, and socially accepted, they are more inclined to develop self-regulation skills and to be motivated intrinsically, as opposed to extrinsically, toward positive behaviour. Accordingly, this is likely to bring about feelings of well-being and satisfaction in children. Consideration of these goals is especially relevant in the current context where although children's rights are advocated, they still face pervasive threats to safety in their communities. In particular, in terms of threats, many children in this context identified their lack of mobility and ability to explore their environments and to play with friends, which hindered their basic need for autonomy (Ryan and Deci 2000), and right to participation. Thomson and Philo (2004) highlight that the literature points to how children inhabit a local geography which is exceedingly discerned regarding 'permissions and sanctions', resulting in children being acutely aware of their 'spatial ranges' and 'territorial limits' – particularly when engaging in places which are outside the bounds of home. With their research similarly conducted across three diverse communities, affording perspectives on the influence of social class on the 'social geographies of children's play', Thomson and Philo (2004) distinguish between 'disordered spaces' and 'idle spaces' wherein play is made sense of more as a 'state of being' than an activity.

The threats against children in their communities and the disparate levels of mobility and well-being owing to this, at a broader level concerns the issue of children's rights. With South Africa as a signatory, and having ratified the UNCRC, the endeavour is to better all children's lives, and not in terms of a hierarchy of SES. Appended to this, is the reality of South Africa having one of the highest levels of inequality in the world (Bosch et al. 2010). While children's rights has been a pertinent issue on the agenda at a national level, with several legislations implemented to counter the violence and abuse against children (see Savahl et al. 2015c; September and Dinbabo 2008; September and Savahl 2009), there is still widespread violence against children. The South African government has thus given precedence to children's well-being as a key development goal (September and Dinbabo 2008). As Savahl et al. (2015c) indicate, these progressions in legislation should translate into children being protected from abuse and exploitation, and advancing children's socio-economic rights, yet this is far from being met, and is evident in the increasing levels of crimes against children each year.

Montserrat and Casas 2006; see also Dinisman et al. 2012; Montserrat et al. 2015; Navarro et al. 2015) point to the significance of including children from marginalised groups and those enduring social disadvantage (such as children in care), in research, as they offer unique perspectives on their well-being. While children are afforded rights and privileges in law and policies in South Africa, they still constitute a vulnerable population. When conducting research with children, special care and attention is vital. It is incumbent on researchers to consider children's agency and children's rights in relation to the potential harms and benefits of the proposed research study. Emerging researchers should be aware of the notion of 'acknowledgment of competencies' and provide special consideration of the age and maturity of child participants, and children's vulnerability to exploitation in their interaction with adults – the differential power relationship between adult researcher and child participant. Decisions involving children in research should be guided by the overarching principle of the 'Best Interests of the Child', reflected in Section 28 (Ch.2) of the Constitution, Section 7 of the Children's Act of 2005 and Article 3.1 of the UNCRC.

15.8. Conclusion

The recent upsurge in terms of interest and research in the field of children's SWB has the potential to determine the QoL of populations, and in so doing, use this data to make cross-national comparisons (Casas and Rees 2015). They note that "Such comparisons have huge potential to highlight differences in QoL, and the underlying factors associated with those differences, which will be valuable to national and international policy makers" (Casas and Rees 2015, p.50).

South Africa, however, lags behind most developed countries and some developing African countries (such as Algeria, see Tiliouine et al. 2006; and Ethiopia, see Mekonen 2009, 2010) in collecting consistent, national data, to track children's SWB. The field is still in its infancy in this context, yet the research which has been conducted shows some interesting results (see Savahl et al. 2015a).

It is accepted that children's well-being is influenced by their environment, as well as their position, and resources. Children's environments are not static but variable, as it is "but a set of dynamic factors, producing different outcomes for different groups of children." (Ben-Arieh and Frønes 2007, p. 250). This consideration is particularly significant in relation to the social inequality in South Africa, and how these differing conditions impact children's realities, and how they make sense of their lives. In addition to the legislative endeavours to protect children, many organisations and initiatives have been established in the country to promote children's well-being. Among the most renowned publications reporting on children's well-being (in terms of objective measures) is the South African Child Gauge (compiled by the Children's Institute of the University of Cape Town), as well as sporadic publications from the United Nations Children's Fund, and collaborating partners such as the Department of Social Development and the former Department of Women, Children, and People with Disabilities. The stark disparity between the results of objective and subjective indicators of children's well-being in this context evinces the struggle which theorists have encountered in attempting to reconcile these two fields since Easterlin's (1974) work on income and happiness.

In capacitating emerging researchers in terms of theoretical and methodological considerations of children's QoL there are innumerable content topics to consider. Five key components are proposed to be covered in an introductory syllabus for emerging researchers namely: contextualising children and childhood in South Africa; children's QOL and inequalities; theories of children's SWB; methodological considerations, and children's rights and SWB. The syllabus should include rich discussion activities on factors influencing children's QoL and SWB, and manners in which to enhance children's QoL.

Teaching and training emerging researchers on SWB and QoL, can be both scholarly and intellectual (Diener and Scollon 2014). Therefore, the intended contribution of this chapter is to provide a frame and foray for other researchers and emerging scholars to conducting research on QoL with children, particularly in a developing context as South Africa. The goal of preparing emerging researchers in this field of study is to continue working toward improving the lives of children across all spheres.

References

Adams, S., & Savahl, S. (2015). Children's perceptions of the natural environment: A South African perspective. *Children's Geographies, 13*(2), 196–211.

Adams, S., & Savahl, S. (2017a). Children's discourses of natural spaces: Considerations for children's subjective well-being. *Child Indicators Research, 10*(2), 423–446.

Adams, S., & Savahl, S. (2017b). Nature as children's space: A systematic review. *Journal of Environmental Education, 48*(5), 291–321.

Adams, S., & Savahl, S. (2018). Children's recreational engagement with nature in South Africa: Implications for children's subjective well-being. In L. R. R. de la Vega & W. N. Toscano (Eds.), *Handbook of leisure, physical activity, sports, recreation and quality of life* (pp. 71–95). Dordrecht: Springer.

Adams, S., & Savahl, S., & Fattore, T. (2017). Children's representations of nature using photovoice and community mapping: Perspectives from South Africa. Int J Qual Stud Health Well Being. https://doi.org/10.1080/17482631.2017.1333900.

Amsden, J., & VanWynsberghe, R. (2005). Community mapping as a research tool with youth. *Action Research, 3*(4), 357–381.

Andresen, S., Diehm, I., Sander, U., & Ziegler, H. (Eds.). (2010). *Children and the good life: New challenges for research on children.* Dortrecht: Springer.

Ben-Arieh, A. (2008). The child indicators movement: Past, present, and future. *Child Indicators Research, 1*(1), 3–16.

Ben-Arieh, A. (2009). From child welfare to children well-being: The child indicators perspective. In S. B. Kamerman, S. Phipps, & A. Ben-Arieh (Eds.), *From child welfare to children Well-being: An international perspective on knowledge in the service of making policy* (pp. 9–22). Dordrecht: Springer.

Ben-Arieh, A. (2010). Developing indicators for child well-being in a changing context. In C. McAuley & W. Rose (Eds.), *Child well-being: Understanding children's lives* (pp. 129–142). London: Jessica Kingsley Publishers.

Ben-Arieh, A., & Frønes, I. (2007). Indicators of children's well-being: What should be measured and why? *Social Indicators Research, 84*(3), 249–250.

Benninger, E., & Savahl, S. (2016). The use of visual methods to explore how children construct and assign meaning to the "self" within two urban communities in the Western Cape, South Africa. *International Journal of Qualitative Studies on Health and Well-Being, 11*(1), 31251.

Benninger, E., & Savahl, S. (2017a). Children's discursive constructions of the 'self'. *Child Indicators Research, 10*(4), 899–927.

Benninger, E., & Savahl, S. (2017b). The Children's Delphi: Considerations for developing a programme for promoting children's selfconcept and Well-being. *Child & Family Social Work, 22*(2), 1094–1103. https://doi.org/10.1111/cfs.12329.

Biggeri, M., Ballet, J., & Comim, F. (Eds.). (2011). *Children and the capability approach.* London: Palgrave Macmillan.

Bosch, A., Roussouw, J., Claassens, T., & du Plessis, B. (2010). *A second look at measuring inequality in South Africa: A modified Gini coefficient. School of Development Studies,* Working paper (58). University of Kwazulu-Natal.

Bradshaw, J. (2015). Subjective well-being and social policy: Can nations make their children happier? *Child Indicators Research, 8*(1), 227–241. https://doi.org/10.1007/s12187-014-9283-1.

Brickman, P., & Campbell, D. T. (1971). Hedonic relativism and planning the good society. In *Adaptation-level Theory* (pp. 287–305). New York: Academic.

Burton, P., & Leoschut, L. (2013). *School violence in South Africa: Results of the 2012 national school violence study.* Claremont: Centre for Justice and Crime Prevention.

Casas, F. (2011). Subjective social indicators and child and adolescent well-being. *Child Indicators Research, 4*(4), 555–575.

Casas, F. (2016). Children, adolescents and quality of life: The social sciences perspective over two decades. In *A life devoted to quality of life* (pp. 3–21). Cham: Springer.

Casas, F., & Rees, G. (2015). Measures of children's subjective well-being: Analysis of the potential for cross-national comparisons. *Child Indicators Research, 8*(1), 49–69.

Casas, F., Sarriera, J. C., Abs, D., Coenders, G., Alfaro, J., Saforcada, E., & Tonon, G. (2012). Subjective indicators of personal well-being among adolescents. Performance and results for different scales in Latin-language speaking countries: A contribution to the international debate. *Child Indicators Research, 5*(1), 1–28.

Chawla, L. (2007). Childhood experiences associated with care for the natural world: A theoretical framework for empirical results. *Children Youth and Environments, 17*(4), 144–170.

Chawla, L., & Hart, R. A. (1995). The roots of environmental concern. *NAMTA Journal, 20*(1), 148–157.

Clark, A. (2005). Ways of seeing: Using the mosaic approach to listen to young children's perspectives. In A. Clark, Kjørholt, & P. Moss (Eds.), *Beyond listening: Children's perspectives on early childhood services* (pp. 29–49). Bristol: Policy Press.

Clark, A., & Moss, P. (2012). *Listening to young children: The MOSAIC approach* (2nd Revised ed.). London: National Children's Bureau.

Comim, F., Ballet, J., Biggeri, M., & Iervese, V. (2011). Introduction – Theoretical foundations and the book's roadmap. In *Children and the capability approach* (pp. 3–21). London: Palgrave Macmillan.

Conti, G. & Heckman, J. J. (2012). The economics of child Well-being. IZA Discussion Paper No. 6930. Available at SSRN: http://ssrn.com/abstract=2164659.

Corsaro, W. (1992). Interpretive reproduction in children's peer cultures. *Social Psychology Quarterly, 55*, 160–177.

Cummins, R. A. (1995). *The comprehensive quality of life scale: Theory and development: Health outcomes and quality of life measurement*. Canberra: Institute of Health and Welfare.

Cummins, R. A. (1996). The domains of life satisfaction: An attempt to order chaos. *Social Indicators Research, 38*(3), 303–328.

Cummins, R. A. (2003). Normative life satisfaction: Measurement issues and a homeostatic model. *Social Indicators Research, 64*(2), 225–256.

Cummins, R. A. (2010). Subjective wellbeing, homeostatically protected mood and depression: A synthesis. *Journal of Happiness Studies, 11*(1), 1–17.

Cummins, R. A. (2014). Understanding the well-being of children and adolescents through homeostatic theory. In A. Ben-Arieh, F. Casas, I. Frønes, & J. E. Korbin (Eds.), *Handbook of child well-being: Theories, methods and policies in global perspective* (pp. 635–662). Dordrecht: Springer.

Dang, A. T. (2014). Amartya Sen's capability approach: A framework for well-being evaluation and policy analysis? *Review of Social Economy, 72*(4), 460–484.

Dawes, A., Bray, R., & Van der Merwe, A. (2007). *Monitoring child well-being: A South African rights-based approach*. Cape Town: HRSC press.

Deci, E. L., & Ryan, R. M. (1985). *Intrinsic motivation and self-determination in human behavior*. New York: Plenum.

Deci, E. L., & Ryan, R. M. (2008a). Hedonia, eudaimonia, and well-being: An introduction. *Journal of Happiness Studies, 9*(1), 1–11.

Deci, E. L., & Ryan, R. M. (2008b). Self-determination theory: A macro theory of human motivation, development, and health. *Canadian Psychology/Psychologie Canadienne, 49*(3), 182.

Department of Basic Education. (2016). *Annual report*. Pretoria: Department of Basic Education. Retrieved from http://www.education.gov.za.

Diener, E. (1984). Subjective well-being. *Psychological Bulletin, 95*(3), 542–575.

Diener, E. (2000). Subjective well-being: The science of happiness and a proposal for a national index. *American Psychologist, 55*, 34–43. https://doi.org/10.1037//0003-066X.55.1.34.

Diener, E. (2012). New findings and future directions for subjective well-being research. *American Psychologist, 67*, 591–597. https://doi.org/10.1037/a0029541.

Diener, E., & Scollon, C. N. (2014). The what, why, when, and how of teaching the science of subjective well-being. *Teaching of Psychology, 41*(2), 175–183.

Diener, E., Lucas, R. E., & Scollon, C. N. (2006). Beyond the hedonic treadmill: Revising the adaptation theory of well-being. *American Psychologist, 61*(4), 305–314. https://doi.org/10.1037/0003-066X.61.4.305.

Dinisman, T., Montserrat, C., & Casas, F. (2012). The subjective well-being of Spanish adolescents: Variations according to different living arrangements. *Children and Youth Services Review, 34*(12), 2374–2380.

Durayappah, A. (2011). The 3P model: A general theory of subjective well-being. *Journal of Happiness Studies, 12*(4), 681–716.

Easterlin, R. A. (1974). Does economic growth improve the human lot? Some empirical evidence. In *Nations and households in economic growth* (pp. 89–125). New York: Academic.

Fattore, T., Fegter, S., & Hunner-Kreisel, C. (2018). Children's understandings of Well-being in global and local contexts: Theoretical and methodological considerations for a multinational qualitative study. *Child Indicators Research*. https://doi.org/10.1007/s12187-018-9594-8.

Fattore, T., Mason, J., & Watson, E. (2007). Children's conceptualisation(s) of their well-being. *Social Indicators Research, 80*, 5–29.

Fattore, T., Mason, J., & Watson, E. (2012). Locating the child centrally as subject in research: Towards a child interpretation of well-being. *Child Indicators Research, 5*(3), 423–435.

Fattore, T., Mason, J., & Watson, E. (2017). *Children's understandings of well-being: Towards a child standpoint.* Dordrecht: Springer.

Fegter, S., & Richter, M. (2014). Capability approach as a framework for research on children's well-being. In A. Ben-Arieh, F. Casas, I. Frones, & J. E. Korbin (Eds.), *Handbook of child well-being: Theories, methods and policies in global perspective* (pp. 739–758). Dordrecht: Springer.

Gilman, R., & Huebner, S. (2003). A review of life satisfaction research with children and adolescents. *School Psychology Quarterly, 18*(2), 192–205.

Green, C. J. (2015). Toward young children as active researchers: A critical review of the methodologies and methods in early childhood environmental education. *The Journal of Environmental Education, 46*(4), 207. https://doi.org/10.1080/00958964.2015.1050345.

Haikkola, L., & Rissotto, A. (2007). Legislation, policy and participatory structures as opportunities for children's participation? A comparison of Finland and Italy. *Children Youth and Environments, 17*(4), 352–387.

Hall, K., Woolard, I., Lake, L., & Smith, C. (2012). *South African child gauge.* Cape Town: Children's Institute. University of Cape Town.

Hammaberg, T. (1995). Foreword. In J. R. Himes (Ed.), *Implementing the convention on the rights of the child: Resource mobilization in low-income countries* (pp. v–xiii). Dordrecht: Kluwer.

Hart, R. A. (1984). The geography of children and children's geographies. In T. Saarinen, D. Seamon, & J. L. Sell (Eds.), *Environmental perception and behavior: An inventory and prospect* (Research Paper No. 209) (pp. 99–129). Chicago: Department of Geography, University of Chicago.

Hart, R. A. (1992). *Children's participation: From Tokenism to Citizenship.* Florence: UNICEF.

Hart, R. A. (1994). Children's role in primary environmental care. *Childhood, 2*, 92–102.

Himes, J. R. (1993). *The United Nations convention on the rights of the child: Three essays on the challenge of implementation* (No. inness 93/2).

Howie, S. J., Combrinck, C., Roux, K., Tshele, M., Mokoena, G. M., & McLeod Palane, N. (2017). *PIRLS literacy 2016 progress in international reading literacy study 2016: South African children's reading literacy achievement.* Pretoria: Centre for Evaluation and Assessment.

International Wellbeing Group. (2006). *Personal Wellbeing Index* (4th ed.). Melbourne: Australian Centre on Quality of Life, Deakin University. www.deakin.edu.au/research/acqol/instruments/wellbeing-index/.

James, A., & Prout, A. (Eds.). (1990). *Constructing and re-constructing childhood.* Basingstoke: Falmer Press.

Jamieson, L., Berry, L., & Lake, L. (2017a). *South African child gauge*. Cape Town: Children's Institute, University of Cape Town.

Jamieson, J. P., Hangen, E. J., Lee, H. Y., & Yeager, D. S. (2017b). Capitalizing on appraisal processes to improve affective responses to social stress. *Emotion Review, 10*(1), 30–39.

Kopnina, H. N. (2011). Applying the new ecological paradigm scale in the case of environmental education: Qualitative analysis of the ecological world view of Dutch children. *Journal of Peace Education, 5*, 15.

Langhout, R. D., & Thomas, E. (2010). Imagining participatory action research in collaboration with children: An introduction. *American Journal of Community Psychology, 46*(1–2), 60–66.

Lloyd, K., & Emerson, L. (2017). (Re) examining the relationship between children's subjective wellbeing and their perceptions of participation rights. *Child Indicators Research, 10*(3), 591–608.

Malone, K. (2016). Reconsidering children's encounters with nature and place using posthumanism. *Australian Journal of Environmental Education, 32*, 42–56.

Mathews, S., & Benvenuti, P. (2014). Violence against children in South Africa: Developing a prevention agenda. *South African Child Gauge, 1*, 26–34.

Mathews, S., & Martin, L. J. (2016). Developing an understanding of fatal child abuse and neglect: Results from the South African child death review pilot study. *South African Medical Journal, 106*(12), 1160–1163.

McKendrick, J. H. (2014). Geographies of children's well-being: In, of and for space. In A. Ben-Arieh, F. Casas, I. Frones, & J. E. Korbin (Eds.), *Handbook of child Well-being: Theories, methods and policies in global perspective* (pp. 279–300). Dordrecht: Springer.

Mekonen, Y. (2009). *Governance and child wellbeing: How to measure government performance*. Addis Ababa: The African Child Policy Forum.

Mekonen, Y. (2010). Measuring government performance in realising child rights and child well-being: The approach and indicators. *Child Indicators Research, 3*(2), 205–241.

Minkkinen, J. (2013). The structural model of child well-being. *Child Indicators Research, 6*(3), 547–558.

Møller, V. (1997). South Africa's emergent 'Social Indicators Movement'. *Social Indicators Research, 41*(1–3), 1–14.

Møller, V. (2013a). South African quality of life trends over three decades, 1980–2010. *Social Indicators Research, 113*(3), 915–940.

Møller, V. (2013b). Valerie Møller: A Pioneer in South African quality of life research. *Applied Research in Quality of Life, 8*(3), 409–410.

Møller, V., & Roberts, B. (2014). South Africa, quality of life. In *Encyclopaedia of quality of life and well-being research* (pp. 6218–6223). London: Springer.

Møller, V., & Schlemmer, L. (1982). *Attitudes toward beach integration: A comparative study of black and white reactions to multiracial beaches in Durban*. Durban: Centre for Applied Social Sciences, University of Natal.

Møller, V., & Schlemmer, L. (1983). Quality of life in South Africa: Towards an instrument for the assessment of quality of life and basic needs. *Social Indicators Research, 12*(3), 225–279.

Møller, V., & Schlemmer, L. (1989). South African quality of life: A research note. *Social Indicators Research, 21*(3), 279–291.

Montserrat, C., & Casas, F. (2006). Kinship foster care from the perspective of quality of life: Research on the satisfaction of the stakeholders. *Applied Research in Quality of Life, 1*(3), 227–237.

Montserrat, C., Casas, F., & Moura, J. F. (2015). Children's subjective well-being in disadvantaged situations. In *Theoretical and empirical insights into child and family poverty* (pp. 111–126). Dordrecht: Springer.

Moore, R. C. (1986). *Childhood's domain*. London: Croom Helm.

Moses, S. (2008). Children and participation in South Africa: An overview. *International Journal of Children's Rights, 16*, 327–342.

Navarro, D., Montserrat, C., Malo, S., González, M., Casas, F., & Crous, G. (2015). Subjective well-being: What do adolescents say? *Child & Family Social Work, 22*(1), 175–184. https://doi.org/10.1111/cfs.12215.

Nussbaum, M. (1988). Nature, function and capability: Aristotle on political distribution. *Oxford Studies in Ancient Philosophy, 1*, 145–184.

Nussbaum, M. C. (2000). *Women and human development: The capabilities approach.* Cambridge: Cambridge University Press.

Pollard, E. L., & Lee, P. D. (2003). Child well-being: A systematic review of the literature. *Social Indicators Research, 61*(1), 59–78.

Raghavan, R., & Alexandrova, A. (2015). Toward a theory of child Well-being. *Social Indicators Research, 121*(3), 887–902.

Rees, G., & Main, G. (Eds.). (2015). *Children's views on their lives and well-being in 15 countries: A report on the Children's world's survey, 2013–14.* Children's Worlds.

Richter, L., Mathews, S., Kagura, J., & Nonterah, E. (2018). A longitudinal perspective on violence in the lives of South African children from the birth to twenty plus cohort study in Johannesburg-Soweto. *South African Medical Journal, 108*(3), 181–186.

Ryan, R. M., & Deci, E. L. (2000). Intrinsic and extrinsic motivations: Classic definitions and new directions. *Contemporary Educational Psychology, 25*(1), 54–67.

Sancar, F. H., & Severcan, Y. C. (2010). Children's places: Rural–urban comparisons using participatory photography in the Bodrum peninsula, Turkey. *Journal of Urban Design, 15*(3), 293–324.

Savahl, S. (2010). *Ideological constructions of childhood.* Unpublished Doctoral Dissertation. Bellville: University of the Western Cape.

Savahl, S., Adams, S., Isaacs, S., September, R., Hendricks, G., & Noordien, Z. (2015a). Subjective Well-being amongst a sample of south African children: A descriptive study. *Child Indicators Research, 8*(1), 211–226.

Savahl, S., Casas, F., & Adams, S. (2015b). Validation of the Children's Hope scale amongst a sample of adolescents in the Western cape region of South Africa. *Child Indicators Research, 9*(3), 701–713.

Savahl, S., Malcolm, C., Slembrouk, S., Adams, S., Willenberg, I. A., & September, R. (2015c). Discourses on Well-being. *Child Indicators Research, 8*(4), 747–766.

Savahl, S., Casas, F., & Adams, S. (2017). Children's subjective well-being: Multi-group analysis among a sample of children from two socio-economic status groups in the Western Cape, South Africa. *Child Indicators Research, 10*(2), 473–488.

Savahl, S., Montserrat, C., Casas, F., Adams, S., Tiliouine, H., Benninger, E., & Jackson, K. (2018). Children's experiences of bullying victimization and the influence on their subjective well-being: A multinational comparison. *Child Development*, 1–18.

Savahl, S., Adams, S., Benninger, E., Florence, M., Jackson, K., Manuel, D., Mpilo, M., Bawa, U., & Isobell, D. (2019). Researching children's subjective well-being in South Africa: Considerations for method, theory and social policy. In I. Eloff (Ed.), *Quality-of-life in African societies*. Dordrecht: Springer.

Seligman, M. (2011). *Flourish: A visionary new understanding of happiness and Well-being.* New York: Simon & Schuster.

Sen, A. (1985). Well-being, agency and freedom: The Dewey lectures 1984. *The Journal of Philosophy, 82*(4), 169–221.

Sen, A. K. (1993). Capability and well-being. In M. Nussbaum & A. Sen (Eds.), *The quality of life* (pp. 30–53). Oxford: Oxford University Press.

Sen, A. (2005). Human rights and capabilities. *Journal of Human Development, 6*(2), 151–166. https://doi.org/10.1080/14649880500120491.

Sen, A. K. (2007). Children and human rights. *Indian Journal of Human Development, 2*(1), 1–18.

September, R., & Dinbabo, M. (2008). Gearing up for implementation: A new Children's act for South Africa. *Practice, 20*(2), 113–122.

September, R., & Savahl, S. (2009). Children's perspectives on child well-being. *Social Work Practitioner/Researcher, 21*(1), 23–40.

South African Police Services. (2017). *SAPS annual crime statistics 2016/2017*. Pretoria: South African Police Services.

Statistics South Africa. (2017). *Mid-year population statistics 2017*. Pretoria: Statistics South Africa.

Statistics South Africa. (2018). *General household survey*. Pretoria, Statistics SA.

Stoecklin, D., & Bonvin, J. M. (2014). *Children's rights and the capability approach* (Children's Well-Being: Indicators and Research). Dordrecht: Springer.

Strack, R. W., Magill, C., & McDonagh, K. (2004). Engaging youth through photovoice. *Health Promotion Practice, 5*(1), 49–58.

Thomson, J. L., & Philo, C. (2004). Playful spaces? A social geography of children's play in Livingston, Scotland. *Children's Geographies, 2*(1), 111–130.

Tiliouine, H., Cummins, R. A., & Davern, M. (2006). Measuring wellbeing in developing countries: The case of Algeria. *Social Indicators Research, 75*(1), 1–30.

UNICEF Office of Research. (2007). *Child poverty in perspective: An overview of child well-being in rich countries, Innocenti report card 7*. Florence: UNICEF Office of Research.

United Nations Development Programme. (2018). *Human development indices and indicators: Statistical update*. New York: United Nations Development Programme.

United Nations General Assembly. (1989). *Convention on the Rights of the Child*. United Nations, Treaty Series, vol. 1577, p. 3, available at: http://www.refworld.org/docid/3ae6b38f0.html. Accessed 6 Mar 2016.

Wang, C., & Burris, M. A. (1994). Empowerment through photo novella: Portraits of participation. *Health Education Quarterly, 21*(2), 171–186.

Wang, C., & Burris, M. A. (1997). Photovoice: Concept, methodology, and use for participatory needs assessment. *Health Education & Behavior, 24*(3), 369–387.

Weinstein, N., & Ryan, R. M. (2010). When helping helps: Autonomous motivation for prosocial behavior and its influence on well-being for the helper and recipient. *Journal of Personality and Social Psychology, 98*(2), 222.

World Bank. (2018). *The World Bank annual report 2018 (English)*. Washington, DC: World Bank Group. http://documents.worldbank.org/curated/en/630671538158537244/The-World-Bank-Annual-Report-2018.

World Health Organization. (1946). *Constitution of World Health Organization*, from: http://www.opbw.org/int_inst/health_docs/WHO-CONSTITUTION.pdf

Zuch, M., Mathews, C., De Koker, P., Mtshizana, Y., & Mason-Jones, A. (2013). Evaluation of a Photovoice pilot project for school safety in South Africa. *Children Youth and Environments, 23*(1), 180–197.

Sabirah Adams is senior lecturer and research psychologist specialising in the disciplines of social and positive psychology, based at the Language Development Group, Centre for Higher Education Development, at the University of Cape Town, South Africa. Her research interests are in the area of quality of life of children and adolescents, with a specific focus on children's subjective well-being and flourishing, developing subjective well-being indicators, participatory child research and children's rights. She is a member of the International Society for Child Indicators. She is the principal investigator of the Children's Worlds: International Survey on Children's Well-Being (South Africa), and the Multinational Qualitative Study on Children's Understandings of Well-Being – Global and Local Contexts (South Africa). She is the consultant editorial assistant of the journal Neuropsychoanalysis.

Shazly Savahl is an associate professor and research psychologist specialising in the disciplines of social and positive psychology, based in Child and Family Studies and the Department of Psychology at the University of the Western Cape, South Africa. His research interests are in the area of quality of life of children and adolescents, with a specific focus on children's subjective well-being and flourishing, developing subjective well-being indicators, participatory child research and children's rights. He is a member of the International Society for Child Indicators. He is the principal investigator of the Children's Worlds: International Survey on Children's Well-Being (South Africa), and the Multinational Qualitative Study on Children's Understandings of Well-Being – Global and Local Contexts (South Africa).

Maria Florence is a senior lecturer and researcher, based at the Department of Psychology at the University of the Western Cape, South Africa. Her research interests include quantitative methodology measurement design and validation, youth risk behaviour, women's health, and substance use in low socio-economic status communities. This work is conducted collaboratively across South African institutions as well as internationally with researchers in Europe and the United States.

Kyle Jackson is a research psychologist and counsellor, based at the Department of Psychology at the University of the Western Cape, South Africa. He is currently a doctoral student at the University of the Western Cape. His research interests include masculinity and fatherhood and child well-being. He is a project member of the Children's Worlds: International Survey on Children's Well-Being (South Africa).

Donnay Manuel is researcher based at the Department of Psychology at the University of the Western Cape, South Africa, with a focus in the areas of children's subjective well-being and quality of life, adolescents' subjective well-being, career aspirations and bullying. She is a project member of the *Children's Worlds: International Survey on Children's Well-Being* (South Africa).

Mulalo Mpilo is researcher, based at the Department of Psychology at the University of the Western Cape, South Africa, with a focus in the areas of children's subjective well-being and quality of life, adolescents' subjective well-being, career aspirations and bullying. She is a project member of the *Children's Worlds: International Survey on Children's Well-Being*.

Deborah Isobell is a registered research psychologist and counsellor. She is currently a doctoral candidate at the University of the Western Cape and Ghent University. Her research interests include substitute addictions and recovery, research translation and participatory research methods.

Printed by Printforce, the Netherlands